Current Controversies in Perinatology V

Guest Editors

MICHAEL R. UHING, MD
ROBERT KLIEGMAN, MD

CLINICS IN PERINATOLOGY

www.perinatology.theclinics.com

March 2009 • Volume 36 • Number 1

SAUNDERS an imprint of ELSEVIER, Inc.

W.B. SAUNDERS COMPANY
A Division of Elsevier Inc.

Elsevier, Inc. • 1600 John F. Kennedy Blvd. • Suite 1800 • Philadelphia, PA 19103-2899

http://www.theclinics.com

CLINICS IN PERINATOLOGY Volume 36, Number 1
March 2009 ISSN 0095-5108, ISBN-10: 1-4160-5802-8, ISBN-13: 978-1-4160-5802-1

Editor: Carla Holloway
Developmental Editor: Donald Mumford

Clinics in Perinatology (ISSN 0095-5108) is published in quarterly by Elsevier Inc., 360 Park Avenue South, New York, NY 10010-1710. Months of issue are March, June, September, and December. Business and Editorial offices: 1600 John F. Kennedy Blvd., Suite 1800, Philadelphia, PA 19103-2899. Customer Service Office: 6277 Sea Harbor Drive, Orlando, FL 32887-4800. Periodicals postage paid at New York, NY and additional mailing offices. Subscription prices are $217.00 per year (US individuals), $321.00 per year (US institutions), $255.00 per year (Canadian individuals), $408.00 per year (Canadian institutions), $314.00 per year (foreign individuals), $408.00 per year (foreign institutions) $105.00 per year (US students), and $153.00 per year (Canadian and foreign students). Foreign air speed delivery is included in all Clinics subscription prices. All prices are subject to change without notice. **POSTMASTER:** Send address changes to *Clinics in Perinatology*; Elsevier Periodicals Customer Service, 11830 Westline Industrial Drive, St. Louis, MO 63146. Customer Service (orders, claims, online, change of address): Elsevier Periodicals Customer Service, 11830 Westline Industrial Drive, St. Louis, MO 63146. Tel: 1-800-654-2452 (U.S. and Canada); 314-453-7041 (outside U.S. and Canada). Fax: 314-453-5170. E-mail: journalscustomerservice-usa@elsevier.com (for print support); journalsonlinesupport-usa@elsevier.com (for online support).

Reprints. For copies of 100 or more, of articles in this publication, please contact the Commercial Reprints Department, Elsevier Inc., 360 Park Avenue South, New York, NY 10010-1710. Tel. (212) 633-3812; Fax: (212) 482-1935; email: reprints@elsevier.com.

Clinics in Perinatology is also pubilshed in Spanish by McGraw-Hill Interamericana Editores S.A., P.O. Box 5-237, 06500 Mexico D.F., Mexico.

Clinics in Perinatology is covered in *MEDLINE/PubMed (Index Medicus) Current Contents, Excepta Medica, BIOSIS and ISI/BIOMED.*

Printed and bound in the United Kingdom
Transferred to Digital Print 2011

Contributors

GUEST EDITORS

MICHAEL R. UHING, MD
Associate Professor of Pediatrics, Division of Neonatology, Medical College of Wisconsin; Director, Neonatal Intensive Care Unit, Children's Hospital of Wisconsin, Milwaukee, Wisconsin

ROBERT KLIEGMAN, MD
Professor and Chair, Department of Pediatrics, Medical College of Wisconsin, Milwaukee, Wisconsin

AUTHORS

NANDINI ARUL, MD
Assistant Professor of Pediatrics, Division of Neonatology, Medical College of Wisconsin; Division of Neonatology, Department of Pediatrics, Milwaukee, Wisconsin

ALAN R. BARNETTE, MD
Clinical Fellow of Pediatrics, Division of Newborn Medicine, Washington University School of Medicine, St. Louis, Missouri

K.J. BARRINGTON, MBChB, MRCP, FRCP
Professor of Pediatrics, Department of Pediatrics, CHU-Ste Justine, Ste-Justine Hospital, University of Montreal, Montreal, Quebec, Canada

ULRICH BROECKEL, MD
Associate Professor and Chief, Section of Genomic Pediatrics; Associate Director, Children's Research Institute; Director, Individualized Medicine Institute, Medical College of Wisconsin, Milwaukee, Wisconsin

JAMES W. COLLINS, Jr., MD, MPH
Professor of Pediatrics, Department of Pediatrics, Northwestern University's Feinberg School of Medicine, Chicago, Illinois

UTPALA (SHONU) G. DAS, MD
Assistant Professor of Pediatrics/Neonatology, Medical College of Wisconsin, Milwaukee, Wisconsin

RICHARD J. DAVID, MD
Professor of Pediatrics, Department of Pediatrics, University of Illinois at Chicago, Chicago, Illinois

E.M. DEMPSEY, MBBCh, FRCPI
Neonatologist, Department of Neonatology, Cork University Maternity Hospital, Cork, Ireland

RICHARD A. EHRENKRANZ, MD
Professor of Pediatrics and Obstetrics, Gynecology and Reproductive Sciences, Division of Perinatal Medicine, Department of Pediatrics, Yale University School of Medicine, New Haven, Connecticut

JEFFERY S. GARLAND, MD
Wheaton Franciscan Health Care, St. Joseph Hospital; Clinical Assistant Professor, Department of Pediatrics, Medical College of Wisconsin; Clinical Associate Professor, Department of Pediatrics, University of Wisconsin School of Medicine and Public Health, Milwaukee, Wisconsin

MICHAEL K. GEORGIEFF, MD
Professor of Pediatrics and Child Development, Division of Neonatology, University of Minnesota; Director, Center for Neurobehavioral Development, University of Minnesota, Minneapolis, Minnesota

PRAVEEN S. GODAY, MBBS, CNSP
Assistant Professor of Pediatrics, Division of Pediatric Gastroenterology and Nutrition, Medical College of Wisconsin, Milwaukee, Wisconsin

R. WHIT HALL, MD
Professor of Pediatrics, Division of Neonatology, University of Arkansas for Medical Sciences, Little Rock, Arkansas

TERRIE E. INDER, MBChB, MD, FRACP
Associate Professor of Pediatrics, Divisions of Newborn Medicine, Neurology, and Radiology, Washington University School of Medicine, St. Louis, Missouri

ALAN H. JOBE, MD, PhD
Division of Pulmonary Biology, Cincinnati Children's Hospital, University of Cincinnati, Cincinnati, Ohio

G. GANESH KONDURI, MD
Professor of Pediatrics; Director, Division of Neonatology, Medical College of Wisconsin; Division of Neonatology, Department of Pediatrics, Milwaukee, Wisconsin

KAREN MARESSO, MPH
Research Associate, Section of Genomic Pediatrics, Children's Research Institute, Medical College of Wisconsin, Milwaukee, Wisconsin

KYLE O. MOUNTS, MD, MPH
Assistant Clinical Professor, Department of Pediatrics, Medical College of Wisconsin, Milwaukee; Assistant Clinical Professor, Department of Pediatrics, University of Wisconsin-Madison, Madison; Division of Neonatology, Wheaton Franciscan Healthcare St. Joseph, Milwaukee, Wisconsin

RAGHAVENDRA RAO, MD
Assistant Professor of Pediatrics, Division of Neonatology, University of Minnesota; Center for Neurobehavioral Development, University of Minnesota, Minneapolis, Minnesota

ROLLA M. SHBAROU, MD
Assistant Professor of Pediatrics, Division of Neurology, University of Arkansas for Medical Sciences, Arkansas Children's Hospital, Little Rock, Arkansas

JEAN M. SILVESTRI, MD
Associate Professor of Pediatrics, Department of Pediatrics, Rush University Medical Center; Clinical Director, Neonatal Intensive Care Unit, Rush Children's Hospital, Chicago, Illinois

NEELESH A. TIPNIS, MD
Assistant Professor of Pediatrics, Division of Pediatric Gastroenterology and Nutrition, Department of Pediatrics, Children's Hospital of Wisconsin and the Medical College of Wisconsin, Milwaukee, Wisconsin

SAJANI M. TIPNIS, MD
Assistant Professor of Pediatrics, Division of Neonatology, Department of Pediatrics, Children's Hospital of Wisconsin and the Medical College of Wisconsin, Milwaukee, Wisconsin

MICHAEL R. UHING, MD
Associate Professor of Pediatrics, Division of Neonatology, Medical College of Wisconsin; Director, Neonatal Intensive Care Unit, Children's Hospital of Wisconsin, Milwaukee, Wisconsin

ISABELLE VON KOHORN, MD
Clinical Fellow, Division of Perinatal Medicine, Department of Pediatrics, Yale University School of Medicine, New Haven, Connecticut

Contents

Preface xv

Michael R. Uhing and Robert Kliegman

Errata xvii

Strategies to Prevent Bacterial and Fungal Infection in the Neonatal Intensive Care Unit 1

Jeffery S. Garland and Michael R. Uhing

Hospital-acquired infections are one of the leading causes of preventable morbidity and mortality in neonatal intensive care units (NICUs). Device-related infections, such as catheter-associated blood stream infections (CABSIs) and ventilator-associated pneumonia (VAP), are the most common nosocomial infections. This review examines the pathogenesis of CABSIs and methods, widely accepted and novel, that can be used to help prevent them. Strategies to prevent fungal infections, which are often associated with the presence of a central venous catheter, are also reviewed. Finally, the dilemmas in the diagnosis and prevention of VAP in the NICU are discussed.

Drugs of Choice for Sedation and Analgesia in the Neonatal ICU 15

R. Whit Hall and Rolla M. Shbarou

Painful procedures in the neonatal ICU are common, undertreated, and lead to adverse consequences. The drugs most commonly used to treat neonatal pain include the opiates, benzodiazepines, barbiturates, ketamine, propofol, acetaminophen, and local and topical anesthetics. This article discusses the indications for and advantages and disadvantages of the commonly used analgesic drugs. Guidance and references for drugs and dosing for specific neonatal procedures are provided.

Iron Therapy for Preterm Infants 27

Raghavendra Rao and Michael K. Georgieff

Preterm infants are at risk for both iron deficiency and iron overload. The role of iron in multiple organ functions suggests that iron supplementation is essential for the preterm infant. Conversely, the potential for iron overload and the poorly developed antioxidant measures in the preterm infant argue against indiscriminate iron supplementation in this population. This

Prospective trials of intervention for hypotension and circulatory compromise are urgently required.

Although there is a large body of literature describing infants who experience apnea of prematurity and apparent life-threatening events, there is no consensus regarding the use of home monitoring. This article focuses on issues that affect decision making regarding the use of home monitors in these two groups of infants and reviews existing data to guide a decision to discontinue monitoring at hospital discharge or to prescribe monitoring in the home.

Short bowel syndrome (SBS) is the most common cause of intestinal failure. This article discusses the prognostic factors that predict weaning from parenteral nutrition in SBS. The article also delineates an approach to enteral feeding in SBS.

Since the late 1980s recombinant human erythropoietin (r-EPO) has been studied as an alternative to packed red blood cell (RBC) transfusion for the treatment of anemia of prematurity in very low birth weight infants. Initial trials and reports focused on r-EPO's ability to prevent or treat anemia of prematurity with the goal of eliminating RBC transfusion but achieved limited success. New concerns about the safety of r-EPO administration have emerged. Past cost–benefit analyses of r-EPO administration versus transfusion for the treatment of anemia of prematurity have been nearly balanced. Autologous transfusion, blood-sparing technologies, changes in RBC transfusion technique and safety, and further elucidation of the risk–benefit ratio of r-EPO therapy may change the cost–benefit analysis.

Ischemic perinatal stroke (IPS) occurs in 1 of 2300 to 5000 live births. It is an under-recognized cause of significant long-term disabilities, including hemiplegic cerebral palsy, epilepsy, cognitive delays, and behavioral impairments. The pathophysiology is complex and multifactorial, involving maternal, fetal, placental, and neonatal factors. Knowledge and interventions are emerging to facilitate early diagnosis and treatment of IPS. Early treatment may translate into improved long-term neurodevelopmental outcomes.

The Role of Genomics in the Neonatal ICU **189**

Karen Maresso and Ulrich Broeckel

Results of both the Human Genome and International HapMap Projects have provided the technology and resources necessary to enable fundamental advances through the study of DNA sequence variation in almost all fields of medicine, including neonatology. Genome-wide association studies are now practical, and the first of these studies are appearing in the literature. This article provides the reader with an overview of the issues in technology and study design relating to genome-wide association studies and summarizes the current state of association studies in neonatal ICU populations with a brief review of the relevant literature. Future recommendations for genomic association studies in neonatal ICU populations are also provided.

Index **205**

GOAL STATEMENT

The goal of *Clinics in Perinatology* is to keep practicing neonatologists and maternal-fetal medicine specialists up to date with current clinical practice in perinatology by providing timely articles reviewing the state of the art in patient care.

ACCREDITATION

The *Clinics in Perinatology* is planned and implemented in accordance with the Essential Areas and Policies of the Accreditation Council for Continuing Medical Education (ACCME) through the joint sponsorship of the University of Virginia School of Medicine and Elsevier. The University of Virginia School of Medicine is accredited by the ACCME to provide continuing medical education for physicians.

The University of Virginia School of Medicine designates this educational activity for a maximum of 60 *AMA PRA Category 1 Credits*™. Physicians should only claim credit commensurate with the extent of their participation in the activity.

The American Medical Association has determined that physicians not licensed in the US who participate in this CME activity are eligible for *AMA PRA Category 1 Credits*™.

Credit can be earned by reading the text material, taking the CME examination online at http://www.theclinics.com/home/cme, and completing the evaluation. After taking the test, you will be required to review any and all incorrect answers. Following completion of the test and evaluation, your credit will be awarded and you may print your certificate.

FACULTY DISCLOSURE/CONFLICT OF INTEREST

The University of Virginia School of Medicine, as an ACCME accredited provider, endorses and strives to comply with the Accreditation Council for Continuing Medical Education (ACCME) Standards of Commercial Support, Commonwealth of Virginia statutes, University of Virginia policies and procedures, and associated federal and private regulations and guidelines on the need for disclosure and monitoring of proprietary and financial interests that may affect the scientific integrity and balance of content delivered in continuing medical education activities under our auspices.

The University of Virginia School of Medicine requires that all CME activities accredited through this institution be developed independently and be scientifically rigorous, balanced and objective in the presentation/discussion of its content, theories and practices.

All authors/editors participating in an accredited CME activity are expected to disclose to the readers relevant financial relationships with commercial entities occurring within the past 12 months (such as grants or research support, employee, consultant, stock holder, member of speakers bureau, etc.). The University of Virginia School of Medicine will employ appropriate mechanisms to resolve potential conflicts of interest to maintain the standards of fair and balanced education to the reader. Questions about specific strategies can be directed to the Office of Continuing Medical Education, University of Virginia School of Medicine, Charlottesville, Virginia.

The faculty and staff of the University of Virginia Office of Continuing Medical Education have no financial affiliations to disclose.

The authors/editors listed below have identified no professional or financial affiliations for themselves or their spouse/partner:

Nandini Arul, MD; Robert Boyle, MD (Test Author); Alan R. Barnette, MD; K. J. Barrington, MBChB, MRCP, FRCP; Ulrich Broeckel, MD; James W. Collins, Jr., MD, MPH; Utpala "Shonu" G. Das, MD; Richard J. David, MD; E. M. Dempsey, MBBCh, FRCPI; Richard A. Ehrenkranz, MD; Jeffery S. Garland, MD; Michael K. Georgieff, MD; Praveen S. Goday, MBBS, CNSP; Richard Whit Hall, MD; Carla Holloway (Acquisitions Editor); Terrie E. Inder, MBChB, MD, FRACP; Robert Kleigman, MD (Guest Editor); G. Ganesh Konduri, MD; Karen Maresso, MPH; Kyle O. Mounts, MD, MPH; Raghavendra Rao, MD; Rolla M. Shbarou, MD; Jean M. Silvestri, MD; Sajani M. Tipnis, MD; and Isabelle Von Kohorn, MD.

The authors/editors listed below identified the following professional or financial affiliations for themselves or their spouse/partner:

Alan H. Jobe, MD, PhD has received funding and supply equipment from Fisher and Paykel, has received supply surfactant from Chiesi Pharm, and has received supplies from Amgen, Inc.
Neelesh A. Tipnis, MD has received funding from Wyeth Pharmaceuticals.
Michael R. Uhing, MD (Guest Editor) is employed by Medi-Flex, Inc.

Disclosure of Discussion of Non-FDA Approved Uses for Pharmaceutical Products and/or Medical Devices.
The University of Virginia School of Medicine, as an ACCME provider, requires that all faculty presenters identify and disclose any off-label uses for pharmaceutical and medical device products. The University of Virginia School of Medicine recommends that each physician fully review all the available data on new products or procedures prior to clinical use.

TO ENROLL

To enroll in the *Clinics in Perinatology* Continuing Medical Education program, call customer service at 1-800-654-2452 or visit us online at www.theclinics.com/home/cme. The CME program is available to subscribers for an additional fee of $195.00.

FORTHCOMING ISSUES

June 2009

Fetal Surgery

Hanmin Lee, MD, *Guest Editor*

September 2009

Fetal and Neonatal Neurology

Adré du Plessis, MD, *Guest Editor*

RECENT ISSUES

December 2008

Neuroprotection in the Newborn

Alan R. Spitzer, MD, Robert D. White, MD, *Guest Editors*

September 2008

Cesarean Delivery: Its Impact on the Mother and Newborn—Part II

Lucky Jain, MD, MBA, Ronald Wapner, MD, *Guest Editors*

June 2008

Cesarean Delivery: Its impact on the Mother and Newborn—Part I

Lucky Jain, MD, MBA, Ronald Wapner, MD, *Guest Editors*

RELATED INTEREST

2008 Year Book of Neonatal and Perinatal Medicine
Avroy A. Fanaroff, *Editor-in-Chief*
www.eclips.consult.com

Clinics in Perinatology, September 2004 (Volume 31, Issue 3)
Current Controversies in Perinatal Medicine IV
Arthur I. Eidelman, MD, and Robert M. Kliegman, MD, *Guest Editors*
www.perinatology.theclinics.com

Preface

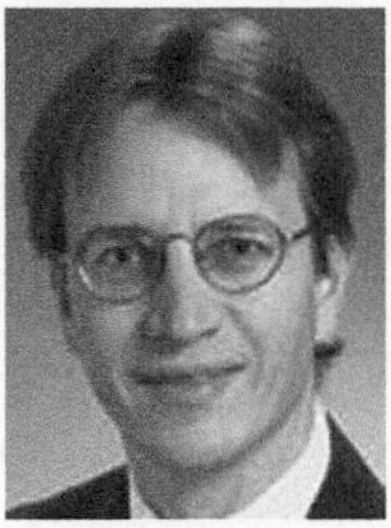

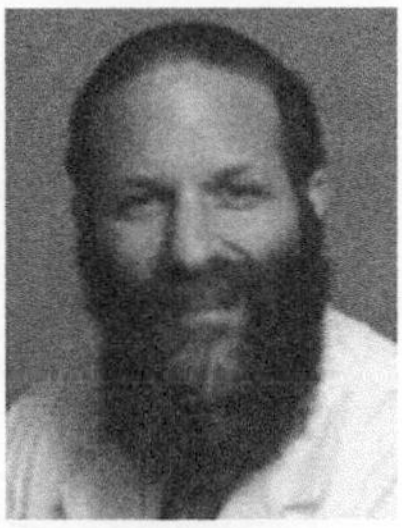

Michael R. Uhing, MD Robert Kliegman, MD
Guest Editors

Clinicians caring for neonates often are drawn to new and novel therapies in an attempt to improve outcomes. These new therapies undergo extensive evidence-based reviews and discussions before their introduction into the nursery. The older, more common therapies in the neonatal intensive care unit (NICU) are frequently not questioned, despite the fact that the evidence for their introduction may have been weak in the first place or that new evidence has emerged suggesting their role may have changed. Examples of therapies or practices extensively used in all NICUs include treatment of gastroesophageal reflux, use of home apnea monitoring, treatment of anemia, pain management, and nutritional support of the preterm infant. Discussions with colleagues around the world, and even within individual institutions, reveal considerable practice variation. For this issue of *Clinics in Perinatology* on "controversies," we chose to focus on these more common concerns facing clinicians caring for neonates. Interestingly, many of these topics have been reviewed in previous issues. Either the initial controversies surrounding each topic remain unresolved or new ones have emerged as knowledge has been obtained.

The final article on the role of genomics in the NICU may seem out of place in an issue dedicated to the more common topics, but we feel that this will significantly impact the care of all infants in the NICU in the near future. Genomic testing will likely be extensively used to predict outcome or affect the choice of medical therapy. As genomic testing becomes more common place, it is important that clinicians are aware of the issue involved.

We wish to thank the contributors to this issue. Each of them is an expert in their field and offers a unique perspective. The goal of each of article is to provide a thorough review of the topic, concentrating on the important controversial issues. We challenged each author to offer conclusions and/or recommendations based on the current available evidence and their extensive experience. We realize that the very nature of controversy makes this a truly difficult task, however, each author has risen to the challenge and provided an excellent review.

Clin Perinatol 36 (2009) xv–xvi
doi:10.1016/j.clp.2008.11.002 perinatology.theclinics.com
0095-5108/08/$ – see front matter

We hope that this issue stimulates you to review your practices and to conduct research to resolve many of the remaining unanswered questions.

Michael R. Uhing, MD
Department of Pediatrics
Section of Neonatology
Medical College of Wisconsin
Children's Corporate Center
PO Box 1997
Milwaukee, WI 53201

Robert Kliegman, MD
Department of Pediatrics
Section of Neonatology
Medical College of Wisconsin
Children's Corporate Center
PO Box 1997
Milwaukee, WI 53201

E-mail addresses:
muhing@mcw.edu (M.R. Uhing)
rkliegma@mcw.edu (R. Kliegman)

Errata

The author of the article "Cesarean Delivery and Its Impact on the Anomalous Infant," which appears in the June 2008 issue of *Clinics in Perinatology* (Volume 35, Issue 2), would like to amend the paragraph on page 402 under the heading "Hydrops." The paragraph should read:

Fetal hydrops results from a variety of causes in addition to the aforementioned masses, including congenital heart disease or arrhythmias, twin-twin transfusion, chromosomal abnormalities, hematologic abnormalities (immune and nonimmune anemia), congenital viral infections, and congenital chylothorax [64]. The literature on mode of delivery for fetal hydrops is insufficient to recommend one mode of delivery over the other, though in certain cases, cesarean delivery may avoid abdominal dystocia and reduce trauma to edematous and friable fetal tissues. Interventions should be individualized to the specific situation.

The authors of the article "Cytokines and Perinatal Brain Damage," which appears in the December 2008 issue of *Clinics in Perinatology* (Volume 35, Issue 4), would like to add the following acknowledgement of funding support to their article:

During the writing of this paper, the authors received support from the NIH (1 U01 NS 40069-01A2), the Susan B. Saltonstall Fund, the Richard Saltonstall Foundation, and the European Union (NEOBRAIN; LSHM-CT-2006-036534).

Clin Perinatol 36 (2009) xvii
doi:10.1016/j.clp.2008.11.001

Strategies to Prevent Bacterial and Fungal Infection in the Neonatal Intensive Care Unit

Jeffery S. Garland, MD[a,b,c,*], Michael R. Uhing, MD[d]

KEYWORDS

- Central venous catheter • Ventilator-associated pneumonia
- Fluconazole • Catheter-associated blood stream infection

Hospital-acquired infections occur in 7% to 24% of patients admitted to the neonatal intensive care unit (NICU) and lead to increases in length of stay, hospital cost, risk for neurologic impairment, and mortality.[1–7] Blood stream infections (BSIs) and pneumonia are most often associated with the use of central venous catheters (CVCs) and mechanical ventilation and account for up to 55% and 30% of NICU infections, respectively.[8] Gram-positive organisms are responsible for 70% of all BSI infections and 80% of all catheter-associated blood stream infections (CABSIs).[1,9] Gram-negative organisms account for just 18% of BSIs but for most ventilator-associated pneumonia (VAP).[1,10–12] Fungi account for up to 15% of BSIs in the NICU.[1,11,13]

Reporting agencies and outcome reports are now focused on device-related hospital-acquired infections, such as CABSIs and VAP, because these are the most common preventable nosocomial infections in the NICU.[14] Therefore, this review focuses primarily on these device-related infections. In addition, because invasive fungal infections account for a significant proportion of BSIs in the NICU and are often associated with the presence of CVCs, prevention strategies for fungal infections are examined.

Drs. Garland and Uhing have received research support from Medi-Flex, Inc. for the study of chlorhexidine gluconate.

[a] Wheaton Franciscan Health Care, St. Joseph Hospital, 3070 North 51st Street, Suite 309 Milwaukee, WI 53210, USA

[b] Department of Pediatrics, Medical College of Wisconsin, WI, USA

[c] Department of Pediatrics, University of Wisconsin School of Medicine and Public Health, WI, USA

[d] Division of Neonatology, Medical College of Wisconsin, Department of Pediatrics, Children's Corporate Center, Suite C410, PO Box 1997, Milwaukee, WI 53201–1997, USA

* Corresponding author. 3070 North 51 Street, Suite 309, Milwaukee, WI.

E-mail address: 53210.jsgarland@hotmail.com (J.S. Garland).

Clin Perinatol 36 (2009) 1–13

doi:10.1016/j.clp.2008.09.005 perinatology.theclinics.com

CATHETER-ASSOCIATED BLOODSTREAM INFECTIONS

One of the most important risk factors for a hospital-acquired BSI among critically ill neonates is the presence of a CVC.[1,15] In the National Hospital Safety Network (NHSN) survey, the rate of CABSIs was 4.4 to 6.4 per 1000 catheter-days among neonates weighing less than 1000 g.[14] Garland and colleagues,[9] in a large randomized trial of neonates with CVCs, noted that gram-positive organisms caused 79% of CABSIs, of which 83% were coagulase-negative Staphylococcus (CONS).

For the purpose of this review, the definition of a CABSI developed by the Centers for Disease Control and Prevention (CDC) is used, as defined by the following criteria: (1) the presence of a recognized pathogen isolated from at least one blood culture or a known skin pathogen from two blood cultures, (2) one or more clinical signs of infection, (3) the presence of an intravascular catheter when the BSI was diagnosed, and (4) no other documented primary site of infection. Such a definition is likely to overestimate the rate of CVC infections in neonates but serves as a practical and effective means to monitor the incidence of CABSIs in the NICU. References to catheter-related blood stream infections (CRBSIs) are occasionally made in this review. The criteria for the diagnosis of a CRBSI are similar to those for a CABSI, with the caveat that the catheter tip or hub is cultured and colonized with the same organism grown from the blood. Because the catheter hub or tip is rarely cultured in clinical practice, CABSI is more appropriate.

An understanding of the pathogenesis of CABSIs is essential so as to devise effective strategies for their prevention. Most CABSIs derive from extraluminal or intraluminal contamination of the catheter (**Fig. 1**). Extraluminal colonization of the intracutaneous tract is responsible for most CRBSIs in adults with short-term CVCs.[16,17] Contamination of the catheter tract occurs at the time of catheter insertion or within the first week of catheterization when the catheter is most mobile and can slide in and out of the insertion site, drawing organisms that are colonizing the skin into the catheter tract and down along the external surface of the catheter by capillary action. BSIs may follow when organisms are then released from the biofilm on the implanted portion of the catheter.

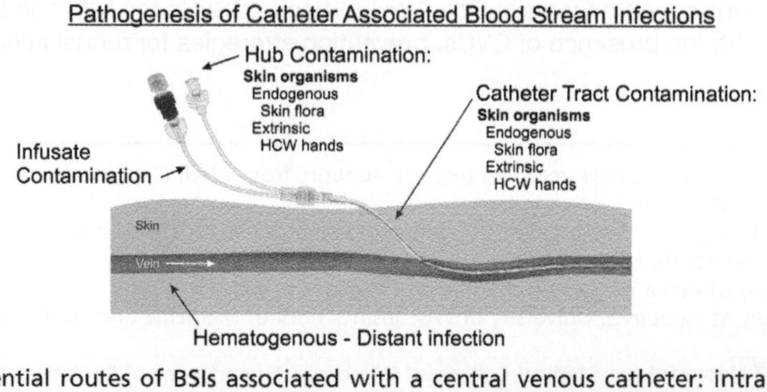

Fig. 1. Potential routes of BSIs associated with a central venous catheter: intraluminal, by contamination of the intravenous fluids or the catheter hub, and extraluminal, by contamination with local skin or health care worker (HCW) hand flora or from a distant unrelated site by way of a hematogenous route. (*Adapted from* Garland JS, Alex CP, Sevallius JM, et al. Cohort study of the pathogenesis and molecular epidemiology of catheter-related bloodstream infection in neonates with peripherally inserted central venous catheters. Infect Control Hosp Epidemiol 2008;29:244; with permission.)

Intraluminal contamination occurs primarily when the catheter hub becomes colonized and is responsible for CABSIs when central venous catheterization is prolonged.[16,18,19] Neonatal CVCs are routinely in place for more than 7 days; thus, most CABSIs are derived from intraluminal colonization after hub manipulation and contamination. Among neonates with primarily surgically placed CVCs, Salzman and colleagues[20] noted that in 10 of 28 episodes of CRBSIs, the same microorganism grown from the blood was grown from the catheter hub before the onset of BSI symptoms. In a prospective cohort of 357 patients with CVCs, Mahieu and colleagues[21] showed that the frequency of catheter manipulations was directly related to the risk for development of a CABSI. Recently, Garland and colleagues[22] used molecular epidemiology to examine the pathogenesis of neonatal catheter-related BSIs caused by CONS. Concordance between the organism grown from the catheter hub, catheter tip, and isolates from the blood was established using molecular subtyping by pulse-field gel electrophoresis. Ten (67%) of 15 catheter-related BSIs were considered intraluminally acquired, 3 (20%) of which were extraluminally acquired and 2 of which were of indeterminate origin. In a previous trial (n = 700) of CVCs, Garland and colleagues[9] found that just 3.5% of CRBSIs were associated with a colonized catheter tip. In both trials, the CVCs were in place for longer than 15 days.

Prevention of Catheter-Associated Blood Stream Infections

A multifaceted approach to prevent CABSIs is necessary because most infections can originate from two sources (contaminated catheter tract or hub). The 2002 Hospital Infection Control Practices Advisory Committee CDC Guidelines of Prevention of Intravascular Device-Related Infections provide a set of guidelines for all aspects of vascular care.[23] Most deal with adult and pediatric devices. Recently, several neonatal time-sequence trials have shown a reduction in neonatal CABSIs when "bundles" of the guidelines were incorporated into clinical practice.[7,24–26] By adopting CDC guidelines specific to neonates and extrapolating appropriate adult guidelines, a multifaceted approach can be developed to reduce CABSIs among neonates. Such an approach should include ongoing surveillance, staff education, a trained team of caregivers for catheter insertion and care, and strategies designed to prevent extraluminally and intraluminally acquired BSIs. Novel technologies may prove effective in units with high rates of CABSIs despite stringent compliance with infection control guidelines.

Surveillance

The CDC and the Joint Commission on Accreditation of Healthcare Organizations recommend routine monitoring of the incidence of CABSIs in the NICU and expressing the rate as CABSIs per 1000 catheter-days.[23] Continuously monitoring CABSI incidence allows for earlier detection of changes in infection rates, along with changes in unit practice. A recent multicenter cohort study performed by Schwab and colleagues[27] illustrates the importance of surveillance for neonatal BSIs. These researchers were able to show a 24% reduction in BSIs over a 3-year period among NICUs that were members of a surveillance network. The results of the surveillance-alone program are comparable to those of Bloom and colleagues,[26] who noted a 46% reduction in hospital-acquired infections after introduction of a comprehensive quality management program, along with a surveillance program. It is not likely that simple surveillance decreased the incidence of hospital-acquired infections in study NICUs; however, by knowing the local incidence of BSIs and comparing it with the network incidence, it is likely that poorly performing institutions took internal steps to reduce their infection rates. Networks similar to the NHSN offer opportunities for nurseries to track their CABSI incidence continuously against national rates so that unit practice changes can be more thoroughly evaluated.

Preventing Extraluminal Catheter Contamination

Proper hand hygiene, aseptic catheter insertion, and a well-applied sterile dressing help to prevent extraluminal colonization at the time of insertion and during the first week of catheterization. Because most hospital-acquired infections in the NICU, especially gram-positive organisms,[28] are transmitted on the hands of caregivers, hand hygiene has been singled out as the most important procedure for their prevention.[29,30] Although hand hygiene is a simple inexpensive procedure, compliance among health care workers is rarely 100%. Several studies have demonstrated that interventions to improve hand-washing compliance can effectively reduce hospital-acquired infections among neonates. Pessoa-Silva and colleagues[31] used a multifaceted hand hygiene education program to improve compliance among NICU caregivers and successfully reduced hospital-acquired infections among very low birth weight (VLBW) neonates. Similarly, Won and colleagues[32] and Lam and colleagues[33] showed a reduction in hospital-acquired infections in level III NICUs as hand hygiene compliance improved. Adequate hand hygiene before CVC placement should begin when entering the NICU. On entering the NICU, medical caregivers should perform a 3-minute scrub of their hands and arms with an antiseptic soap to a point above the elbow. Hands should be decontaminated with an alcohol-based hand rub or antiseptic soap before donning sterile gloves for CVC insertion.

Maximal sterile barrier precautions (eg, cap, mask, sterile gown, sterile gloves, large sterile drapes) should be used during CVC insertion.[34] Although povidone-iodine has been the most widely used antiseptic for cleansing potential CVC sites before insertion, chlorhexidine gluconate in an alcohol base is now recommended along with povidone-iodine as an effective antiseptic for the skin preparation before catheter placement for patients older than 2 months of age.[23] Chlorhexidine gluconate is currently not approved by the US Food and Drug Administration for use in neonates. Garland and colleagues[35] showed that 0.5% chlorhexidine gluconate in a 70% alcohol solution reduced colonization of neonatal peripheral intravenous catheters when compared with a 10% povidone-iodine scrub before catheter insertion; however, the rates of CRBSIs were similar. A chlorhexidine-impregnated gauze reduced CVC colonization among neonates when compared with a 10% povidone-iodine scrub before CVC placement.[9] Unlike adult studies, however, in which the impregnated gauze effectively reduced the rate of CRBSIs when compared with a povidone-iodine scrub, CRBSIs (catheter tip positive for the organism grown in the blood: 3.8% versus 3.2%; $P = 0.65$) and non-CRBSIs (BSIs without a source and a sterile catheter tip culture: 15.2% versus 14.3%; $P = 0.69$) rates were similar among treatment groups. Contact dermatitis occurred in 15% of neonates who weighed less than 1000 g, limiting the usefulness of this dressing in neonates. Differences between neonatal and adult results may partially be explained by the fact that neonatal CVCs were in situ longer than adult catheters (17.7 ± 0.9 days versus 3.8 ± 3 days); thus, extraluminal contamination likely played a smaller role in the pathogenesis of CRBSIs in neonates.[16]

After the position of the catheter is documented, it should be fixed with a clear semipermeable dressing. The catheter insertion site should be recleansed and redressed on a weekly basis.[36] In at least one quasiexperimental time-sequence study, weekly dressing changes, bundled with other accepted preventative guidelines, reduced the incidence of CABSIs in a NICU.[7] Current CDC guidelines suggest that the risk for catheter dislodgement may outweigh the benefits of dressing changes in neonates. During a multicenter randomized trial to assess the efficacy of a chlorhexidine-impregnated catheter, just one catheter was dislodged during more than 1200 scheduled dressing changes.[9] Over the past 5 years in two busy level III NICUs using a two-person dressing change technique, the authors have not lost a catheter.

Preventing Intraluminal Contamination

Meticulous hub care is an important aspect of preventing CABSIs in neonates whose catheters remain in place longer than 1 week. Daily hub entry for medication administration should be limited. One port of a bifuse or trifuse extension set attached to the catheter should be used exclusively for parenteral nutrition and lipid emulsions. Medications can be administered using a closed medication system through a separate port.[7] Intravenous tubing changes should be done with aseptic techniques. The entry port of the hub or needleless devices should be disinfected for at least 10 seconds with an antiseptic before entry. Most units currently use alcohol wipes. Recently, 0.5% chlorhexidine gluconate in a 70% alcohol solution has been shown to be more effective than alcohol alone in decontaminating needleless entry ports.[37] The incidence of CABSIs was not assessed during the trial; thus, it is not known whether the more effective external hub decontamination with the use of chlorhexidine necessarily results in lower CABSI rates.

Removal of the CVC is the most effective means of reducing CVC hub manipulation. While the catheter is in place, daily catheter management goals should focus on whether or not the catheter is required and, if required, how hub manipulations can be minimized. Removing catheters when enteral feedings reach 100 mL/kg/d can reduce days of catheterization. Transitioning intravenous medications to an enteral route or to a peripheral intravenous catheter when possible can also help to reduce daily hub manipulations.

Antibiotic Lock Prophylaxis

The efficacy of a prophylactic antibiotic lock solution has been demonstrated in pediatric patients.[38] Garland and colleagues[39] assessed the efficacy of a vancomycin (25 μg/mL)-heparin lock solution for the prevention of CRBSIs in ill neonates. Percutaneously placed CVCs of study neonates (n = 42) were locked twice daily with the vancomycin-heparin lock solution for 20 or 60 minutes, depending on enteral intake. Controls (n = 43) were locked with a heparin solution. The vancomycin-lock group had significantly fewer CRBSIs. No vancomycin-resistant organisms were recovered from study or nonstudy neonates during the trial. Vancomycin was not detected in the blood of neonates in the vancomycin-heparin lock group during the trial. At least one episode of hypoglycemia (whole blood glucose ≤45 mg/dL) occurred at the end of a dwell period in 19% of study infants. In a follow-up time-sequence quasiexperimental trial in two level III NICUs, neonates (n = 191) whose catheters were locked twice daily with a vancomycin-heparin lock solution for 10 or 20 minutes, depending on enteral intake, were less likely to have CABSIs from gram-positive organisms (7% versus 13%, odds ratio = 0.61, 95% confidence interval: 0.33–1.1) than historic controls (n = 288), although the results did not reach statistical significance.[40] Total days of systemic vancomycin therapy per 1000 catheter-days were significantly less in lock-treated neonates ($P<0.001$). Only 3% of neonates developed an episode of hypoglycemia at the end of the dwell period. Hypoglycemia episodes were asymptomatic and resolved immediately with reinstitution of intravenous fluids. Vancomycin-resistant organisms have not been isolated in any of the units. In a meta-analysis done by Safdar and Maki[41] of seven randomized trials involving 463 patients, risk for CRBSIs was reduced in patients whose CVCs were locked with a vancomycin-heparin solution.

In a recent randomized trial of a fusidic acid (4 mg/mL)–heparin lock solution, treated neonates were less likely to develop CRBSIs than control neonates (6.6 versus 24.9 per 1000 catheter-days; *P*<0.01).[42] Fusidic acid is not available in the United States.

More data are needed, especially from randomized studies that prospectively assess the impact on nosocomial colonization by drug-resistant microorganisms, before routine use of antibiotic lock solutions can be recommended. The CDC does not currently recommend the routine use of antibiotic lock solutions because of concerns for the development of resistant organisms. The use of antibiotic lock solutions may be considered in units in which the rate of CABSIs remains elevated even after strict adherence to established published catheter care guidelines.

Treatment of Line-Related Infections

Treatment for CABSIs begins with documentation that a BSI truly exists. Obtaining two peripheral blood cultures from separate sites after cleansing the sites thoroughly with an antiseptic is routinely done in pediatric patients and adult patients to ensure adequate sampling. Blood cultures are often difficult to obtain from neonates, prompting caregivers to rely on a single blood culture before initiating antibiotics for a presumptive BSI. Obtaining two blood cultures before antibiotic treatment may help to reduce antibiotic exposure after a potentially contaminated culture.[43] In a time-sequence cohort study, Garland and colleagues[40] obtained a single blood culture from neonates with CVCs before initiating antibiotic coverage with a semisynthetic penicillin and gentamicin. If the culture grew CONS, a second blood culture was done and vancomycin was substituted for semisynthetic penicillin. If the newborn was doing well and the second blood culture was sterile, antibiotics were discontinued. The incidence of CABSIs was lowered, and days of systemic vancomycin per 1000 catheter-days were significantly less after initiation of this management strategy and the vancomycin-lock protocol.

Antibiotic treatment through the CVC can effectively clear most CABSIs attributable to CONS. If the blood is not sterile after several days of systemic vancomycin, the catheter should be removed.[44,45] In one case series of neonates with Enterobacteriaceae, 45% of the neonates were effectively treated with appropriate antibiotics through the CVC.[46] Benjamin and colleagues[45] found that just 37% of neonates with gram-negative BSIs could retain their CVC without infection-related complications, however, and recommend removal of the CVC when the CABSI was caused by a gram-negative organism or *Staphylococcus aureus*. CVCs should be removed when a fungal CABSI occurs.

PREVENTION OF INVASIVE FUNGAL INFECTIONS

In a retrospective case-controlled study, colonization of the CVC with *Candida* species was the most important risk factor for the development of invasive *Candida* infection.[47] Other risk factors for an invasive fungal infection include lower birth weight/gestation,[48–52] abdominal surgery or pathologic findings,[13,49,51,53,54] H_2 blocker exposure,[49] lipid,[49] antibiotic exposure,[13,47,49] increased length of mechanical ventilation, and increased length of stay.[49]

Multiple studies have shown the efficacy of fluconazole prophylaxis to prevent fungal colonization and invasive disease.[50,55–61] A recent Cochrane meta-analysis showed a significant reduction in invasive fungal disease in VLBW infants with fluconazole prophylaxis.[62] The reviewers noted that the rate of invasive fungal disease was higher than previously reported in several of the studies' control groups, however. Risk for death before hospital discharge trended lower with fluconazole prophylaxis, but the difference was not statistically significant.

Various dosing regimens have been studied. Fluconazole doses range from 3 to 6 mg/kg per dose with initial dosing intervals varying from every third day to twice weekly. In most studies, the dosing interval decreases from twice weekly to every other day after 2 weeks of treatment and then to daily 2 weeks later. Kaufman and colleagues[56] compared a dosing regimen of twice weekly for the entire 6 weeks and a regimen with increasing frequency, such as that described previously, and found no difference between the two regimens. Therefore, this simpler regimen decreases exposure to fluconazole, minimizing the treatment risks while maintaining efficacy for the prevention of fungal infection.

There are several concerns regarding widespread use of fluconazole to prevent fungal disease in VLBW infants. Whenever prophylactic antibiotic use is widespread, there are concerns about the development of resistant organisms. Most studies have not found a change in organism resistance patterns in nurseries after the introduction of fluconazole prophylaxis into the unit.[51,55,57–60,63] Sarvikivi and colleagues[64] did find the emergence of a fluconazole-resistant strain of *Candida parapsilosis* in Finland after 10 years of fluconazole prophylaxis. Therefore, with more widespread and long-term use of fluconazole, resistant strains may begin to develop.

Hepatotoxicity is also a concern with fluconazole prophylaxis. In extremely low birth weight (ELBW) infants, cholestasis may occur with fluconazole prophylaxis.[50] In a retrospective analysis of a shorter course of prophylaxis in a targeted high-risk population, cholestasis did not occur.[51] In this study, however, the high threshold to meet the criteria for cholestasis, a direct bilirubin level greater than 5 mg/dL, probably led to an underestimation of the incidence. Other studies have reported transient elevations in serum transaminase concentrations but have not found long-term hepatotoxicity.[57,59] Fluconazole inhibits CYP 450 enzymes, and therefore may interfere with the metabolism of barbiturates, phenytoin, theophylline, and caffeine.

Strict adherence to infection control guidelines and CDC recommendations for CVC care are necessary before considering the implementation of any unit-wide targeted or comprehensive prophylactic fluconazole treatment protocol. Because of the potential benefits of fluconazole prophylaxis, it may be reasonable to target only those neonates who have multiple risk factors for the development of invasive fungal disease. Such an approach has been shown to minimize risk and preserve efficacy.[50,51,60]

VENTILATOR-ASSOCIATED PNEUMONIA

The incidence of VAP in NICUs varies from 0 to 15.7 episodes per 1000 ventilator-days.[14,65,66] Risk factors include lower gestational age, lower birth weight, duration of mechanical ventilation, number of reintubations, opiate use, and endotracheal suctioning.[10,14,65–67]

The major controversy regarding VAP in the NICU is the criteria used to make the diagnosis.[68] The CDC and NHSN have established stringent clinical criteria for the diagnosis of VAP that include all the following: mechanical ventilation within 48 hours before onset of infection; worsening gas exchange with increased oxygen or ventilation requirements; two or more chest radiographs showing new infiltrates, consolidation, cavitation, or pneumatoceles; and at least three signs and symptoms, such as temperature instability, change in respiratory secretions, abnormal leukocyte count, wheezing, tachypnea, cough, and abnormal heart rate. These criteria are not specific to neonates, particularly VLBW infants with bronchopulmonary dysplasia, and have not been validated in the neonatal population. Signs and symptoms of VAP are open to subjective interpretation because they often overlap with other disease processes. VLBW infants with pneumonia seldom develop cough, rhonchi, fever, or wheezing. Interpretation of radiographs in VLBW infants with underlying chronic lung disease is also difficult.[12] Finally, the lack of a uniform surveillance method dramatically affects the reported incidence of VAP.[69,70] Despite these difficulties, the incidence of VAP in the NICU is monitored by the NHSN and, more frequently, by many other public and private reporting agencies.

Although not included in the diagnostic criteria for VAP, tracheal aspirate cultures and Gram stains are often included in the evaluation of patients. These tests have a low sensitivity, specificity, and positive predictive value because it is difficult to distinguish between tracheal colonization and a true respiratory tract infection.[71] The presence of white blood cells in the tracheal aspirate fluid has been used to help differentiate between colonization and infection. In a retrospective cohort study, 92% of neonates with VAP in the NICU had purulent tracheal aspirates (>25 leukocytes per high-power field), whereas only 53% had a positive tracheal culture.[10] In VLBW infants, however, VAP occurs in 7% of preterm infants without purulent tracheal aspirates and in just 5% of infants with purulent aspirates.[72] Most VLBW infants with purulent tracheal aspirates are asymptomatic, whereas leukocytes are absent in 58% of culture-positive tracheal aspirates.[72] When a positive tracheal aspirate culture is associated with VAP, gram-negative organisms, especially *Pseudomonas*, *Escherichia coli*, and *Klebsiella*, are most common.[10–12] The "gold standard" for diagnosis involves lung biopsy, which is not practical in neonates. Other invasive testing using bronchoalveolar lavage or a protected specimen brush improves diagnostic accuracy in adults and older pediatric patients but is also not practical in the neonatal population.[67]

The CDC and American Thoracic Society have published guidelines for prevention of health care–associated pneumonia.[73,74] Several studies show that implementation of these practices reduces VAP in adults.[75–79] The Institute for Healthcare Improvement has modified the recommendations for pediatric patients. Specific recommendations include elevation of the head of the bed of a neonate 15° to 30° to prevent aspiration of enteral feedings, daily assessment extubation readiness to reduce the length of mechanical ventilation, age-appropriate comprehensive mouth care to reduce oropharyngeal colonization, preventing ventilator circuit condensation by draining water away from the patient every 2 to 4 hours and using heated circuits, changing ventilator circuits and in-line suction catheters only when they are visibly soiled, and storage of oral suction devices in a clean nonsealed plastic bag when not in use.[80] In a time-sequence experimental study done in children, the rate of VAP was reduced after the implementation of these guidelines.[81]

Only a few of the recommendations have been studied in neonates. In time-sequenced cohort studies, reducing days of mechanical ventilation in preterm infants by using a high-flow nasal cannula device[82] or traditional nasal continuous positive airway pressure[83] significantly decreased the incidence of VAP. Increasing hand hygiene compliance in a NICU from 43% to 80% during a time-sequence quasiexperimental trial reduced respiratory infections from 3.35 to 1.09 per 1000 patient-days.[32] In a prospective randomized trial, increasing the interval between ventilator circuit changes has not been shown to increase the incidence of VAP in preterm infants.[84]

Although definitive evidence for the use of specific VAP prevention measures is lacking in neonates, most recommendations are biologically plausible and easy to implement. To determine if preventative strategies can truly reduce neonatal VAP, however, diagnostic criteria and surveillance methods that are applicable to the neonatal population need to be established.

SUMMARY

Device-related infections (CABSIs or VAP) are the most common type of hospital-acquired infections in neonates. Prevention of CABSIs requires a multifaceted approach that should concentrate on the prevention of extraluminal and intraluminal catheter contamination. Implementation of an antibiotic lock solution or prophylactic fluconazole protocol to prevent CABSIs should be considered only after ensuring strict adherence to established published catheter care guidelines. Although most strategies to prevent VAP among neonatal patients are biologically plausible and easily implemented, better diagnostic criteria and surveillance techniques for VAP in the neonatal population need to be established before the effectiveness of these strategies can be assessed.

REFERENCES

1. Stoll BJ, Hansen N, Fanaroff AA, et al. Late-onset sepsis in very low birth weight neonates: the experience of the NICHD neonatal research network. Pediatrics 2002;110(2 Pt 1):285–91.
2. Mahieu LM, Buitenweg N, Beutels P, et al. Additional hospital stay and charges due to hospital-acquired infections in a neonatal intensive care unit. J Hosp Infect 2001;47(3):223–9.
3. Stoll BJ, Hansen NI, Adams-Chapman I, et al. Neurodevelopmental and growth impairment among extremely low-birth-weight infants with neonatal infection. J Am Med Assoc 2004;292(19):2357–65.
4. Aziz K, McMillan DD, Andrews W, et al. Variations in rates of nosocomial infection among Canadian neonatal intensive care units may be practice-related. Available at: http://www.pubmedcentral.nih.gov/articlerender.fcgi?tool=pubmed&pubmedid=16004613. Accessed November 7, 2008.
5. Gray JE, Richardson DK, McCormick MC, et al. Coagulase-negative staphylococcal bacteremia among very low birth weight infants: relation to admission illness severity, resource use, and outcome. Pediatrics 1995;95(2):225–30.
6. Horbar JD, Rogowski J, Plsek PE, et al. Collaborative quality improvement for neonatal intensive care. NIC/Q Project Investigators of the Vermont Oxford Network. Pediatrics 2001;107(1):14–22.
7. Aly H, Herson V, Duncan A, et al. Is bloodstream infection preventable among premature infants? A tale of two cities. Pediatrics 2005;115(6):1513–8.
8. Borghesi A, Stronati M. Strategies for the prevention of hospital-acquired infections in the neonatal intensive care unit. J Hosp Infect 2008;68(4):293–300.
9. Garland JS, Alex CP, Mueller CD, et al. A randomized trial comparing povidone-iodine to a chlorhexidine gluconate-impregnated dressing for prevention of central venous catheter infections in neonates. Pediatrics 2001;107(6):1431–6.
10. Yuan TM, Chen LH, Yu HM. Risk factors and outcomes for ventilator-associated pneumonia in neonatal intensive care unit patients. J Perinat Med 2007;35(4):334–8.
11. Su BH, Hsieh HY, Chiu HY, et al. Nosocomial infection in a neonatal intensive care unit: a prospective study in Taiwan. Am J Infect Control 2007;35(3):190–5.
12. Cordero L, Ayers LW, Miller RR, et al. Surveillance of ventilator-associated pneumonia in very-low-birth-weight infants. Am J Infect Control 2002;30(1):32–9.
13. Feja KN, Wu F, Roberts K, et al. Risk factors for candidemia in critically ill infants: a matched case-control study. J Pediatr 2005;147(2):156–61.
14. Edwards JR, Peterson KD, Andrus ML, et al. National healthcare safety network (NHSN) report, data summary for 2006, issued June 2007. Am J Infect Control 2007;35(5):290–301.

15. Perlman SE, Saiman L, Larson EL. Risk factors for late-onset health care-associated bloodstream infections in patients in neonatal intensive care units. Am J Infect Control 2007;35(3):177–82.
16. Safdar N, Maki DG. The pathogenesis of catheter-related bloodstream infection with noncuffed short-term central venous catheters. Intensive Care Med 2004;30(1):62–7.
17. Maki DG, Stolz SM, Wheeler S, et al. Prevention of central venous catheter-related bloodstream infection by use of an antiseptic-impregnated catheter. A randomized, controlled trial. Ann Intern Med 1997;127(4):257–66.
18. Raad I, Costerton W, Sabharwal U, et al. Ultrastructural analysis of indwelling vascular catheters: a quantitative relationship between luminal colonization and duration of placement. J Infect Dis 1993;168(2):400–7.
19. Sitges-Serra A, Puig P, Linares J, et al. Hub colonization as the initial step in an outbreak of catheter-related sepsis due to coagulase negative staphylococci during parenteral nutrition. JPEN J Parenter Enteral Nutr 1984;8(6):668–72.
20. Salzman MB, Isenberg HD, Shapiro JF, et al. A prospective study of the catheter hub as the portal of entry for microorganisms causing catheter-related sepsis in neonates. J Infect Dis 1993;167(2):487–90.
21. Mahieu LM, De Dooy JJ, Lenaerts AE, et al. Catheter manipulations and the risk of catheter-associated bloodstream infection int neonatal intensive care unit patients. J Hosp Infect 2001;48(1):20–6.
22. Garland JS, Alex CP, Sevallius JM, et al. Cohort study of the pathogenesis and molecular epidemiology of catheter-related bloodstream infection in neonates with peripherally inserted central venous catheters. Infect Control Hosp Epidemiol 2008;29(3):243–9.
23. O'Grady NP, Alexander M, Dellinger EP, et al. Guidelines for the prevention of intravascular catheter-related infections. Am J Infect Control 2002;30(8):476–89.
24. Andersen C, Hart J, Vemgal P, et al. Prospective evaluation of a multi-factorial prevention strategy on the impact of nosocomial infection in very-low-birthweight infants. J Hosp Infect 2005;61(2):162–7.
25. Kilbride HW, Wirtschafter DD, Powers RJ, et al. Implementation of evidence-based potentially better practices to decrease nosocomial infections. Pediatrics 2003;111(4 Pt 2):e519–33.
26. Bloom BT, Craddock A, Delmore PM, et al. Reducing acquired infections in the NICU: observing and implementing meaningful differences in process between high and low acquired infection rate centers. J Perinatol 2003;23(6):489–92.
27. Schwab F, Geffers C, Barwolff S, et al. Reducing neonatal nosocomial bloodstream infections through participation in a national surveillance system. J Hosp Infect 2007;65(4):319–25.
28. Larson EL, Cimiotti JP, Haas J, et al. Gram-negative bacilli associated with catheter-associated and non-catheter-associated bloodstream infections and hand carriage by healthcare workers in neonatal intensive care units. Pediatr Crit Care Med 2005;6(4):457–61.
29. Steere AC, Mallison GF. Handwashing practices for the prevention of nosocomial infections. Ann Intern Med 1975;83(5):683–90.
30. Daschner FD. Useful and useless hygienic techniques in intensive care units. Intensive Care Med 1985;11(6):280–3.
31. Pessoa-Silva CL, Hugonnet S, Pfister R, et al. Reduction of health care associated infection risk in neonates by successful hand hygiene promotion. Pediatrics 2007; 120(2):e382–90.
32. Won SP, Chou HC, Hsieh WS, et al. Handwashing program for the prevention of nosocomial infections in a neonatal intensive care unit. Infect Control Hosp Epidemiol 2004;25(9):742–6.

33. Lam BC, Lee J, Lau YL. Hand hygiene practices in a neonatal intensive care unit: a multimodal intervention and impact on nosocomial infection. Pediatrics 2004; 114(5):e565–71.
34. Raad II, Hohn DC, Gilbreath BJ, et al. Prevention of central venous catheter-related infections by using maximal sterile barrier precautions during insertion. Infect Control Hosp Epidemiol 1994;15(4 Pt 1):231–8.
35. Garland JS, Buck RK, Maloney P, et al. Comparison of 10% povidone-iodine and 0.5% chlorhexidine gluconate for the prevention of peripheral intravenous catheter colonization in neonates: a prospective trial. Pediatr Infect Dis J 1995;14(6): 510–6.
36. Laura R, Degl'Innocenti M, Mocali M, et al. Comparison of two different time interval protocols for central venous catheter dressing in bone marrow transplant patients: results of a randomized, multicenter study. The Italian Nurse Bone Marrow Transplant Group (GITMO). Haematologica 2000;85(3):275–9.
37. Casey AL, Worthington T, Lambert PA, et al. A randomized, prospective clinical trial to assess the potential infection risk associated with the PosiFlow needleless connector. J Hosp Infect 2003;54(4):288–93.
38. Henrickson KJ, Axtell RA, Hoover SM, et al. Prevention of central venous catheter-related infections and thrombotic events in immunocompromised children by the use of vancomycin/ciprofloxacin/heparin flush solution: a randomized, multicenter, double-blind trial. J Clin Oncol 2000;18(6):1269–78.
39. Garland JS, Alex CP, Henrickson KJ, et al. A vancomycin-heparin lock solution for prevention of nosocomial bloodstream infection in critically ill neonates with peripherally inserted central venous catheters: a prospective, randomized trial. Pediatrics 2005;116(2):e198–205.
40. Garland JS, Kannenberg SM, Porter DM, et al. Reducing PICC-related bloodstream infections (CRBSI) and systemic vancomycin use in VLBW neonates with routine use of a vancomycin/heparin lock solution. [abstract]. Pediatr Res 2004;55(4 (Part 2)):392A.
41. Safdar N, Maki DG. Use of vancomycin-containing lock or flush solutions for prevention of bloodstream infection associated with central venous access devices: a meta-analysis of prospective, randomized trials. Clin Infect Dis 2006;43(4): 474–84.
42. Filippi L, Pezzati M, Di Amario S, et al. Fusidic acid and heparin lock solution for the prevention of catheter-related bloodstream infections in critically ill neonates: a retrospective study and a prospective, randomized trial. Pediatr Crit Care Med 2007;8(6):556–62.
43. Struthers S, Underhill H, Albersheim S, et al. A comparison of two versus one blood culture in the diagnosis and treatment of coagulase-negative Staphylococcus in the neonatal intensive care unit. J Perinatol 2002;22(7):547–9.
44. Nistala K, Nicholl R. Should preterm neonates with a central venous catheter and coagulase negative staphylococcal bacteraemia be treated without removal of the catheter? Arch Dis Child 2003;88(5):458–9.
45. Benjamin DK Jr, Miller W, Garges H, et al. Bacteremia, central catheters, and neonates: when to pull the line. Pediatrics 2001;107(6):1272–6.
46. Nazemi KJ, Buescher ES, Kelly RE Jr, et al. Central venous catheter removal versus in situ treatment in neonates with Enterobacteriaceae bacteremia. Pediatrics 2003;111(3):e269–74.
47. Manzoni P, Farina D, Leonessa M, et al. Risk factors for progression to invasive fungal infection in preterm neonates with fungal colonization. Pediatrics 2006; 118(6):2359–64.

48. Farmaki E, Evdoridou J, Pouliou T, et al. Fungal colonization in the neonatal intensive care unit: risk factors, drug susceptibility, and association with invasive fungal infections. Am J Perinatol 2007;24(2):127–35.
49. Saiman L, Ludington E, Pfaller M, et al. Risk factors for candidemia in Neonatal Intensive Care Unit patients. The National Epidemiology of Mycosis Survey Study Group. Pediatr Infect Dis J 2000;19(4):319–24.
50. Aghai ZH, Mudduluru M, Nakhla TA, et al. Fluconazole prophylaxis in extremely low birth weight infants: association with cholestasis. J Perinatol 2006;26(9):550–5.
51. Uko S, Soghier LM, Vega M, et al. Targeted short-term fluconazole prophylaxis among very low birth weight and extremely low birth weight infants. Pediatrics 2006;117(4):1243–52.
52. Johnsson H, Ewald U. The rate of candidaemia in preterm infants born at a gestational age of 23–28 weeks is inversely correlated to gestational age. Acta Paediatr 2004;93(7):954–8.
53. Coates EW, Karlowicz MG, Croitoru DP, et al. Distinctive distribution of pathogens associated with peritonitis in neonates with focal intestinal perforation compared with necrotizing enterocolitis. Pediatrics 2005;116(2):e241–6.
54. Adderson EE, Pappin A, Pavia AT. Spontaneous intestinal perforation in premature infants: a distinct clinical entity associated with systemic candidiasis. J Pediatr Surg 1998;33(10):1463–7.
55. Kaufman D, Boyle R, Hazen KC, et al. Fluconazole prophylaxis against fungal colonization and infection in preterm infants. N Engl J Med 2001;345(23):1660–6.
56. Kaufman D, Boyle R, Hazen KC, et al. Twice weekly fluconazole prophylaxis for prevention of invasive Candida infection in high-risk infants of <1000 grams birth weight. J Pediatr 2005;147(2):172–9.
57. Kicklighter SD, Springer SC, Cox T, et al. Fluconazole for prophylaxis against candidal rectal colonization in the very low birth weight infant. Pediatrics 2001;107(2):293–8.
58. Manzoni P, Arisio R, Mostert M, et al. Prophylactic fluconazole is effective in preventing fungal colonization and fungal systemic infections in preterm neonates: a single-center, 6-year, retrospective cohort study. Pediatrics 2006;117(1):e22–32.
59. Manzoni P, Stolfi I, Pugni L, et al. A multicenter, randomized trial of prophylactic fluconazole in preterm neonates. N Engl J Med 2007;356(24):2483–95.
60. McCrossan BA, McHenry E, O'Neill F, et al. Selective fluconazole prophylaxis in high-risk babies to reduce invasive fungal infection. Arch Dis Child Fetal Neonatal Ed 2007;92(6):F454–8.
61. Bertini G, Perugi S, Dani C, et al. Fluconazole prophylaxis prevents invasive fungal infection in high-risk, very low birth weight infants. J Pediatr 2005;147(2):162–5.
62. Clerihew L, Austin N, McGuire W. Prophylactic systemic antifungal agents to prevent mortality and morbidity in very low birth weight infants. Cochrane Database Syst Rev 2007;(4):CD003850.
63. Fridkin SK, Kaufman D, Edwards JR, et al. Changing incidence of Candida bloodstream infections among NICU patients in the United States: 1995–2004. Pediatrics 2006;117(5):1680–7.
64. Sarvikivi E, Lyytikainen O, Soll DR, et al. Emergence of fluconazole resistance in a Candida parapsilosis strain that caused infections in a neonatal intensive care unit. J Clin Microbiol 2005;43(6):2729–35.
65. Apisarnthanarak A, Holzmann-Pazgal G, Hamvas A, et al. Ventilator-associated pneumonia in extremely preterm neonates in a neonatal intensive care unit: characteristics, risk factors, and outcomes. Pediatrics 2003;112(6 Pt 1):1283–9.

66. Stover BH, Shulman ST, Bratcher DF, et al. Nosocomial infection rates in US children's hospitals' neonatal and pediatric intensive care units. Am J Infect Control 2001;29(3):152–7.
67. Foglia E, Meier MD, Elward A. Ventilator-associated pneumonia in neonatal and pediatric intensive care unit patients. Clin Microbiol Rev 2007;20(3):409–25 [table of contents].
68. Baltimore RS. The difficulty of diagnosing ventilator-associated pneumonia. Pediatrics 2003;112(6 Pt 1):1420–1.
69. Eggimann P, Hugonnet S, Sax H, et al. Ventilator-associated pneumonia: caveats for benchmarking. Intensive Care Med 2003;29(11):2086–9.
70. Langley JM, Bradley JS. Defining pneumonia in critically ill infants and children. Pediatr Crit Care Med 2005;6(3 Suppl):S9–13.
71. Evans ME, Schaffner W, Federspiel CF, et al. Sensitivity, specificity, and predictive value of body surface cultures in a neonatal intensive care unit. J Am Med Assoc 1988;259(2):248–52.
72. Cordero L, Sananes M, Dedhiya P, et al. Purulence and gram-negative bacilli in tracheal aspirates of mechanically ventilated very low birth weight infants. J Perinatol 2001;21(6):376–81.
73. Tablan OC, Anderson LJ, Besser R, et al. Guidelines for preventing health-care–associated pneumonia, 2003: recommendations of CDC and the Healthcare Infection Control Practices Advisory Committee. MMWR Recomm Rep 2004;53(RR-3):1–36.
74. Guidelines for the management of adults with hospital-acquired, ventilator-associated, and healthcare-associated pneumonia. Am J Respir Crit Care Med 2005; 171(4):388–416.
75. Kollef MH. Prevention of hospital-associated pneumonia and ventilator-associated pneumonia. Crit Care Med 2004;32(6):1396–405.
76. Gastmeier P, Geffers C. Prevention of ventilator-associated pneumonia: analysis of studies published since 2004. J Hosp Infect 2007;67(1):1–8.
77. Omrane R, Eid J, Perreault MM, et al. Impact of a protocol for prevention of ventilator-associated pneumonia. Ann Pharmacother 2007;41(9):1390–6.
78. Resar R, Pronovost P, Haraden C, et al. Using a bundle approach to improve ventilator care processes and reduce ventilator-associated pneumonia. Jt Comm J Qual Patient Saf 2005;31(5):243–8.
79. Lorente L, Blot S, Rello J. Evidence on measures for the prevention of ventilator-associated pneumonia. Eur Respir J 2007;30(6):1193–207.
80. Pediatric Affinity Group. How-to-guide pediatric supplement: ventilator associated pneumonia. Institute for Healthcare Improvement. Available at: http://www.nichq.org/NR/rdonlyres/8425AC41-EE37-4D0F-A3BA-27CFC3AD9045/5520/VAP.pdf. Accessed November 9, 2008.
81. Curley MA, Schwalenstocker E, Deshpande JK, et al. Tailoring the Institute for Health Care Improvement 100,000 Lives Campaign to pediatric settings: the example of ventilator-associated pneumonia. Pediatr Clin North Am 2006;53(6): 1231–51.
82. Holleman-Duray D, Kaupie D, Weiss MG. Heated humidified high-flow nasal cannula: use and a neonatal early extubation protocol. J Perinatol 2007;27(12):776–81.
83. Hentschel J, Brungger B, Studi K, et al. Prospective surveillance of nosocomial infections in a Swiss NICU: low risk of pneumonia on nasal continuous positive airway pressure? Infection 2005;33(5–6):350–5.
84. Makhoul IR, Kassis I, Berant M, et al. Frequency of change of ventilator circuit in premature infants: impact on ventilator-associated pneumonia. Pediatr Crit Care Med 2001;2(2):127–32.

Drugs of Choice for Sedation and Analgesia in the Neonatal ICU

R. Whit Hall, MD[a,*], Rolla M. Shbarou, MD[b]

KEYWORDS

• Pain • Infant • Newborn • Premature • Analgesia • Sedation
• Opiate • Benzodiazepine • Barbituate

Before 1980, pain in the newborn period was infrequently recognized or treated.[1] The reference standard of pain assessment is self reporting which clearly is not possible in the newborn period; thus, clinicians can measure pain only indirectly. Animal and human studies have documented that neonatal pain is associated with both short- and- long term consequences.[2,3] Further, the enhanced survival of extremely low birth weight babies makes them more susceptible to the effects of pain and stress because of increased exposure. Indeed, one study documented that neonates under 32 weeks' gestation were exposed to 10 to 15 painful procedures per day, and most of these procedures were untreated.[4] Unfortunately, this problem continues. A recent study by Carbajol and colleagues[5] has documented the increased occurrence and lack of treatment of neonatal pain in almost 80% of newborns in intensive care!

Analgesia and sedation in the neonatal ICU (NICU) has been fraught with controversy because of concern about the safety of these drugs in the neonatal population, the lack of adequate pharmacokinetic and pharmacodynamic data in this population, difficulty in assessing pain, and lack of long-term neurodevelopmental assessment of survivors for the pain experienced in the neonatal period.[6–9] Legitimate concern about safety has led to more governance for moderate sedation privileges for clinicians caring for neonates as well as more emphasis on obtaining consent for sedation,[10] creating roadblocks to giving sedation to neonates undergoing painful procedures. Further, individual differences and decreased morphine metabolism in neonates of younger gestational age may lead to the rapid development of tolerance as well as to the accumulation of the drug in extremely preterm neonates.[11] Thus, the use of

The author's (RWH) work was supported in part by funding from The Center for Translational Neuroscience by grant # RR 020,146 from the National Institutes of Health.
[a] Division of Neonatology, University of Arkansas for Medical Sciences, Slot 512B, 4301 W Markham, Little Rock, AR 72205, USA
[b] Division of Neurology, University of Arkansas for Medical Sciences, Arkansas Children's Hospital, Slot 512, 800 Marshall Street, Little Rock, AR 72202, USA
* Corresponding author.
E-mail address: hallrichardw@uams.edu (R.W. Hall).

Clin Perinatol 36 (2009) 15–26
doi:10.1016/j.clp.2008.09.007 perinatology.theclinics.com

sedation and analgesia in the neonatal population, although extremely important, must be done safely and effectively.

OPIOIDS

Opioids are used commonly in modern NICUs.[12] They provide relief from procedural pain (eg, medication before intubation)[13–15] and from chronic pain (eg, pain caused by necrotizing enterocolitis[16] or ventilation).[17–19] Several studies and reviews have concluded that opioids should be used selectively. A recent Cochrane review found insufficient evidence to recommend routine use of opioids in mechanically ventilated newborns.[19] The Cochrane review looked at pain scales and found an overall significant effect on pain in the treatment group. No significant effects were seen the treatment group with respect to neonatal mortality, duration of ventilation, short-term or long-term neurodevelopmental outcome, incidence of severe intraventricular hemorrhage (IVH), any IVH, or periventricular leukomalacia (PVL). Given the likely long-term adverse consequences associated with the chronic pain and stress of mechanical ventilation, it is reassuring that short-term adverse effects of analgesia are not more common in the opioid-treated groups.

Morphine

Morphine is the most frequently used opioid analgesic in patients of all ages and is the drug most commonly used for analgesia in ventilated neonates.[12] Morphine has a slow onset of analgesia. Its mean onset of action is 5 minutes, and the peak effect is at 15 minutes. It is metabolized in the liver into two active compounds, morphine-3-glucuronide and morphine-6-glucuronide. The former is an opioid antagonist, and the latter is a potent analgesic. Preterm infants mostly produce morphine-3-glucuronide, which explains why the infant develops tolerance after 3 to 4 days of morphine therapy.[20] Side effects of morphine include hypotension in neonates who have pre-existing hypotension and a gestational age less than 26 weeks,[21] prolonged need for assisted ventilation, and increased time to reach full feeds.[17,18] Others have suggested that morphine may have a specific effect on pulmonary mechanics, possibly resulting from some as yet undefined direct toxicity such as histamine release and/or bronchospasm.[22] There is even controversy as to whether morphine is effective in the treatment of acute pain.[23]

A randomized, controlled trial conducted in the Netherlands compared the analgesic effect of morphine versus placebo infusions for a duration of 7 days in 150 newborns who received mechanical ventilation. The findings of the study suggested that routine morphine infusion in preterm newborns who received ventilatory support neither improved pain relief nor protected against poor neurologic outcome (defined as severe IVH, PVL, or death within 28 days).[17]

The NEurologic Outcomes and Preemptive Analgesia in Neonates (NEOPAIN) trial included ventilated preterm neonates from 16 centers in the United States and Europe. It compared the effect of morphine versus placebo infusions, following a loading dose, on the neurologic outcomes of the ventilated neonates. The results suggested that continuous morphine infusion did not reduce early neurologic injury in ventilated preterm neonates. The poor neurologic outcome was defined as severe IVH, PVL, or death.[18,24] Hypotension occurred more frequently in the morphine group than the placebo group.

One study assessed the long-term outcome at age 5 to 6 years of prematurely born children (< 34 weeks' gestation) who by randomization received morphine in the neonatal period to facilitate mechanical ventilation. This study looked at children from two trials. The first included 95 infants who were assigned randomly to receive morphine alone, pancuronium alone, or both morphine and pancuronium. The second trial included 21 infants who received morphine and 20 infants who received placebo. Each child was assessed using three scales: the full-scale Weschler Preschool and Primary Scale of Intelligence, the Movement Assessment Battery for Children, and the Child Behavior Checklist. No adverse effects on intelligence, motor function, or behavior were found in the children treated with morphine.[25]

Fentanyl

Fentanyl is an opioid analgesic that is 50 to 100 times more potent than morphine.[26] It is used frequently because it provides rapid analgesia.[27] It may be used as a slow intravenous push every 2 to 4 hours or as a continuous infusion. Tolerance may develop, and withdrawal symptoms may occur after 5 or more days of continuous infusion.[26] In a blinded, randomized, controlled trial, a single dose of fentanyl given to ventilated preterm newborns significantly reduced pain behaviors and changes in heart rate. It also increased growth hormone levels.[28] In another study, fentanyl provided the same pain relief as morphine but with fewer side effects.[29] In other studies, fentanyl use resulted in lower heart rates and lower behavioral stress scores and pain scores than seen with placebo; however, the infants receiving fentanyl required higher ventilator rates and peak inspiratory pressures at 24 hours.[30] Fentanyl also may be used transdermally in patients who have limited intravenous access.

Side effects of fentanyl include bradycardia, chest wall rigidity, and opioid tolerance after prolonged therapy.[27]

Methadone

Methadone is a potent analgesic with a rapid onset of action and prolonged effect.[27] It has minimal side effects, high enteral bioavailability, and a low cost.

Other Opiates

Other opiates include the short-acting drugs sulfentanil, alfentanil, and remifentanil. All are useful for short procedures such as intubation. Sulfentanil and alfentanil are metabolized by the liver, which is immature in preterm neonates, resulting in increased drug levels with repeated infusions, especially in preterm neonates.[31] Remifentanil, on the other hand, is cleared rapidly by plasma esterases and is unaffected by the maturity of the liver enzyme system, making it attractive for short neonatal surgery or other procedures when rapid recovery is anticipated.[31]

BENZODIAZEPINES

The benzodiazepines are anxietolytic drugs that have limited analgesic effect but are commonly used in NICUs to produce sedation and muscle relaxation and to provide amnesia (in older patients). This class of drugs inhibits gamma aminobutyric acid A receptors.[32] The main complications include myoclonic jerking, excessive sedation, respiratory depression, and occasional hypotension.

Midazolam

The most commonly used benzodiazepine in the NICU is midazolam. When administered with morphine, it provides better sedation than morphine alone in ventilated patients, without adverse effects.[33] The minimal effective dose for most neonates is 200 μg/kg with a maintenance dose of 100 μg /kg/h.[34] It can be given orally, although in neonates the bioavailability of oral midazolam is only half that of intravenous midazolam.[35] Intranasal midazolam has been shown to be effective for fundoscopic examinations in older children, but this mode of delivery has not been tested in neonates.[36] One recent review found no apparent clinical benefit of midazolam compared with opiates in mechanically ventilated neonates.[37] Further, midazolam was associated with worse short-term adverse effects (death, severe IVH, or PVL) in the NOPAIN trial compared with morphine alone.[38] In summary, midazolam seems to provide sedative effects in mechanically ventilated neonates, but it should be used with caution because of reported adverse effects, particularly when used alone.

Lorazepam

Lorazepam is a longer-acting benzodiazepine that frequently is used in preterm neonates. Its duration of action is 8 to 12 hours. It also is an effective anticonvulsant for neonates refractory to phenobarbital. Unfortunately, one of its main side effects is myoclonic jerking, which mimics seizure activity.[12,39] It has been shown (along with morphine) to adhere to the tubing in patients treated with extracorporeal membrane oxygenation (ECMO), increasing dosing requirements by 50% in those patients.[40]

BARBITURATES

Barbiturates are used commonly in neonates for sedation and analgesic effects, despite a lack of evidence for pain relief.[12]

Phenobarbital

Phenobarbital usually is considered the drug of choice for seizure control. Despite minimal animal evidence for antinociception, it often is used for analgesia.[41] It also is used in conjunction with opioids for sedation,[18] although there is little recent evidence that it is effective. Classically, phenobarbital has been used for neonatal abstinence syndrome, but recent work by Ebner and colleagues[42] has demonstrated that opiates shorten the time required for treatment. Because of its anticonvulsant effects, however, phenobarbital is an attractive adjunct for patients who have seizures.

Thiopental

Thiopental is a short-acting barbiturate used for anesthetic induction. It is used sparingly in the NICU, but one randomized, controlled trial showed a decreased time needed for intubation and maintenance of heart rate and blood pressure with thiopental compared with placebo during nasotracheal intubation.[43]

Chloral Hydrate

Chloral hydrate is used for hypnosis when sedation but not analgesia is required for certain procedures such as MRI. Apnea and bradycardia may occur in ex-preterm infants undergoing procedural sedation with doses as little as 30 mg/kg. Side effects were inversely related to gestational age.[44] The usual dose is 50 to 100 mg/kg. A dose of 75 mg/kg administered orally is more efficacious than a 0.2-mg/kg dose of intravenous midazolam and has comparable side effects (apnea, bradycardia).[45]

KETAMINE

Ketamine is a dissociative anesthetic used for anesthesia, analgesia, and sedation. It causes bronchodilation and mild increases in blood pressure and heart rate.[46] Cerebral blood flow is relatively unaffected with ketamine, making it an attractive choice for some unstable hypotensive neonates requiring procedures such as cannulation for ECMO.[47] Animal studies have raised concern about the neurodegenerative effects of ketamine[48,49] although ketamine in clinically relevant doses is neuroprotective in the presence of inflammatory pain.[20] Nevertheless, extrapolating animal to human data is problematic at best, and there has been no credible evidence that ketamine is detrimental to the developing human brain in the presence of pain.[50] Clearly, more study is needed to determine the safety and efficacy of this anesthetic.

PROPOFOL

Propofol has become popular as an anesthetic agent for young children, but it has not been studied extensively in neonates.[51–53] One study compared propofol with morphine, atropine, and suxamethonium for intubation and found that propofol led to shorter intubation times, higher oxygen saturations, and less trauma than the combination regimen in neonates.[54] Propofol should be used with caution in young infants, however, because clearance is inversely related to neonatal and postmenstrual age. Thus with intermittent bolus or continuous administration this drug can accumulate in young immature neonates, leading to toxicity.[55]

ACETAMINOPHEN

Acetaminophen acts by inhibiting the cyclo-oxygenase (COX) enzymes in the brain and has been well studied in newborns.[16] It is useful for mild pain, in conjunction with other pain relief, or after circumcision.[56]

LOCAL ANESTHETICS

Lidocaine

Lidocaine inhibits axonal transmission by blocking Na^+ channels. Lidocaine is used commonly for penile blocks for circumcisions. In this circumstance, its use has demonstrated effectiveness in decreasing pain response to immunizations as long as 4 months after circumcision compared with neonates who received placebo.[57] The ring block has been shown to be a more effective than a dorsal penile root block or eutectic mixture of local anesthetics (EMLA) cream in relieving the pain of circumcision.[58]

Topical Anesthetics

Topical anesthetics have demonstrated effectiveness for certain types of procedural pain such as venipuncture,[59] lumbar puncture,[60] or immunizations.[61] Complications include methemoglobinemia and transient skin rashes.[62] In preterm neonates with thin skin, the concern for methemoglobinemia is accentuated.

Unfortunately, topical anesthetics are not effective in providing pain relief for the heel prick, one of the most common skin-breaking procedures, because of increased skin thickness.[63] Newer topical anesthetics include 4% tetracaine and 4% liposomal lidocaine. Although the newer agents have a shorter onset of action, they are no more effective in pain relief.

COMMON PROCEDURES

Common neonatal procedures and advantages and disadvantages of drug therapy are summarized in **Table 1**.

Table 1
Summary of procedures and treatment

Procedure	Drugs	Advantages of Treatment	Disadvantages of Treatment	Comments
Mechanical ventilation[17–19,29]	Fentanyl (1–3 μg/kg) Morphine (0.1 mg/kg) Midazolam (0.1–0.2 mg/kg)	Improved ventilator synchrony, lower pain scores	Prolonged time on assisted ventilation, prolonged time to full feeds, increased bladder catheterization, hypotension	Use sedation as needed, not preemptively; midazolam was associated with adverse short-term effects in NOPAIN trial.
Circumcision[58,62]	Lidocaine (1 mL) EMLA	Less pain response up to 4 months post-procedure	Allergic reaction, bruising at injection site	Ring block is more effective than dorsal penile nerve root block.
Heel lance[63]	Sucrose	Shorter crying, reduced changes in heart rate	None	EMLA cream is not effective.
Venipuncture, arterial puncture, lumbar puncture[60,61]	Topical anesthetic (EMLA) Sucrose	Lower Premature Infant Pain Profile scores, less crying	Local reaction, rare methemoglobinemia	Other nonpharmacologic treatments are effective.
Intubation[14,15,54,69,70]	Morphine (0.1 mg/kg) Fentanyl (1–3 μg g/kg) Remifentanil (1 mg/kg) Midazolam (0.2 mg/kg) Propofol (2–6 mg/kg) Ketamine (1 mg/kg) Suxamethonium (2 mg/kg)	Shorter time to intubation, less trauma, less desaturation, better maintenance of vital signs	None	There is no accepted premedication. Opiates are the class most common used.

More invasive procedures (eg, cannulation for ECMO)[71,72]	Propofol (2–6 mg/kg) Ketamine (1 mg/kg) Fentanyl (1–3 mcg/kg)	Maintenance of cardiovascular stability	Questionable neurotoxicity with ketamine	Ketamine may be neuroprotective.
Postsurgical pain[73]	Fentanyl (1–3 μg g/kg) Morphine (0.1 mg/kg) Acetaminophen (15 mg/kg)	Lowered neuroendocrine response, faster recovery	Respiratory depression, hypotension with opiates	Use acetaminophen only for mild pain.
Endotracheal suctioning[34,74]	Midazolam (0.2 mg/kg) Morphine (0.1 mg/kg) Fentanyl (1–3 μg/kg)	Anxietolytic	Respiratory depression, hypotension, dependence	Pain usually is not treated.
Imaging (MRI)[45]	Chloral hydrate (50–100 mg/kg)	Sedation	Respiratory depression, hypotension	Chloral hydrate provides sedation only.

FUTURE DIRECTIONS

Nonsteroidal Anti-Inflammatory Drugs

Nonsteroidal anti-inflammatory drugs (NSAIDS) are used extensively for pain relief in children and adults, but they are used mainly for patent ductus arteriosus (PDA) closure in neonates. They act by inhibiting the COX-1 and COX-2 enzymes responsible for converting arachidonic acid into prostaglandins, thus producing their analgesic, antipyretic, and anti-inflammatory effects.[27] The analgesic effects of NSAIDS have not been studied in neonates, although both ibuprofen and indomethacin have been studied for use in PDA closure. Concern about side effects of renal dysfunction, platelet adhesiveness, and pulmonary hypertension have limited their study for this indication.[37,64,65] Ibuprofen, however, has demonstrated beneficial effects on cerebral circulation in human studies[66] as well as beneficial effects on the development of chronic lung disease in baboon experiments,[67] making it an attractive analgesic in preterm neonates. Nonpharmacologic approaches such as acupuncture, massage therapy, sucrose, and music are also safe and effective.[68]

ACKNOWLEDGMENTS

The authors thank Diana Hershberger for assistance in preparing this manuscript.

REFERENCES

1. Anand KJ, Hall RW. Controversies in neonatal pain: an introduction. Semin Perinatol 2007;31(5):273–4.
2. Anand KJ, Hickey PR. Pain and its effects in the human neonate and fetus. N Engl J Med 1987;317(21):1321–9.
3. Fumagalli F, Molteni R, Racagni G, et al. Stress during development: impact on neuroplasticity and relevance to psychopathology. Prog Neurobiol 2007;81(4): 197–217.
4. Barker DP, Rutter N. Exposure to invasive procedures in neonatal intensive care unit admissions. Arch Dis Child Fetal Neonatal Ed 1995;72(1):F47–8.
5. Carbajal R, Rousset A, Danan C, et al. Epidemiology and treatment of painful procedures in neonates in intensive care units. JAMA 2008;300(1):60–70.
6. Jacqz-Aigrain E, Burtin P. Clinical pharmacology of sedatives in neonates. Clin Pharm 1996;31(6):423–43.
7. Anand KJ, Aranda JV, Verde CB, et al. Summary proceedings from the neonatal pain-control group. Pediatrics 2006;117(3 Pt 2):S9–S22.
8. Ranger M, Johnston CC, Anand KJ. Current controversies regarding pain assessment in neonates. Semin Perinatol 2007;31(5):283–8.
9. Whitfield MF, Grunau RE. Behavior, pain perception, and the extremely low-birth weight survivor. Clin Perinatol 2000;27(2):363–79.
10. American Academy of Pediatrics, American Academy of Pediatric Dentistry, Charles J, et al. Guidelines for monitoring and management of pediatric patients during and after sedation for diagnostic and therapeutic procedures: an update. Pediatrics 2006;118(6):2587–602.
11. Saarenmaa E, Neuvonen PJ, Roseberg P, et al. Morphine clearance and effects in newborn infants in relation to gestational age. Clin Pharmacol Ther 2000;68(2): 160–6.
12. Hall RW, Boyle E, Young T. Do ventilated neonates require pain management? Semin Perinatol 2007;31(5):289–97.

13. Whyte S, Birrell G, Wyllie J. Premedication before intubation in UK neonatal units. Arch Dis Child Fetal Neonatal Ed 2000;82(1):F38–41 [see comment].
14. Roberts KD, Leone TA, Edwards WH, et al. Premedication for nonemergent neonatal intubations: a randomized, controlled trial comparing atropine and fentanyl to atropine, fentanyl, and mivacurium. Pediatrics 2006;118(4):1583–91.
15. Sarkar S, Schumacher RE, Baumgart S, et al. Are newborns receiving premedication before elective intubation? J Perinatol 2006;26(5):286–9.
16. Menon G, Anand KJ, McIntosh N. Practical approach to analgesia and sedation in the neonatal intensive care unit. Semin Perinatol 1998;22(5):417–24.
17. Simons SH, van Dijk M, van Lingen RA, et al. Routine morphine infusion in preterm newborns who received ventilatory support: a randomized controlled trial. JAMA 2003;290(18):2419–27.
18. Anand KJ, Hall RW, Desai N, et al. Effects of morphine analgesia in ventilated preterm neonates: primary outcomes from the NEOPAIN randomised trial. Lancet 2004;363(9422):1673–82 [see comment].
19. Bellu R, de Waal KA, Zanini R. Opioids for neonates receiving mechanical ventilation. [update of Cochrane Database Syst Rev. 2005;(1):CD004212; PMID: 15674933]. Cochrane Database Syst Rev 2008;(1):CD004212.
20. Anand KJ. Pharmacological approaches to the management of pain in the neonatal intensive care unit. J Perinatol 2007;27(Suppl. 1):S4–11.
21. Hall RWKS, Barton BA, Kaiser JR, et al. Morphine, hypotension, and adverse outcomes in preterm neonates: who's to blame? Pediatrics 2005;115(5): 1351–9.
22. Levene M. Morphine sedation in ventilated newborns: who are we treating? Pediatrics 2005;116(2):492–3 [comment].
23. Carbajal R, Lenclen R, Jugie M, et al. Morphine does not provide adequate analgesia for acute procedural pain among preterm neonates. Pediatrics 2005; 115(6):1494–500.
24. Bhandari V, Bergqvist LL, Kronsberg SS, et al. Morphine administration and short-term pulmonary outcomes among ventilated preterm infants. Pediatrics 2005;116(2):352–9 [see comment].
25. MacGregor R, Evans D, sugden D, et al. Outcome at 5–6 years of prematurely born children who received morphine as neonates. Arch Dis Child Fetal Neonatal Ed 1998 Jul;79(1):F40–3.
26. Mitchell A, Brooks S, Roane D. The premature infant and painful procedures. Pain Manag Nurs 2000;1(2):58–65.
27. Anand KJ, Hall RW. Pharmacological therapy for analgesia and sedation in the newborn. [erratum appears in Arch Dis Child Fetal Neonatal Ed 2007 Mar;92(2):F156 Note: dosage error in text]. Arch Dis Child Fetal Neonatal Ed 2006;91(6):F448–53.
28. Guinsburg R, Kopelman BL, Anand KJ, et al. Physiological, hormonal, and behavioral responses to a single fentanyl dose in intubated and ventilated preterm neonates. J Pediatr 1998;132(6):954–9.
29. Saarenmaa E, Huttunen P, Leppaluoto J, et al. Advantages of fentanyl over morphine in analgesia for ventilated newborn infants after birth: a randomized trial. J Pediatr 1999;134(2):144–50 [see comment].
30. Orsini AJ, Leef KH, Costarino A, et al. Routine use of fentanyl infusions for pain and stress reduction in infants with respiratory distress syndrome. J Pediatr 1996;129(1):140–5 [see comment].
31. Berde CB, Jaksic T, Lynn AM, et al. Anesthesia and analgesia during and after surgery in neonates. Clin Ther 2005;27(6):900–21.

32. Blumer JL. Clinical pharmacology of midazolam in infants and children. Clin Pharm 1998;35(1):37–47.
33. Arya V, Ramji S. Midazolam sedation in mechanically ventilated newborns: a double blind randomized placebo controlled trial. Indian Pediatr 2001;38(9):967–72 [see comment].
34. Treluyer JM, Zohar S, Rey E, et al. Minimum effective dose of midazolam for sedation of mechanically ventilated neonates. J Clin Pharm Ther 2005;30(5): 479–85.
35. de Wildt SN, Kearns GL, Hop WC, et al. Pharmacokinetics and metabolism of oral midazolam in preterm infants. Br J Clin Pharmacol 2002;53(4):390–2.
36. Altintas O, Karabas VL, Demirci G, et al. Evaluation of intranasal midazolam in refraction and fundus examination of young children with strabismus. J Pediatr Ophthalmol Strabismus 2005;43(6):355–9.
37. Aranda JV, Carlo W, Hummel P, et al. Analgesia and sedation during mechanical ventilation in neonates. Clin Ther 2005;27(6):877–99.
38. Anand KJ, Baton BA, McIntosh N, et al. Analgesia and sedation in preterm neonates who require ventilatory support: results from the NOPAIN trial. Neonatal Outcome and Prolonged Analgesia in Neonates. [erratum appears in Arch Pediatr Adolesc Med 1999 Aug;153(8):895]. Arch Pediatr Adolesc Med 1999; 153(4):331–8.
39. Chess PR, D'Angio CT. Clonic movements following lorazepam administration in full-term infants. Arch Pediatr Adolesc Med 1998;152(1):98–9.
40. Bhatt-Meht V, Annich G. Sedative clearance during extracorporeal membrane oxygenation. Perfusion 2005;20(6):309–15.
41. Gonzalez-Darder JM, Ortega-Alvaro A, Ruz-Franzi I, et al. Antinociceptive effects of phenobarbital in "tail-flick" test and deafferentation pain. Anesth Analg 1992; 75(1):81–6.
42. Ebner N, Rohrmeister K, Winklbaur B, et al. Management of neonatal abstinence syndrome in neonates born to opioid maintained women. Drug Alcohol Depend 2007;87(2–3):131–8.
43. Bhutada A, Sahni R, Rastogi S, et al. Randomised controlled trial of thiopental for intubation in neonates. Arch Dis Child Fetal Neonatal Ed 2000;82(1):F34–7 [see comment].
44. Allegaert K, Daniels H, Naulaers G, et al. Pharmacodynamics of chloral hydrate in former preterm infants. Eur J Pediatr 2005;164(7):403–7.
45. McCarver-May DG, Kang J, Aouthmany M, et al. Comparison of chloral hydrate and midazolam for sedation of neonates for neuroimaging studies. J Pediatr 1996;128(4):573–6 [see comment].
46. Friesen RH, Henry DB. Cardiovascular changes in preterm neonates receiving isoflurane, halothane, fentanyl, and ketamine. Anesthesiology 1986;64(2): 238–42.
47. Betremieux P, Carre P, Pladys P, et al. Doppler ultrasound assessment of the effects of ketamine on neonatal cerebral circulation. Dev Pharmacol Ther 1993; 20(1–2):9–13.
48. Young C, Jevtovic-Todorovic V, Qin YQ, et al. Potential of ketamine and midazolam, individually or in combination, to induce apoptotic neurodegeneration in the infant mouse brain. Br J Pharmacol 2005;146(2):189–97.
49. Olney JW, Young C, wozniak DF, et al. Anesthesia-induced developmental neuroapoptosis. Does it happen in humans? Anesthesiology 2004;101(2):273–5 [see comment].

50. Bhutta AT, Venkatesan AK, Rovnaghi CR, et al. Anaesthetic neurotoxicity in rodents: is the ketamine controversy real? Acta Paediatr 2007;96(11):1554–6.
51. Disma N, Astuto M, Rizzo G, et al. Propofol sedation with fentanyl or midazolam during oesophagogastroduodenoscopy in children. Eur J Anaesthesiol 2005; 22(11):848–52.
52. Rigby-Jones AE, Nolan JA, Priston MJ, et al. Pharmacokinetics of propofol infusions in critically ill neonates, infants, and children in an intensive care unit. Anesthesiology 2002;97(6):1393–400.
53. Jenkins IA, Playfor SD, Bevan C, et al. Current United Kingdom sedation practice in pediatric intensive care. Paediatr Anaesth 2007;17(7):675–83.
54. Ghanta S, Abdel-Latif ME, Lui K, et al. Propofol compared with the morphine, atropine, and suxamethonium regimen as induction agents for neonatal endotracheal intubation: a randomized, controlled trial. Pediatrics 2007;119(6): e1248–55 [see comment].
55. Allegaert K, Peeters MY, Verbesselt T, et al. Inter-individual variability in propofol pharmacokinetics in preterm and term neonates. Br J Anaesth 2007;99(6):864–70.
56. Howard CR, Howard FM, Weitzman ML. Acetaminophen analgesia in neonatal circumcision: the effect on pain. Pediatrics 1994;93(4):641–6.
57. Taddio A, Katz J, Ilersich AL, et al. Effect of neonatal circumcision on pain response during subsequent routine vaccination. Lancet 1997;349(9052): 599–603 [see comment].
58. Lander J, Brady-Fryer B, Metcalfe JB, et al. Comparison of ring block, dorsal penile nerve block, and topical anesthesia for neonatal circumcision: a randomized controlled trial. JAMA 1997;278(24):2157–62 [see comment].
59. Garcia OC, Reichberg S, Brion LP, et al. Topical anesthesia for line insertion in very low birth weight infants. J Perinatol 1997;17(6):477–80.
60. Kaur G, Gupta P, Kumar A. A randomized trial of eutectic mixture of local anesthetics during lumbar puncture in newborns. Arch Pediatr Adolesc Med 2003; 157(11):1065–70.
61. Gradin M, Eriksson M, Holmqvist G, et al. Pain reduction at venipuncture in newborns: oral glucose compared with local anesthetic cream. Pediatrics 2002; 110(6):1053–7 [see comment].
62. Taddio A, Stevens B, Craig K, et al. Efficacy and safety of lidocaine-prilocaine cream for pain during circumcision. N Engl J Med 1997;336(17):1197–201 [see comment].
63. Larsson BA, Norman M, Bjerring P, et al. Regional variations in skin perfusion and skin thickness may contribute to varying efficacy of topical, local anaesthetics in neonates. Paediatr Anaesth 1996;6(2):107–10.
64. Allegaert K, Cossey V, DeBeer A, et al. The impact of ibuprofen on renal clearance in preterm infants is independent of the gestational age. Pediatr Nephrol 2005;20(6):740–3.
65. Ohlsson A, Walia R, Shah S. Ibuprofen for the treatment of patent ductus arteriosus in preterm and/or low birth weight infants. [update of Cochrane Database Syst Rev. 2005;(4):CD003481; PMID: 16235321]. Cochrane Database Syst Rev 2008;(1):CD003481.
66. Naulaers G, Delanghe G, Allegaert K, et al. Ibuprofen and cerebral oxygenation and circulation. Arch Dis Child Fetal Neonatal Ed 2005;90(1):F75–6.
67. McCurnin D, Seidner S, Chang LY, et al. Ibuprofen-induced patent ductus arteriosus closure: physiologic, histologic, and biochemical effects on the premature lung. Pediatrics 2008;121(5):945–56.

68. Golianu B, Krane E, Seybold J, et al. Non-pharmacological techniques for pain management in neonates. Semin Perinatol 2007;31(5):318–22.
69. Pereira e Silva Y, Gomez RS, Barbosa RF, et al. Remifentanil for sedation and analgesia in a preterm neonate with respiratory distress syndrome. Paediatr Anaesth 2005;15(11):993–6 [see comment].
70. Knolle E, Oehmke MJ, Gustorff B, et al. Target-controlled infusion of propofol for fibreoptic intubation. Eur J Anaesthesiol 2003;20(7):565–9.
71. Singh A, Girotra S, Mehta Y, et al. Total intravenous anesthesia with ketamine for pediatric interventional cardiac procedures. J Cardiothorac Vasc Anesth 2000; 14(1):36–9.
72. Oklu E, Bulutcu FS, Yalcin Y, et al. Which anesthetic agent alters the hemodynamic status during pediatric catheterization? Comparison of propofol versus ketamine. J Cardiothorac Vasc Anesth 2003;17(6):686–90 [see comment].
73. Bouwmeester JJ, Hop WC, van Dijk M, et al. Postoperative pain in the neonate: age-related differences in morphine requirements and metabolism. Intensive Care Med 2003;29(11):2009–15.
74. Simons SH, van Dijk M, Anand KS, et al. Do we still hurt newborn babies? A prospective study of procedural pain and analgesia in neonates. Arch Pediatr Adolesc Med 2003;157(11):1058–64.

Iron Therapy for Preterm Infants

Raghavendra Rao, MD[a,b,*], Michael K. Georgieff, MD[a,b]

KEYWORDS

- Guidelines • Infant • Iron • Iron overload
- Premature • Therapy

The need for iron therapy in preterm infants has been debated at least since the 1950s.[1] The essential role of iron in various tissue functions and their propensity to develop iron deficiency suggest that iron supplementation is essential to the preterm infants. Conversely, the pro-oxidant role of non–protein-bound iron and the poorly developed antioxidant measures in preterm infants caution against aggressive iron supplementation in this population. It is not surprising that there are wide variations in iron supplementation practices among neonatal units.[2]

RISK OF IRON DEFICIENCY IN PRETERM INFANTS

Between 25% and 85% of preterm infants develop evidence of iron deficiency during infancy.[3–8] Unlike full-term infants, in whom the condition typically occurs during the second half of infancy, preterm infants are at risk for developing iron deficiency during their first 6 postnatal months.[5–9] Gestationally more premature and smaller preterm infants are at greater risk for developing iron deficiency at an earlier age.[5,9,10] Iron deficiency is more common in preterm infants from developing countries[4] and in those consuming human milk exclusively without supplementation.

Factors Predisposing to Iron Deficiency

A number of factors combine to predispose the premature infant to negative iron balance. Iron is accumulated mostly during the third trimester of gestation.[11] Total body iron and hemoglobin contents and serum and storage iron concentrations are lower in preterm infants.[11–13] Conditions such as severe maternal iron deficiency,[14] intrauterine growth restriction,[12,15,16] and chronic blood loss during gestation can compromise fetal iron endowment further.

This work was supported by grant HD 29421-14 from the National Institutes of Health.
[a] Division of Neonatology, Department of Pediatrics, University of Minnesota, Mayo Mail Code 39, 420 Delaware Street, SE, Minneapolis, MN 55455, USA
[b] Center for Neurobehavioral Development, University of Minnesota, Mayo Mail Code 507, 420 Delaware Street, SE, Minneapolis, MN 55455, USA
* Corresponding author. Division of Neonatology, Mayo Mail Code 39, 420 Delaware Street, SE, Minneapolis, MN 55455.
E-mail address: raoxx017@umn.edu (R. Rao).

Clin Perinatol 36 (2009) 27–42
doi:10.1016/j.clp.2008.09.013 perinatology.theclinics.com
0095-5108/08/$ – see front matter

Postnatally, the meager iron stores can be depleted rapidly during the first 6 to 8 weeks, coinciding with the onset of erythropoiesis and rapid catch-up growth.[1,5,15] The hemoglobin nadir is lower and occurs earlier in more premature (gestational age 28–32 weeks) infants than in those born at a gestational age of 33 to 36 weeks.[3] Beginning at 9 weeks and continuing until 12 months of age, however, hemoglobin concentrations are comparable in the two gestational age groups,[3] suggesting the need for a more robust erythropoiesis and therefore a greater iron requirement in the more prematurely born infants.

Tissue iron stores are depleted sooner in the preterm infants demonstrating the greatest growth velocity,[15] especially in more immature preterm infants who demonstrate the most rapid catch-up growth.[1] Interestingly, the iron status at birth does not influence the postnatal growth rate,[17] signifying that preterm infants will grow whether they are iron replete or not at birth. The high rate of postnatal catch-up growth with its attendant increases in blood volume and hemoglobin mass requires additional iron. Unless augmented by external sources, the endogenous iron stores of preterm infants at birth meet their iron demands only until the doubling of the birth weight at approximately 2 to 3 months of age.[18] Chronic gastrointestinal hemorrhage and clinical practices such as uncompensated phlebotomy losses and inadequate iron supplementation further deplete iron stores and increase iron requirements.

Consequences of Iron Deficiency

The effects of iron deficiency are pervasive and involve multiple organ systems. Poor physical growth, gastrointestinal disturbances, thyroid dysfunction, altered immunity, and temperature instability have been attributed to iron deficiency in very low birth weight (VLBW, birth weight < 1500 g) infants.[19] Anemia typically is a late sign and suggests significant depletion of iron stores. A major concern of early iron deficiency is its effect on the developing brain.

Potential effects of iron deficiency on neurodevelopment

Dietary iron deficiency during early infancy is associated with long-term neurodevelopmental impairments that seem to be irreversible in spite of iron supplementation (reviewed in).[20] Long-term cognitive abnormalities also have been demonstrated in full-term infants who have iron deficiency in the neonatal period.[13,21]

A limited number of studies suggest that early iron deficiency in preterm infants also may affect neurologic function and neurodevelopment adversely. Compared with nonanemic, iron-replete infants, preterm infants who had anemia (hemoglobin $\leq$ 10 g/dL) and low iron stores (serum ferritin $\leq$ 76 μg/L) had an increased number of abnormal neurologic reflexes at a postmenstrual age of 37 weeks.[22] A recent study demonstrated more mild neurologic abnormalities, such as broad gait, dysdiadochokinesis, or dysmetria at 5 years of age in preterm infants who received iron supplementation from 2 months of age than in those who received iron supplementation from 2 weeks after birth.[23] A trend toward poorer cognitive performance also was present in those supplemented late.[23] Thus, early iron deficiency seems to affect neurodevelopment adversely in preterm infants. Interestingly, unlike the cognitive deficits that tend to predominate in full-term infants who have neonatal iron deficiency,[13,21] motor deficits seem to predominate in preterm infants.

RISK OF IRON OVERLOAD IN PRETERM INFANTS

In the absence of genetic conditions, such as congenital hemochromatosis, iatrogenic factors are responsible for excessive iron accumulation in preterm infants. There are, however, no specific data on the incidence of iron overload caused by nutritional iron therapy in preterm infants.

Factors Predisposing to Iron Overload

Multiple erythrocyte transfusions may lead to excess iron accumulation in preterm infants. Approximately 80% of VLBW and 95% of extremely low birth weight (ELBW, birth weight < 1000 g) infants receive erythrocyte transfusions during their hospitalization.[24] The mean life span of transfused erythrocytes is shorter in preterm infants than in adults.[25] The accelerated breakdown of erythrocytes may lead to excess iron accumulation[26] and a need for repeated transfusions. Each milliliter of transfused packed erythrocytes potentially delivers 0.5 to 1.0 mg of iron to the body.[27,28] Elevated serum iron and ferritin concentrations and liver iron concentration are common after multiple transfusions in preterm infants.[29–31] Preterm infants who have received multiple transfusions may maintain iron stores without iron supplementation up to 6 months of life.[30,32,33]

Although the serum iron concentration increases transiently after the intravenous administration of iron in preterm infants,[34] there are no data indicating that this practice leads to iron overload at commonly used dosages. Similarly, there is no evidence for excess iron accumulation with enteral iron administration at the doses typically used for supplementation.[35,36]

Consequences of Iron Excess in Preterm Infants

As with iron deficiency, excess iron accumulation potentially affects multiple organ systems. Large doses of enteral iron administration were associated with hemolysis in preterm infants who had vitamin E deficiency.[37] This nutritional deficiency is rare at present. There is an association between multiple erythrocyte transfusions and retinopathy of prematurity (ROP)[29,38] and bronchopulmonary dysplasia (BPD).[30,39] The incidence and severity of both conditions correlate with the number and volume of erythrocyte transfusions.[29,30] Although it is tempting to speculate that transfusion-related iron overload may be involved in the pathogenesis of these conditions, other studies have failed to provide such evidence.[40]

Oxidative stress mediated by non–protein-bound ("free") iron in the presence of poor antioxidant capabilities has been postulated to initiate or potentiate the progression of BPD and ROP through the generation of reactive oxygen species.[30,39] Multiple studies have demonstrated that the milieu in preterm infants is conducive for iron to exist in the pro-oxidant ferrous state and for the formation of reactive oxygen species.[3,26,39] Additionally, although ferritin iron is protein bound, there is potential for the release of free iron from ferritin during oxidative stress.[41]

Nevertheless, assigning a direct causative role for iron in BPD and ROP has been problematic. Infants developing these multifactorial conditions tend to be more premature and sicker and thus more likely to receive multiple transfusions. It has yet to be established in vivo that iron is directly involved with oxidative stress in preterm infants.[27,30,38,42] Increased serum iron concentration following multiple transfusions was not associated with lipid peroxidation in preterm infants who had BPD,[30] nor was increased hepatic iron concentration in multiply transfused preterm infants associated with hepatocyte injury.[31] Unfortunately, most of the assessments have been short term and assessed oxidative stress soon after a single transfusion[27] or after enteral iron administration of short duration.[42,43] Long-term studies are necessary to assess conclusively the risk of oxidative stress and tissue injury with cumulative doses of iron administration in preterm infants.

Potential effects of iron overload on neurodevelopment

Iron overload is postulated in the pathogenesis of ischemic brain injury and many neurodegenerative disorders in adults.[44] Similarly, increased non–protein-bound iron and lipid peroxidation products have been demonstrated in the cerebrospinal fluid of newborn infants who have birth asphyxia.[45] These are non-nutritional effects of iron. Parkinson-like neurodegeneration in adulthood has been demonstrated in mice following enteral administration of large doses of iron (approximately 40 times that present in own mother's milk) during the lactation period.[46] Although this animal study is of concern, long-term neurodevelopmental deficits caused by iron supplementation at typical doses have not been demonstrated in human infants.

In summary, the preterm infant is at risk of both iron deficiency and iron overload. Because of the potential adverse impact of iron deficiency on developing organ systems, preventive and therapeutic measures seem to be crucial. Conversely, the potential for organ injury with excess iron suggests that iron therapy should be instituted carefully in preterm infants.

PREVENTIVE MEASURES FOR IRON DEFICIENCY

Determining the Iron Requirements of Preterm Infants

The goal of nutrient delivery to preterm infants is to mimic the intrauterine accretion rate and to maintain normal serum levels.[47] Using this analogy, a preterm infant would require a daily iron intake of 1.6 to 2.0 mg/kg intravenously[48] or 5 to 6 mg/kg enterally, because enteral iron absorption is approximately 30%.[49] Such supplementation is neither practical nor physiologic soon after birth, however. Enteral nutrition is not feasible soon after birth in most VLBW preterm infants. Unlike intrauterine life, growth and erythropoiesis cease soon after birth, and iron requirements are lower under those circumstances. Estimates of daily requirements based on a factorial approach[50] also are likely to be imprecise.[51] Well-executed, randomized, controlled trials probably are the best method to determine the iron requirements of preterm infants. These trials have established the beneficial effect of iron supplementation via fortification of human milk, iron-fortified formula, and medicinal iron in decreasing the risk of iron deficiency.[8,16,51–53] Most studies, however, have evaluated only short-term benefits on hematologic parameters. There is a paucity of information on the long-term effects of iron supplementation on hematologic and nonhematologic parameters, such as growth and neurodevelopment.

ENTERAL IRON SUPPLEMENTATION THROUGH DIET

Fortification of Human Milk

The iron content of human milk is approximately 0.5 mg/L.[54] Although human milk meets the iron requirements of full-term infants during the first 4 to 6 months of life, additional iron is necessary to meet the needs of erythropoiesis and growth of preterm infants.[16] The iron status of preterm infants receiving nonfortified breast milk starts to deteriorate within 1 to 4 months.[7,9,10] Cow milk–based human milk fortifiers that are currently available in the United States contain 3.5 to 14.4 mg/L of iron and deliver 0.7 to 2.2 mg/kg d^{-1} of additional iron if milk consumption is 150 mL/kg d^{-1}. Fortification with an iron-fortified human milk fortifier is associated with fewer erythrocyte transfusions than fortification with a low-iron fortifier.[52] Therefore, additional iron supplementation may be necessary if a low-iron fortifier is used. The currently available human milk–based human milk fortifier in the United States is not fortified with iron and provides only 0.3 mg/kg d^{-1} of iron if daily milk consumption is 150 mL/kg.

Use of Iron-Fortified Formula

Compared with a formula lacking iron, weaning to an iron-fortified formula improves hemoglobin and serum ferritin concentrations in preterm infants.[16] Preterm infants with birth weights below 1800 g will not achieve iron sufficiency on a formula containing 3 mg/L of iron or less.[6] Formulas containing 5 to 9 mg/L of iron seemed to meet the iron requirements of erythropoiesis in healthy preterm infants during the first 6 months of life,[55] but in that study 18% of the infants receiving the 9-mg/L formula and 30% of those receiving the 5-mg/L formula developed iron deficiency (serum ferritin concentration < 10 μg/L) between 4 and 8 months of age. The infant formulas currently available in the United States are fortified with 12.0 to 14.4 mg/L of iron and deliver 1.8 to 2.2 mg/kg d^{-1} when consumed at 150 mL/kg d^{-1}. The discharge formulas have an iron content of 13 mg/L and provide approximately 2 mg/kg d^{-1} of iron.

ENTERAL SUPPLEMENTATION THROUGH MEDICINAL IRON

Enteral administration is used commonly for supplementing iron in preterm infants. There are wide variations in the dose, initiation, and duration of supplementation and in the iron compounds used for enteral supplementation.[2] The recommendations of various pediatric societies[47,56,57] are given in **Table 1**. Iron supplementation is not recommended nor is it necessary during the transition period soon after birth.[56] An exogenous source of 2 to 4 mg/kg d^{-1} of iron is recommended during the period of stable growth, beginning at 4 to 8 weeks and continuing until 12 to 15 months of age (see **Table 1**). Although these recommendations provide useful guidelines for iron therapy in preterm infants, they may not be universally applicable, as discussed in the following sections.

Dosage of Elemental Iron

At least 2 to 4 mg/kg d^{-1} of elemental iron is necessary to prevent iron deficiency in nontransfused VLBW infants.[5,58] With such supplementation, however, the hemoglobin level in preterm infants does not reach that of full-term infants by 9 months of age.[58] Even with 4 to 6 mg/kg d^{-1} of iron supplementation from 2 weeks of age, iron deficiency is found at 2 months of age in approximately 15% of preterm infants with a birth weight less than 1301 g.[8] Preterm infants with lower birth weights and gestational ages demonstrate more robust erythropoiesis and greater growth velocity than their heavier and more mature counterparts.[3] At the same time, their iron endowment at birth is lower. A scaled dosage based on gestational age and/or birth weight may be more appropriate.[56,59] Conversely, approximately 95% of ELBW infants receive erythrocyte transfusions[24] and are likely to have larger iron stores. Therefore, body iron stores also should be taken into consideration when evaluating additional iron supplementation in ELBW infants. Preterm infants who are small-for-gestational age also may benefit from higher doses of iron, because they potentially have lower total body iron concentrations than their appropriate-for-gestation counterparts.[16]

Initiation of Supplementation

The initiation of iron supplementation in preterm infants has been debated since the 1950s[1] and has ranged from 14 days to 10 weeks among the neonatal units.[2] The current recommendation is to begin supplementation between 4 and 8 weeks of age, irrespective of gestational age or birth weight (see **Table 1**).

Beginning supplementation earlier may be prudent for the more immature preterm infants, many of who may be in negative iron balance by 1 month of age.[9,33] Compared with unsupplemented infants or those who first received supplementation between

Table 1
Enteral iron intake recommendations for preterm infants in stable clinical condition

Organization	Recommended Supplementation: Population and Dose ($mg/kg\ d^{-1}$)	Initiation	Duration	Additional Considerations
Committee on Nutrition, American Academy of Pediatrics[47]	Infants on human milk: 2.0 Infants on formula milk: 1.0 During rHuEPO use: up to 6.0	1 month	12 months	Only iron-fortified formulas should be used in formula-fed preterm infants.
Nutrition Committee, Canadian Pediatric Society[56]	Birth weight ≥ 1000 g: 2.0–3.0 Birth weight < 1000 g: 3.0–4.0	6–8 weeks	12 months corrected age	A formula containing 12 mg/L of iron may be used to meet the iron requirements of infants with birth weight ≥ 1000 g. Additional oral iron supplementation is necessary for formula-fed infants with birth weight < 1000 g.
Committee on Nutrition of the Preterm Infant, European Society of Pediatric Gastroenterology and Nutrition[57]	Infants on human milk: 2.0–2.5 (maximum, 15 mg/d) Infants on formula milk: 2.0–2.5 (maximum, 15 mg/d) from all sources	No later than 8 weeks	12–15 months	A formula containing 10–13 mg/L of iron is required to meet the total iron requirement without supplementation. Delay oral iron supplementation until erythrocyte transfusions have ceased.

4 and 8 weeks of age, supplementing 2 to 5 mg/kg d^{-1} of iron from 2 weeks of age reduces the need for erythrocyte transfusions and the risk of iron deficiency between 2 and 6 months of age.[5,8,53] Cumulative iron intake was calculated to be more than three times greater with early supplementation than with late supplementation.[8] Hemoglobin, serum iron, and ferritin concentrations were higher, and serum transferrin receptor concentrations were lower at 2 months of age with early iron supplementation,[8,53] suggesting better iron stores at discharge. Early iron supplementation was tolerated well and was not associated with morbidities. A follow-up study demonstrated a lower incidence of mild motor signs and a trend toward better cognitive function at 5 years of age in those supplemented from age 2 weeks,[23] suggesting potential long-term benefits with early supplementation. The lack of long-term neurologic morbidity also supports the safety of early iron supplementation.

On the other hand, the risk of iron-induced hemolysis in preterm infants who have vitamin E deficiency is maximal during the first 6 weeks of life.[37] Serum iron and ferritin concentrations remain elevated during the first 4 to 6 weeks of life even without supplementation.[3] There is a potential for iron excess with higher doses of supplementation, because enteral iron absorption seems to be poorly regulated during the first month of life in ELBW infants.[9,10,51] Furthermore, supplemental iron is better incorporated into red blood cells when it is administered after the onset of erythropoiesis.[60] These studies support delaying iron supplementation until 4 to 6 weeks.

Duration of Supplementation

The duration of supplementation has varied from 6 to12 months.[2] Most organizations recommend supplementation until 12 to 15 months of age (see **Table 1**). The optimal duration of supplementation has yet to established in randomized, controlled trials.

Choice of Iron Compound for Supplementation

Ferrous sulfate is used commonly for supplementation as well as for fortifying formula. It is inexpensive and widely available. Even though there are theoretic advantages for using non-ionic ferric compounds, studies have not established their superiority over ferrous sulfate in tolerance, efficacy, and complications.[61] Moreover, although ferrous sulfate may be administered once daily,[62] some of the other compounds require more frequent administration,[61] which may compromise compliance.

Route of Supplementation

Parenteral iron administration typically is not used for routine iron supplementation. Because iron is not naturally excreted in stools or urine, almost all the parenterally administered iron would be retained in the body. Intramuscular administration of iron is as efficacious as oral supplementation in ameliorating iron deficiency.[63] Nevertheless, the practice is discouraged because of associated pain and complications.[64] Intravenous iron administration is safe and more effective than enteral iron for supporting erythropoiesis.[28,34,35] Even though iron is accreted at a rate of 1.6 to 2.0 mg/kg d^{-1} during the third trimester,[48] an intravenous dose of 120 μg/kg d^{-1} results in a positive iron balance,[28] probably because of decreased iron requirements soon after birth. Between 18% and 68% of the intravenously administered iron is incorporated into erythrocytes within 2 weeks.[60,65] Intravenous administration also is thought to improve growth in preterm infants receiving recombinant human erythropoietin (rHuEPO).[66] Nevertheless, the transient elevation of malondialdehyde, a marker of lipid peroxidation, at the conclusion of iron infusions[34] cautions against routine supplementation through this route. The need for long-term intravenous access also makes it impractical for most infants.

Iron Supplementation in Special Circumstances

Iron supplementation during recombinant human erythropoietin (rHuEPO) therapy

Administration of rHuEPO promotes erythropoiesis and reduces the need for erythrocyte transfusions in preterm infants (see[67] for a review). Iron supplementation is necessary because rHuEPO administration depletes body iron stores.[35,68] A daily intake of 3 to 8 mg/kg of iron seems to be adequate for supporting erythropoiesis, is well tolerated, and does not seem to be associated with oxidative stress.[35,66,67,69] The Committee on Nutrition of the American Academy of Pediatrics recommends enteral supplementation of 6 mg/kg d^{-1} of elemental iron during rHuEPO administration,[47] but this dose may not be sufficient to support erythropoiesis and maintain iron stores.[70] Simultaneous enteral (9 mg/kg d^{-1}) and parenteral (2 mg/kg d^{-1}) iron administration[34] or continuation of enteral iron therapy beyond rHuEPO administration[66] may be necessary to achieve this goal. Enteral doses as high as 18 to 36 mg/d (approximately 12–24 mg/kg d^{-1}) have been used[71] but do not seem to provide additional benefits and may cause hematochezia.[66]

Intravenous iron supplementation in a dose of 2 to 6 mg/kg or 20 mg/kg weekly may improve erythropoietic response and growth during rHuEPO therapy.[70] Such therapy may be useful in infants who have low serum ferritin levels or in whom enteral nutrition has yet to be established. Intramuscular administration of 1 mg/kg d^{-1} or 12 mg/kg once weekly during rHuEPO therapy also seems to be effective.[67,72] Overall, a prudent approach may be to adjust the iron dose to maintain a serum ferritin concentration greater than 100 μg/L during rHuEPO therapy.[73]

Iron supplementation in preterm infants with elevated serum ferritin concentrations

It is usual for preterm infants to have abnormally high serum ferritin concentrations (> 350 μg/L). These concentrations may result from the storage of excess iron following multiple transfusions (ie, true iron overload) or from the sequestration of iron during periods of inflammation (ie, iron redistribution). There are no specific guidelines for iron supplementation of preterm infants who have high serum ferritin concentrations. The increased risk of mortality and morbidity associated with iron supplementation in iron-replete infants and children[74] and the potential for additional iron accumulation resulting from the poor regulation of intestinal absorption[9,51,74] caution against routine supplementation in these infants. Nevertheless, some preterm infants who have elevated serum ferritin may simultaneously have iron-deficient erythropoiesis,[51] suggesting an inability to release ferritin-bound hepatic iron to the bone marrow. Therefore, it may be prudent to rule out iron-deficient erythropoiesis by determining the zinc protoporphyrin to heme (ZnPP/H) ratio and reticulocyte count[75] in infants who have increased serum ferritin levels and to consider iron supplementation on an individual basis. Preterm infants in whom iron supplementation has been withheld probably will benefit from periodic screening of their iron status, because they may be at risk of iron deficiency during the postdischarge period. A recent study with a small sample size demonstrated evidence of iron deficiency between 6 and 12 months corrected age in approximately 25% of preterm infants who had serum ferritin concentration higher than the 95th percentile of normal at discharge, in spite of receiving 2 to 4 mg/kg d^{-1} of iron.[76]

Postingestion Considerations

Absorption and retention

More than 50% of the iron in human milk and approximately 4% to 12% of the iron in cow milk–based formulas is absorbed.[77] Absorption is better from whey-predominant formula than from casein-based formula. Only 1% to 7% of the iron in soy milk-based formula is absorbed.[77]

The absorption and retention of enterally administered medicinal iron depends on the postnatal age and iron status of the infant. Absorption is better if medicinal iron is supplemented with breast milk or between meals.[49,60] Isotope studies have demonstrated that approximately 25% to 30% of the administered iron is absorbed,[9,49] irrespective of the iron endowment.[51] Approximately 10% to 25% of the iron supplemented between feedings is incorporated into erythrocytes within 2 weeks.[60,65]

Adjuvant therapies to enhance the efficacy of enteral iron supplementation

Ascorbic acid and other organic acids in the diet favor absorption, but there are no specific recommendations for administering these or other nutrients during iron supplementation. Although rHuEPO promotes incorporation of absorbed iron into erythrocytes, it does not enhance enteral iron absorption.[78]

Gastrointestinal tolerance

Iron-fortified infant formulas are well tolerated in full-term infants and may be used as the first feeding when breast milk is not available.[77] Gastrointestinal symptoms, such as cramping, gastroesophageal reflux, and flatulence that are attributed to the ingestion of iron have not been borne out by controlled studies of iron-fortified formulas.[79] Similarly, medicinal iron in doses of 2 to 10 mg/kg d^{-1} is well tolerated by preterm infants,[5,8,42,53] but clinically significant hematochezia without necrotizing enterocolitis occurred in 17% of preterm infants receiving 8 to 16 mg/kg d^{-1} of elemental iron, necessitating cessation of supplementation.[66] Whether hematochezia was caused by iron per se or by other factors (eg, allergy to cow milk protein) was not established. In most instances iron therapy could be resumed on the resolution of hematochezia.[66] Other studies have reported tolerance of 18 to 36 mg/d of iron supplementation without gastrointestinal side effects.[71]

Interaction of iron with other minerals

Because many divalent cations share common transport mechanisms,[80] there is a potential for interaction between iron and other minerals. The effect on zinc and copper has been studied in detail. Zinc supplementation does not seem to impede iron absorption at a ratio of 4:1 in formula.[81] Similarly, 2 mg/kg d^{-1} of iron supplementation had no effect on serum zinc levels[82] or selenium absorption.[83] Iron absorption from fortified breast milk seems to be intact in spite of the high calcium content of the fortifier.[60] Iron supplementation seems to alter copper metabolism, but the clinical relevance of this alteration is unclear at present.[51]

Oxidative stress with enteral iron supplementation

In vitro studies have demonstrated increased free radical and lipid peroxidation products in formula and human milk after the addition of medicinal iron.[84] There are no in vivo studies demonstrating oxidative injury following enteral iron supplementation. Preterm infants between 27 and 34 weeks' gestation had no increase in iron overload or oxidative stress with a formula fortified with 8 mg/L of iron.[85] Enteral iron supplementation in doses of 3 to 10 mg/kg d^{-1} was not associated with markers of oxidative stress in plasma or urine of stable VLBW infants.[42,43] Nevertheless, a threshold dose of iron probably exists beyond which the potential for oxidative stress increases.

OTHER PREVENTIVE MEASURES FOR IRON DEFICIENCY

Delaying the clamping the umbilical cord for 30 to180 seconds after birth improves iron status.[86] Data, however, are insufficient to recommend this practice as a general policy, given the potential impact of a large volume expansion on the fragile cerebral circulation of the preterm infant. Limiting phlebotomy losses, avoiding cow milk, and using iron pots for cooking[4] are other preventive measures that may improve the iron status of preterm infants. Of note, it is not possible to enhance the iron concentration of breast milk with maternal iron supplementation after birth.[54]

SCREENING AND TREATMENT OF IRON DEFICIENCY ANEMIA IN PRETERM INFANTS AFTER DISCHARGE

Timing and Frequency of Screening

Periodic assessment of hemoglobin or hematocrit is recommended for screening the iron nutritional status of full-term infants, with an initial screening between 9 and 12 months of age and a second screening 6 months later (ie, between 15 and 18 months).[87] Although there are no specific recommendations for preterm infants, it is considered prudent to screen them at approximately 4 months.[87] Because many preterm infants develop iron deficiency before that age,[8,15] screening at 2 months or at discharge, whichever is earlier, seems prudent. In one study, serum ferritin below 50 μg/L at 2 months predicted future risk of iron deficiency in preterm infants.[5] Determining the ZnPP/H ratio at the time of discharge may be useful for diagnosing iron-deficient erythropoiesis and the need for additional iron.[75] A recheck of hematologic status at 6 months of age, instead of at the recommended 9 months, also may be beneficial. An individualized follow-up schedule based on the iron status at discharge, growth velocity, type of milk feeding, and dose of iron supplementation would be ideal.

Biomarkers of Iron Nutritional Status

Many laboratory tests are available to assess the iron nutritional status comprehensively (see[88] for a review). Their usefulness in diagnosing iron adequacy or deficiency is limited in preterm infants, however, because gestational age–specific normal values have not been established for most biomarkers.[88] Furthermore, many laboratory markers are confounded by normal developmental changes,[89,90] associated morbidities (eg, inflammation), and therapies (eg, rHuEPO administration and transfusions).

Diagnosis and Treatment of Iron Deficiency

Hemoglobin below the age-specific norm, serum ferritin less than 10 to 12 μg/L, and transferrin saturation less than 10% to 17% have been considered suggestive of iron deficiency anemia in preterm infants during the first 2 to 6 months of life.[5,8,53] A relative increase in the absolute reticulocyte count by more than 50% 1 week after starting iron supplementation also has been considered suggestive of pre-existing iron deficiency.[8] There are no universally accepted treatment protocols for iron deficiency in preterm infants. Oral administration of elemental iron, 3 to 6 mg/kg d^{-1}, for 3 months is recommended in confirmed cases of iron deficiency anemia.[87] A scaled dosing of 3 to 12 mg/kg d^{-1}, adjusted according to the ZnPP/H ratio, has been shown to improve erythropoiesis without causing oxidative stress in preterm infants.[43]

Potential Risk of Neuronal Injury with Rapid Iron Replenishment

Animal studies have demonstrated up-regulation of iron receptors and transporters in the brain regions during fetal and neonatal iron deficiency.[91] Thus, there is a potential for increased cerebral uptake and neuronal injury with excess amounts of iron supplementation.[46] Therefore, rapid correction of iron deficiency using erythrocyte transfusions or large doses of iron should be avoided.

PREVENTIVE AND THERAPEUTIC MEASURES FOR IRON EXCESS

Setting guidelines for erythrocyte transfusions based on specific hematologic parameters potentially would avoid iron excess. There are practical difficulties in adhering to the practice,[40] however, because transfusions often are administered for nonhematologic reasons. Use of rHuEPO in lieu of transfusions may be another strategy. Nevertheless, most studies have demonstrated only a modest decrease in the frequency of erythrocyte transfusions with the use of rHuEPO.[67] Furthermore, a conservative transfusion practice or rHuEPO administration in lieu of transfusion may affect the iron stores after discharge negatively.[32]

There are no specific recommendations for managing preterm infants who have transfusion-related elevated serum ferritin concentrations. Periodic monitoring of the iron status may suffice, because in most instances the increased serum ferritin concentrations normalize spontaneously within 2 months[76] because of a combination of cessation of erythrocyte transfusions, accelerating growth, and regulation of enteral iron absorption.[9] A cocktail of antioxidants and iron chelators has been shown to reduce hepatocyte injury and serum ferritin concentration in neonatal hemochromatosis.[92] Such therapies have not been studied in transfusion-related hyperferritinemia, however, and they may not be necessary, because hepatocyte injury has not been demonstrated with the increased iron deposition in preterm infants.[31] Addition of lactoferrin to formula or human milk decreases the levels of iron-induced oxidative products in vitro.[84] This potential benefit has yet to be established in vivo. There is a theoretic benefit in administering rHuEPO, especially if there is co-existing iron-deficient erythropoiesis, because rHuEPO decreases serum ferritin concentrations without inducing lipid peroxidation or altering antioxidant enzyme activities in preterm infants.[93]

SUMMARY AND FUTURE DIRECTIONS

Iron deficiency and iron excess are significant nutritional problems in the preterm infant. The potential risk of neurodevelopmental impairments caused by iron deficiency warrants frequent screening and preventive measures via the fortification of breast milk or the use of iron-fortified formula. Iron supplementation also seems to be effective and safe. Nevertheless, there are unresolved issues concerning the practice. Iron overload remains a significant concern in multiply transfused sick preterm infants because of their poorly developed antioxidant mechanisms. The management of the preterm infant who has iron overload has not been well studied. Careful monitoring and support during the newborn and postdischarge periods is necessary because of the highly variable iron status of preterm infants. There is a need to develop gestational age–specific laboratory markers for assessing iron nutritional status comprehensively. Most studies on iron status and iron supplementation were conducted before the era of improved survival of smaller and gestationally more immature preterm infants. Well-controlled, randomized trials are necessary to establish iron therapy guidelines for these infants. Research also is necessary to establish the mechanism of absorption and regulation of iron homeostasis during typical development.

ACKNOWLEDGMENT

The authors thank Jennifer L.M. Super, RD, LD, for assistance with the iron content of formula and additives and Caitlyn Nystedt for assistance with manuscript preparation.

REFERENCES

1. Halvorsen S, Seip M. Erythrocyte production and iron stores in premature infants during the first months of life; the anemia of prematurity-etiology, pathogenesis, iron requirement. Acta Paediatr 1956;45(6):600–17.
2. Barclay SM, Lloyd DJ, Duffty P, et al. Iron supplements for preterm or low birth-weight infants. Arch Dis Child 1989;64(11):1621–2.
3. Halliday HL, Lappin TR, McClure G. Iron status of the preterm infant during the first year of life. Biol Neonate 1984;45(5):228–35.
4. Borigato EV, Martinez FE. Iron nutritional status is improved in Brazilian preterm infants fed food cooked in iron pots. J Nutr 1998;128(5):855–9.
5. Lundstrom U, Siimes MA, Dallman PR. At what age does iron supplementation become necessary in low-birth-weight infants? J Pediatr 1977;91(6):878–83.
6. Hall RT, Wheeler RE, Benson J, et al. Feeding iron-fortified premature formula during initial hospitalization to infants less than 1800 grams birth weight. Pediatrics 1993;92(3):409–14.
7. Iwai Y, Takanashi T, Nakao Y, et al. Iron status in low birth weight infants on breast and formula feeding. Eur J Pediatr 1986;145(1–2):63–5.
8. Franz AR, Mihatsch WA, Sander S, et al. Prospective randomized trial of early versus late enteral iron supplementation in infants with a birth weight of less than 1301 grams. Pediatrics 2000;106(4):700–6.
9. Shaw JC. Iron absorption by the premature infant. The effect of transfusion and iron supplements on the serum ferritin levels. Acta Paediatr Scand Suppl 1982; 299:83–9.
10. Dauncey MJ, Davies CG, Shaw JC, et al. The effect of iron supplements and blood transfusion on iron absorption by low birthweight infants fed pasteurized human breast milk. Pediatr Res 1978;12(9):899–904.
11. Widdowson EM, Spray CM. Chemical development *in utero*. Arch Dis Child 1951; 26:205–14.
12. Siimes AS, Siimes MA. Changes in the concentration of ferritin in the serum during fetal life in singletons and twins. Early Hum Dev 1986;13(1):47–52.
13. Siddappa AM, Rao R, Long JD, et al. The assessment of newborn iron stores at birth: a review of the literature and standards for ferritin concentrations. Neonatology 2007;92(2):73–82.
14. Singla PN, Chand S, Agarwal KN. Cord serum and placental tissue iron status in maternal hypoferremia. Am J Clin Nutr 1979;32(7):1462–5.
15. Haga P. Plasma ferritin concentrations in preterm infants in cord blood and during the early anaemia of prematurity. Acta Paediatr Scand 1980;69(5):637–41.
16. Olivares M, Llaguno S, Marin V, et al. Iron status in low-birth-weight infants, small and appropriate for gestational age. A follow-up study. Acta Paediatr 1992; 81(10):824–8.
17. Sichieri R, Fonseca VM, Hoffman D, et al. Lack of association between iron status at birth and growth of preterm infants. Rev Saude Publica 2006;40(4):641–7.
18. Aggett PJ, Barclay S, Whitley JE. Iron for the suckling. Acta Paediatr Scand Suppl 1989;361:96–102.
19. Aggett PJ. Trace elements of the micropremie. Clin Perinatol 2000;27(1):119–29, vi.
20. Lozoff B, Georgieff MK. Iron deficiency and brain development. Semin Pediatr Neurol 2006;13(3):158–65.
21. Tamura T, Goldenberg RL, Hou J, et al. Cord serum ferritin concentrations and mental and psychomotor development of children at five years of age. J Pediatr 2002;140(2):165–70.

22. Armony-Sivan R, Eidelman AI, Lanir A, et al. Iron status and neurobehavioral development of premature infants. J Perinatol 2004;24(12):757–62.
23. Steinmacher J, Pohlandt F, Bode H, et al. Randomized trial of early versus late enteral iron supplementation in infants with a birth weight of less than 1301 grams: neurocognitive development at 5.3 years' corrected age. Pediatrics 2007;120(3):538–46.
24. Widness JA, Seward VJ, Kromer IJ, et al. Changing patterns of red blood cell transfusion in very low birth weight infants. J Pediatr 1996;129(5):680–7.
25. Bard H, Widness JA. The life span of erythrocytes transfused to preterm infants. Pediatr Res 1997;42(1):9–11.
26. Hirano K, Morinobu T, Kim H, et al. Blood transfusion increases radical promoting non-transferrin bound iron in preterm infants. Arch Dis Child Fetal Neonatal Ed 2001;84(3):F188–93.
27. Dani C, Martelli E, Bertini G, et al. Effect of blood transfusions on oxidative stress in preterm infants. Arch Dis Child Fetal Neonatal Ed 2004;89(5):F408–11.
28. Friel JK, Andrews WL, Hall MS, et al. Intravenous iron administration to very-low-birth-weight newborns receiving total and partial parenteral nutrition. JPEN J Parenter Enteral Nutr 1995;19(2):114–8.
29. Inder TE, Clemett RS, Austin NC, et al. High iron status in very low birth weight infants is associated with an increased risk of retinopathy of prematurity. J Pediatr 1997;131(4):541–4.
30. Cooke RW, Drury JA, Yoxall CW, et al. Blood transfusion and chronic lung disease in preterm infants. Eur J Pediatr 1997;156(1):47–50.
31. Ng PC, Lam CW, Lee CH, et al. Hepatic iron storage in very low birthweight infants after multiple blood transfusions. Arch Dis Child Fetal Neonatal Ed 2001;84(2):F101–5.
32. Arad I, Konijn AM, Linder N, et al. Serum ferritin levels in preterm infants after multiple blood transfusions. Am J Perinatol 1988;5(1):40–3.
33. Shaw JC. Trace metal requirements of preterm infants. Acta Paediatr Scand Suppl 1982;296:93–100.
34. Pollak A, Hayde M, Hayn M, et al. Effect of intravenous iron supplementation on erythropoiesis in erythropoietin treated premature infants. Pediatrics 2001;107(1): 78–85.
35. Carnielli VP, Da Riol R, Montini G. Iron supplementation enhances response to high doses of recombinant human erythropoietin in preterm infants. Arch Dis Child Fetal Neonatal Ed 1998;79:F44–8.
36. Shannon KM, Keith JF 3rd, Mentzer WC, et al. Recombinant human erythropoietin stimulates erythropoiesis and reduces erythrocyte transfusions in very low birth weight preterm infants. Pediatrics 1995;95(1):1–8.
37. Melhorn DK, Gross S. Vitamin E-dependent anemia in the premature infant. I. Effects of large doses of medicinal iron. J Pediatr 1971;79(4):569–80.
38. Hesse L, Eberl W, Schlaud M, et al. Blood transfusion. Iron load and retinopathy of prematurity. Eur J Pediatr 1997;156(6):465–70.
39. Silvers KM, Gibson AT, Russell JM, et al. Antioxidant activity, packed cell transfusions, and outcome in premature infants. Arch Dis Child Fetal Neonatal Ed 1998; 78:F214–9.
40. Brooks SE, Marcus DM, Gillis D, et al. The effect of blood transfusion protocol on retinopathy of prematurity: a prospective, randomized study. Pediatrics 1999; 104(3 Pt 1):514–8.
41. Bolann BJ, Ulvik RJ. Release of iron from ferritin by xanthine oxidase. Role of the superoxide radical. Biochem J 1987;243(1):55–9.

42. Braekke K, Bechensteen AG, Halvorsen BL, et al. Oxidative stress markers and antioxidant status after oral iron supplementation to very low birth weight infants. J Pediatr 2007;151(1):23–8.
43. Miller SM, McPherson RJ, Juul SE. Iron sulfate supplementation decreases zinc protoporphyrin to heme ratio in premature infants. J Pediatr 2006;148(1):44–8.
44. Berg D, Youdim MB. Role of iron in neurodegenerative disorders. Top Magn Reson Imaging 2006;17(1):5–17.
45. Shouman BO, Mesbah A, Aly H. Iron metabolism and lipid peroxidation products in infants with hypoxic ischemic encephalopathy. J Perinatol 2008;28:487–91.
46. Kaur D, Peng J, Chinta SJ, et al. Increased murine neonatal iron intake results in Parkinson-like neurodegeneration with age. Neurobiol Aging 2007;28(6): 907–13.
47. American Academy of Pediatrics, Committee on Nutrition. Nutritional needs of the preterm infant. In: Kleinman RE, editor. Pediatric nutrition handbook. 5th edition. Chapel Hill (NC): American Academy of Pediatrics; 2004. p. 23–54.
48. Fletcher J, Suter PE. The transport of iron by the human placenta. Clin Sci 1969; 36(2):209–20.
49. Fomon SJ, Nelson SE, Ziegler EE. Retention of iron by infants [in process citation]. Annu Rev Nutr 2000;20:273–90.
50. Oski FA. Iron deficiency in infancy and childhood [see comments]. N Engl J Med 1993;329(3):190–3.
51. Lonnerdal B, Kelleher SL. Iron metabolism in infants and children. Food Nutr Bull 2007;28(4 Suppl):S491–9.
52. Berseth CL, Van Aerde JE, Gross S, et al. Growth, efficacy, and safety of feeding an iron-fortified human milk fortifier. Pediatrics 2004;114(6):e699–706.
53. Arnon S, Shiff Y, Litmanovitz I, et al. The efficacy and safety of early supplementation of iron polymaltose complex in preterm infants. Am J Perinatol 2007;24(2): 95–100.
54. Dorea JG. Iron and copper in human milk. Nutrition 2000;16(3):209–20.
55. Griffin IJ, Cooke RJ, Reid MM, et al. Iron nutritional status in preterm infants fed formulas fortified with iron. Arch Dis Child Fetal Neonatal Ed 1999;81(1):F45–9.
56. Nutrition Committee, Canadian Pediatric Society. Nutrition needs and feeding of premature infants. Can Med Assoc J 1995;152(11):1765–85.
57. Committee on Nutrition of the Preterm Infant, European Society of Paediatric Gastroenterology and Nutrition. Nutrition and feeding of preterm infants. Acta Paediatr Scand 1987;336(Suppl):1–14.
58. Siimes MA, Jarvenpaa AL. Prevention of anemia and iron deficiency in very low-birth-weight infants. J Pediatr 1982;101(2):277–80.
59. Siimes MA. Iron requirement in low birthweight infants. Acta Paediatr Scand Suppl 1982;296:101–3.
60. McDonald MC, Abrams SA, Schanler RJ. Iron absorption and red blood cell incorporation in premature infants fed an iron-fortified infant formula. Pediatr Res 1998;44(4):507–11.
61. Naude S, Clijsen S, Naulaers G, et al. Iron supplementation in preterm infants: a study comparing the effect and tolerance of a Fe2+ and a nonionic FeIII compound. J Clin Pharmacol 2000;40(12 Pt 2):1447–51.
62. Zlotkin S, Arthur P, Antwi KY, et al. Randomized, controlled trial of single versus 3-times-daily ferrous sulfate drops for treatment of anemia. Pediatrics 2001; 108(3):613–6.
63. Heese HD, Smith S, Watermeyer S, et al. Prevention of iron deficiency in preterm neonates during infancy. S Afr Med J 1990;77(7):339–45.

64. Barry DM, Reeve AW. Increased incidence of gram-negative neonatal sepsis with intramuscular iron administration. Pediatrics 1977;60(6):908–12.
65. Zlotkin SH, Lay DM, Kjarsgaard J, et al. Determination of iron absorption using erythrocyte iron incorporation of two stable isotopes of iron (57Fe and 58Fe) in very low birthweight premature infants. J Pediatr Gastroenterol Nutr 1995;21(2): 190–9.
66. Bader D, Kugelman A, Maor-Rogin N, et al. The role of high-dose oral iron supplementation during erythropoietin therapy for anemia of prematurity. J Perinatol 2001;21(4):215–20.
67. Aher S, Ohlsson A. Late erythropoietin for preventing red blood cell transfusion in preterm and/or low birth weight infants. Cochrane Database Syst Rev 2006;3: CD004868.
68. Fujiu T, Maruyama K, Koizumi T. Oral iron supplementation in preterm infants treated with erythropoietin. Pediatr Int 2004;46(6):635–9.
69. Ridley FC, Harris J, Gottstein R, et al. Is supplementary iron useful when preterm infants are treated with erythropoietin? Arch Dis Child 2006;91(12):1036–8.
70. Meyer MP, Haworth C, Meyer JH, et al. A comparison of oral and intravenous iron supplementation in preterm infants receiving recombinant erythropoietin. J Pediatr 1996;129(2):258–63.
71. Bechensteen AG, Haga P, Halvorsen S, et al. Erythropoietin, protein, and iron supplementation and the prevention of anaemia of prematurity. Arch Dis Child 1993;69(1 Spec No):19–23.
72. Kivivuori SM, Virtanen M, Raivio KO, et al. Oral iron is sufficient for erythropoietin treatment of very low birth-weight infants. Eur J Pediatr Feb 1999;158(2):147–51.
73. Carbonell-Estrany X, Figueras-Aloy J, Alvarez E. Erythropoietin and prematurity—where do we stand? J Perinat Med 2005;33(4):277–86.
74. Domellof M. Iron requirements, absorption and metabolism in infancy and childhood. Curr Opin Clin Nutr Metab Care 2007;10(3):329–35.
75. Winzerling JJ, Kling PJ. Iron-deficient erythropoiesis in premature infants measured by blood zinc protoporphyrin/heme J Pediatr 2001;139(1):134–6.
76. deRegnier R-A, Shah MD, Wiles C, Georgieff MK. First year outcome of hyperferremia in multiply transfused preterm infants [abstract E-PAS2008:633774.6]. In: Abstracts2View Online Program of the Pediatric Academic Societies and Asian Society for Pediatric Research Joint Meeting. Honolulu (HI): 2008. Available at: http://www.abstracts2view.com/pas. Accessed June 10, 2008.
77. American Academy of Pediatrics CoN. Iron fortification of infant formulas. Pediatrics 1999;104(1 Pt 1):119–23.
78. Widness JA, Lombard KA, Ziegler EE, et al. Erythrocyte incorporation and absorption of 58Fe in premature infants treated with erythropoietin. Pediatr Res 1997;41(3):416–23.
79. Nelson SE, Ziegler EE, Copeland AM, et al. Lack of adverse reactions to iron-fortified formula. Pediatrics 1988;81(3):360–4.
80. Garrick MD, Dolan KG, Horbinski C, et al. DMT1: a mammalian transporter for multiple metals. Biometals 2003;16(1):41–54.
81. Friel JK, Serfass RE, Fennessey PV, et al. Elevated intakes of zinc in infant formulas do not interfere with iron absorption in premature infants. J Pediatr Gastroenterol Nutr 1998;27(3):312–6.
82. Salvioli GP, Faldella G, Alessandroni R, et al. Plasma zinc concentrations in iron supplemented low birthweight infants. Arch Dis Child 1986;61(4):346–8.
83. Rudolph N, Preis O, Bitzos EI, et al. Hematologic and selenium status of low-birth-weight infants fed formulas with and without iron. J Pediatr 1981;99(1):57–62.

84. Raghuveer TS, McGuire EM, Martin SM, et al. Lactoferrin in the preterm infants' diet attenuates iron-induced oxidation products. Pediatr Res 2002;52(6):964–72.
85. van Zoeren Grobben D, Moison R, Haasnoot A, et al. Iron containing feeding formula and oxidative stress in preterm infants. Pediatr Res 1998;43:270A.
86. Rabe H, Reynolds G, Diaz-Rossello J. A systematic review and meta-analysis of a brief delay in clamping the umbilical cord of preterm infants. Neonatology 2008; 93(2):138–44.
87. American Academy of Pediatrics, Committee on Nutrition. Iron deficiency. In: Kleinman RE, editor. Pediatric nutrition handbook. 5th edition. Chapel Hill (NC): American Academy of Pediatrics; 2004. p. 299–312.
88. Beard J, deRegnier RA, Shaw MD, et al. Diagnosis of iron deficiency in infants. Lab Med 2007;38(2):103–8.
89. Griffin IJ, Reid MM, McCormick KP, et al. Zinc protoporphyrin/haem ratio and plasma ferritin in preterm infants. Arch Dis Child Fetal Neonatal Ed 2002;87(1): F49–51.
90. Lott DG, Zimmerman MB, Labbe RF, et al. Erythrocyte zinc protoporphyrin is elevated with prematurity and fetal hypoxemia. Pediatrics 2005;116(2):414–22.
91. Siddappa AJ, Rao RB, Wobken JD, et al. Iron deficiency alters iron regulatory protein and iron transport protein expression in the perinatal rat brain. Pediatr Res 2003;53(5):800–7.
92. Flynn DM, Mohan N, McKiernan P, et al. Progress in treatment and outcome for children with neonatal haemochromatosis. Arch Dis Child Fetal Neonatal Ed 2003;88(2):F124–7.
93. Akisu M, Tuzun S, Arslanoglu S, et al. Effect of recombinant human erythropoietin administration on lipid peroxidation and antioxidant enzyme(s) activities in preterm infants. Acta Med Okayama 2001;55(6):357–62.

Inhaled Nitric Oxide for Preterm Neonates

Nandini Arul, MD[a,b,*], G. Ganesh Konduri, MD[a,b]

KEYWORDS

- Preterm infants • Inhaled nitric oxide
- Bronchopulmonary dysplasia • Brain injury
- Pulmonary hypertension

The identification of nitric oxide (NO) as an endothelial-derived vasodilator has led to dramatic advances in the understanding of vascular biology over the past 20 years. Inhaled NO (iNO) was investigated as a pulmonary vasodilator in term neonates with respiratory failure within 4 years of discovery of NO[1,2] iNO is now an approved and established therapy for term and near–term neonates with hypoxic respiratory failure. The introduction of iNO therapy has greatly reduced the need for extracorporeal membrane oxygenation in this group of neonates.[3,4] Hypoxic respiratory failure is also a significant contributor to mortality and morbidity in preterm neonates in the neonatal intensive care unit (NICU). Respiratory failure in preterm neonates, however, has a different cause and clinical course from that occurring in term neonates. The underlying pathologic changes in preterm neonates involve surfactant deficiency, pulmonary immaturity, lung injury with inflammation, oxidant stress, and impaired angiogenesis. Hypoxemia in preterm respiratory failure is often a result of ventilation/perfusion (V/Q) mismatch and intrapulmonary shunting. Pulmonary hypertension can also occur in preterm neonates as a complication of respiratory failure, pulmonary hypoplasia secondary to preterm prolonged rupture of membranes (PPROMs), and oligohydramnios or as a late complication in bronchopulmonary dysplasia (BPD).

Despite improved survival in the era of surfactant therapy and antenatal steroids, BPD and brain injury remain significant adverse outcomes in extremely low birth weight preterm neonates. There is growing interest in the application of iNO as a tool to prevent these adverse outcomes, taking advantage of the beneficial effects of iNO on gas exchange, inflammation, and vascular dysfunction.[5–7] Translational investigations in animal models provided the evidence to consider these beneficial effects as biologically plausible. The history of neonatology is, however, filled with well-intentioned therapies that resulted in significant harm to this vulnerable population. The use of iNO therapy has so far been rightfully limited to controlled clinical trials.

[a] Division of Neonatology, Medical College of Wisconsin, Milwaukee, WI, USA
[b] Division of Neonatology, Department of Pediatrics, Children's Corporate Center, Suite C410, PO Box 1997, Milwaukee, WI 53201–1997, USA
* Corresponding author. Division of Neonatology, Department of Pediatrics, Children's Corporate Center, Suite C410, PO Box 1997, Milwaukee, WI 53201–1997.
E-mail address: narul08@gmail.com (N. Arul).

Clin Perinatol 36 (2009) 43–61
doi:10.1016/j.clp.2008.09.002 perinatology.theclinics.com

The purpose of this review is to briefly outline the biology of NO, the role of NO in lung development, the rationale for its use in preterm infants, and the results of recent clinical trials. This review also discusses the role of iNO in the prevention of BPD and brain injury in addition to the unanswered questions from the clinical studies, and identifies areas of future research with this therapy.

BIOLOGY OF NITRIC OXIDE

NO is synthesized as a byproduct of the conversion of L-arginine to L-citrulline by nitric oxide synthase (NOS).[8,9] NO diffuses rapidly across cell membranes; in the case of blood vessels, it reaches the adjacent smooth muscle cells. NO activates soluble guanylate cyclase and increases cyclic guanosine 3′,5′- monophosphate (cGMP) levels in the vascular smooth muscle cell (**Fig. 1**).[10,11] An increase in cGMP levels is associated with decreased cytosolic calcium and relaxation of smooth muscle.[12] iNO can cause selective vasorelaxation of smooth muscle cells by diffusion from the alveoli.[13] NO is rapidly inactivated by combining with hemoglobin in the blood to form nitrosyl hemoglobin and is then oxidized to methemoglobin and inorganic nitrates and nitrites.[14,15]

There are three isoforms of NOS that differ in the site of expression and regulation of their function. Neuronal NOS (NOS-1, nNOS) is constitutively expressed primarily in the airway epithelium in the lung, and its activity is calcium dependent. Inducible NOS (NOS-2) is present in the airway, vascular smooth muscle, and macrophages; its expression is induced by lipopolysaccharide, cytokines, and other mediators of inflammation, and its activity is calcium independent. Endothelial NOS (NOS-3, eNOS) is constitutively expressed in the vascular endothelium and airway epithelial cells, and its activity is calcium dependent.[14] The levels of eNOS and nNOS proteins show developmental increase in late gestation in primates, sheep, and in rodents.[16,17] There is

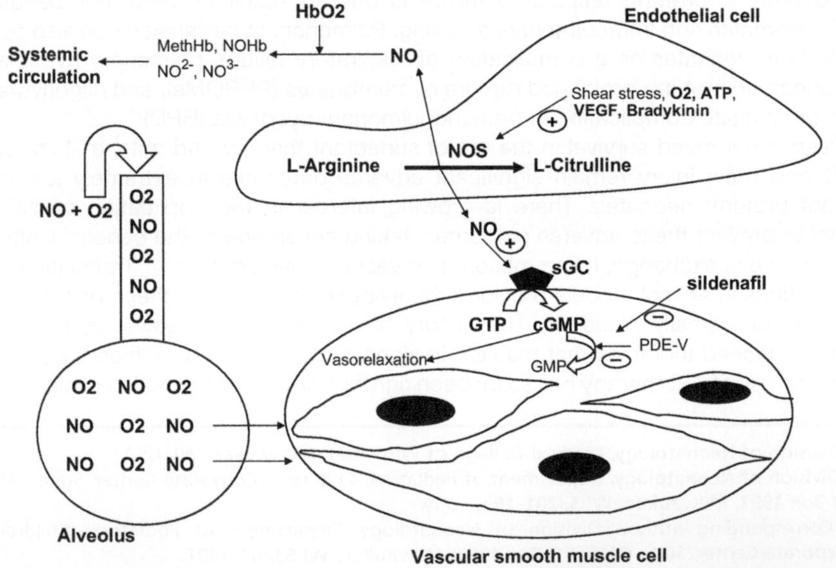

Fig. 1. Mechanism of action of NO. Endogenous NO diffuses from endothelial cells to the smooth muscle cells, whereas iNO diffuses across the alveolus and reaches the smooth muscle cells causing vasorelaxation by means of generation of cGMP. NO is quenched by hemoglobin on reaching the lumen of the pulmonary vessel. GTP, guanosine triphosphate; PDE-V, Phosphodiesterase-V.

sustained basal release of NO in late gestation to maintain pulmonary vascular tone, and developmental increases in NO production occur during late gestation in the primate that may enhance airway and lung function in the immediate postnatal period.[18] The activity of eNOS increases at birth in response to physiologic stimuli like estrogens, shear stress, vascular endothelial growth factor (VEGF), and ATP in addition to pharmacologic stimuli like acetylcholine and bradykinin. NOS activity requires the substrates arginine and oxygen and the cofactors tetrahydrobiopterin (BH4), flavoproteins, heat shock protein 90 (hsp-90), and calmodulin.[19] NOS is an oxidoreductase, and NO production requires an increase in electron flow through the reductase domain, which transfers these electrons to oxygen to generate superoxide (O_2^-) transiently. This occurs in conjunction with oxidation of the terminal amino group of arginine to generate NO and citrulline. Depletion of cofactors hsp-90 and BH4 results in uncoupled activity of eNOS with release of O_2^- radical instead of NO. Increase in NOS-derived O_2^- plays a significant role in impaired vasodilatation in pulmonary hypertension.[20]

ROLE OF NITRIC OXIDE IN LUNG DEVELOPMENT

Early studies in fetal animal models focused on the role of NO in the pulmonary vasodilatation that occurs at birth in response to oxygen and ventilation.[21] NO plays an important physiologic role in lung development, however. Development of lung vasculature and its proper interface with alveolar space are required for the gas exchange function of the lung. Impaired angiogenesis also leads to impaired alveolar maturation.[22] Expression of eNOS is found in vascular endothelial and airway epithelial cells of the developing lung. The timing of eNOS expression has been studied in rat, ovine, and baboon fetal lungs. It is remarkable that in all three species, eNOS mRNA levels progressively increase during the canalicular stage of lung development, suggesting the role of eNOS in parenchymal and vascular development.[16] Experiments using NO donors and inhibitors in an ex vivo fetal rat lung model have demonstrated a major regulatory role for NO in airway branching morphogenesis.[23] NO is a critical downstream and upstream regulator of angiogenic agents like VEGF. NO plays a major role in postnatal angiogenesis, as shown in eNOS knockout mice. Neonatal pups of eNOS knockout mice show signs of respiratory distress and cyanosis, along with hypoplastic lungs containing thickened septa and reduced microvascular endothelial cells.[16] eNOS knockout mice that survive the neonatal period have decreased alveolarization with exposure to mild hypoxia that persists despite recovery in room air. Late rescue treatment with iNO enhances their recovery with alveolar and vascular growth in the distal lung through VEGF signaling.[24–26] These findings suggest that eNOS activity contributes to normal lung development and to recovery of normal growth after chronic hypoxia during the neonatal period. Thus, the NO pathway is critical to proper development and interfacing of the vascular and alveolar components of the lung.

PHYSIOLOGIC BASIS FOR INHALED NITRIC OXIDE THERAPY IN PRETERM INFANTS

There are potential short-term and long-term benefits of iNO in preterm newborns. Short term benefits are (1) selective pulmonary vasodilatation, (2) improvement in V/Q matching, (3) decreased neutrophil accumulation and activation, and (4) improvement in oxygenation in hypoxic respiratory failure.

Long-term benefits are (1) reduced need for oxygen and decrease in oxidant stress, (2) improved surfactant function, (3) decreased airway resistance, and (4) improved lung growth attributable to stimulation of angiogenesis and alveolarization. Several animal and clinical studies have investigated these potential benefits.

Effect of Inhaled Nitric Oxide on Hypoxic Respiratory Failure

Preterm newborns develop hypoxic respiratory failure primarily as a result of V/Q mismatch and intrapulmonary shunting from surfactant deficiency. Early studies have shown that low-dose iNO improves pulmonary blood flow, gas exchange, and pulmonary vascular resistance in mechanically ventilated preterm lambs and human preterm newborns.[27,28] Contribution of significant right-to-left ductal shunt shunting to hypoxemia has been reported in preterm infants.[29] Whether preterm neonates have sufficient musculature in the pulmonary arteries to have persistent pulmonary hypertension (PPHN) is debatable, however. Echocardiographic studies demonstrated pulmonary hypertension secondary to respiratory distress syndrome (RDS), and some studies reported its association with increased mortality in the presurfactant era.[30–33] Recently, Randala and colleagues[34] estimated pulmonary artery pressure (PAP) in the first 4 days of life in healthy term newborns and in preterm newborns with and without RDS by recording ductal Doppler flow velocity and systemic arterial pressure (SAP). At 48 and 72 hours, the PAP-to-SAP ratio was significantly higher in preterm neonates who had RDS than in those who did not have RDS ($P<.05$). Although the number of preterm neonates presenting with PPHN is probably small, PPHN should be considered in neonates who have significant hypoxemia in spite of surfactant therapy and adequate ventilation.[35] Preterm newborns who have PPROM, oligohydramnios, and pulmonary hypoplasia are particularly at increased risk. Kumar and colleagues[36] found that prenatal and postnatal factors independently predictive of pulmonary hypertension in neonates less than 37 weeks of age are PPROM, oligohydramnios, 5-minute Apgar score, pulmonary hypoplasia, and sepsis.

Unlike other vasodilators, which have systemic effects, iNO causes selective dilatation of pulmonary arteries as it diffuses from the alveolar space to the pulmonary artery smooth muscle, where it is quenched by hemoglobin at the luminal side. NO gas is primarily distributed to better ventilated segments of the lung, and improved perfusion of these segments results in improved V/Q match and oxygenation.[37–39] These properties of iNO make it the ideal pulmonary vasodilator for respiratory failure in the neonates. Concerns were expressed about iNO therapy initially because of exposure of airway and alveolar space to a potential oxidant and the direct exposure of vascular smooth muscle to NO from the abluminal side. Recent studies show that NO is normally present in the upper airway from synthesis in the airway mucosa, however, and is inhaled during tidal respiration in neonates. The breath NO levels in the nasal cavity of preterm neonates approach 100 parts per billion (0.1 ppm).[40,41] These data suggest that iNO has a physiologic role in gas exchange and lung protection in neonates.

Effect of Inhaled Nitric Oxide on Lung Injury, Lung Growth, and Lung Function

Chronic lung disease or BPD is associated with an early pulmonary inflammatory response and sequestration of neutrophils.[42] Preterm newborns who have RDS and BPD have increased lung neutrophil counts at 1 week of age compared with newborns who do not have BPD.[43] NO is a major regulator of vascular permeability and neutrophil adhesion in the lung. Inhibition of NO production leads to increased leukocyte rolling and adhesion in various vascular beds.[44] In ventilated preterm lambs, iNO at low doses (5 ppm) decreases pulmonary edema and neutrophil accumulation and improves pulmonary blood flow and gas exchange.[7]

Whether iNO can reduce the oxidant stress that occurs in preterm newborns exposed to high oxygen concentrations was also the subject of several studies. When rat fetal lung tissue in vivo and cultured pulmonary epithelial cells were subjected to greater than 95% oxygen or cytokines, NO inhibited the O_2^--dependent toxicity.[45] Hamon and colleagues[46] assessed oxidative balance in premature newborns who were exposed to low-dose iNO (5 ppm) and assessed their clinical outcome on day 28 of life. Neonates with hypoxemic respiratory failure who were aged less than 32 weeks of gestation were randomized at birth to receive 5 ppm of iNO or placebo. Nonhypoxemic neonates were the reference group. These researchers observed that after 24 hours, blood malondialdehyde (MDA) concentration, an oxidative stress marker, was lower in the iNO group compared with the placebo group and was close to levels measured in the reference group. Plasma glutathione (GSH) concentration, a marker of antioxidant defense, was more stable in the iNO group. On day 28, oxygen need and mortality were associated with a larger increase in MDA, whereas intraventricular hemorrhage (IVH) was associated with a larger initial decrease in GSH.

There is also increasing evidence that deficient endogenous production of NO can contribute to BPD. In the preterm baboon model of BPD, there is a deficiency of the pulmonary nNOS and eNOS activity and enhanced iNOS activity in the first 2 weeks of postnatal life.[47] In ventilated preterm lambs, quantitative immunoblot analysis and semiquantitative immunohistochemistry showed less eNOS protein in the endothelium of small intrapulmonary arteries and epithelium of small airways compared with controls born at term.[48] There was enhanced alveolar development with increased radial alveolar counts in iNO-treated lambs, and eNOS protein did not differ from that of term controls.[49]

In a preterm baboon model of BPD, 14 days of iNO at 5 ppm caused improved lung morphology and compliance and decreased excessive extracellular matrix deposition.[50] In a neonatal rat model, VEGF receptor inhibition reduced eNOS expression and decreased lung vascular growth and alveolarization, and these changes were reversed with iNO treatment.[51] iNO also restores lung structure in eNOS-deficient mice subjected to hypoxia or hyperoxia.

NO has also been shown to induce airway smooth muscle relaxation and reduce tissue and airway components of lung resistance.[52] Bland and colleagues[49] studied the effect of iNO (5–15 ppm) on mechanically ventilated preterm lambs for 3 weeks and found that the pulmonary vascular resistance and expiratory airway resistance were lower and dynamic compliance was better in the iNO-treated group.

NO also has a role in improving surfactant function, as shown in a preterm baboon model of BPD, in which iNO at 5 ppm enhanced surfactant protein function.[53] Hyperoxia-induced surfactant dysfunction in preterm rabbits was mitigated by iNO with preservation of alveolar surfactant function and a decrease in oxidant stress.[54] In these animal models, iNO protects the developing lung by means of several mechanisms, providing a strong rationale for its use in preterm neonates. The proposed effects of iNO on the preterm lung at the saccular or alveolar stage of development are depicted in **Fig. 2**.

Inhaled Nitric Oxide and Neuroprotection

Endogenously produced NO in the brain regulates local blood flow and offers neuroprotection. Whether iNO therapy offers the secondary benefit of neuroprotection is an intriguing possibility.[55,56] Previous studies with NO donors raised the concern of increased permeability of the blood-brain barrier by means of the formation of free radicals like peroxynitrite.[57,58] There are several possible mechanisms for neuroprotection with iNO, such as modulation of circulating neutrophils, monocytes, and

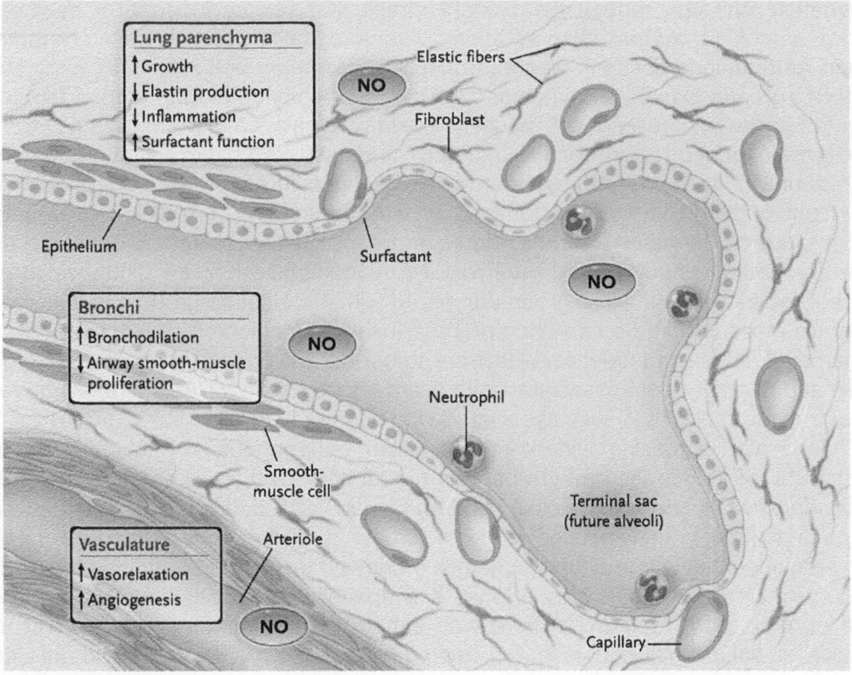

Fig. 2. Potential effects of NO on the developing lung. This figure represents a fetal or preterm lung during the saccular to alveolar stage of development at 25 to 28 weeks of gestation. The potential effects of inducible NO on the developing lung parenchyma, airways, and vasculature are shown. (*From* Martin RJ, Walsh MC. Inhaled nitric oxide for preterm infants—who benefits? N Engl J Med 2005;353:83; with permission. Copyright © 2005, Massachusetts Medical Society.)

platelets as they pass through the lung.[59] A strong association between brain injury and BPD or sepsis is reported, with the systemic inflammatory response and cytokine release probably playing a role.[60] iNO down-regulates lung-derived cytokines and oxidant stress, which may lead to a decrease in brain injury.[61,62]

NO can also combine with sulfur (thiols)-containing proteins to form nitrosothiols, which are considered an endogenous source of NO. They are long-acting stable forms, thereby preventing NO's conversion to toxic radicals.[22] S-nitroso–hemoglobin, for example, resulting from NO-hemoglobin interaction, plays a role in vasodilatation and oxygen delivery in the microcirculation. So, a possible mechanism in neuroprotection may relate to delivery of NO or NO-related metabolites, such as hemoglobin-derived S-nitrosothiol, that account for distant vasodilatory activity.[63,64] Extrapulmonary effects of iNO on reduction of myocardial infarction size and improved left ventricular systolic function have been shown in a murine model.[65] These studies demonstrate that an extrapulmonary vasoprotective effect of iNO is possible.

RESULTS OF RANDOMIZED CONTROLLED CLINICAL TRIALS

Investigation of iNO in term neonates was followed by early case reports of improved oxygenation in preterm neonates with iNO therapy. The major concern with the use of iNO in these babies is an increased incidence of intracranial hemorrhage attributable to inhibition of platelet aggregation by NO.[27,66–68] Although some pilot studies showed an increased IVH rate with iNO, these studies had a small sample size, included critically ill preterm infants, and did not obtain cranial imaging before administering iNO. The efficacy and safety of iNO in this group of babies were tested in three large multicenter trials and a large single-center trial.[59,69–71] To date, the randomized controlled trials (RCTs) have focused on neonates who were ventilated in the immediate postnatal period, thus selecting a high-risk population. The role of iNO therapy in the era of early continuous positive airway pressure (CPAP) use and decreased incidence of BPD remains unanswered from these RCTs. The trials recruited diverse patient populations with differences in severity of illness. The trials also differ in dose, timing, and duration of iNO use; degree of exposure to antenatal steroids; respiratory therapy offered; and definition of BPD. Keeping these limitations in mind, the authors categorized the RCTs into three groups:[72,73]

1. Early prophylactic therapy: trials using iNO in preterm babies requiring mechanical ventilation, less than 72 hours of age, and at risk for BPD, irrespective of disease severity
2. Early rescue therapy: trials using iNO in preterm babies in the first week of life, based on disease severity as measured by the oxygenation index (OI) or a/A ratio
3. Late therapy: trials using iNO in preterm babies requiring mechanical ventilation or CPAP, more than 72 hours of age, and at risk for BPD, irrespective of disease severity

EARLY PROPHYLACTIC THERAPY TRIALS

Schreiber and Colleagues, 2003

This single-center double-blind, controlled trial enrolled 207 newborns, aged 34 weeks or less of gestation, who were mechanically ventilated for RDS.[71] The enrollment was not stratified based on disease severity; the median OI was 6.94. The initial dose of iNO was 10 ppm and weaned to 5 ppm for a total of 7 days. The primary outcome was death or BPD at 36 weeks of postmenstrual age (PMA). A significant reduction in death or BPD was observed in the iNO-treated group compared with controls (48.6% versus 63.7%, relative risk [RR] = 0.76, 95% confidence interval [CI]: 0.60–0.97). Post hoc analysis indicated that a reduction in BPD or death occurred in babies with an OI less than 6.94. The secondary outcome of incidence of severe IVH (grade 3/4) and periventricular leukomalacia (PVL) was significantly lower in the iNO-treated group compared with controls (12.4% versus 23.5%, RR = 0.53, 95% CI: 0.28–0.98; *P* = .04). Although the effect of iNO on BPD was only seen in the less sick subgroup, the beneficial effect of iNO on IVH rates in spite of 56% antenatal steroid use was encouraging. Follow-up of 82% of the survivors to 2 years of corrected age demonstrated a decrease in the incidence of neurodevelopmental impairments in the iNO-treated group (24% iNO versus 46% control, RR = 0.53, 95% CI: 0.33–0.87, number needed to treat [NNT] = 5).[74] This improvement persisted after correction for birth weight, gender, BPD, maternal education, postnatal corticosteroids, and severe IVH or PVL. The beneficial effect of iNO on BPD or death and long-term neurologic outcome may have been amplified by a higher than expected rate of BPD in the control group (63.7%) and enrollment of relatively more mature neonates.[58]

Kinsella and Colleagues, 2006

This multicenter double-blind trial randomized 793 newborns, 34 weeks or less of gestation, within 48 hours of birth, if they required mechanical ventilation.[59] The study subjects received iNO (5 ppm) or a placebo gas for 21 days or until extubation. The median OI at study entry was approximately 5.4 to 5.8. Cranial ultrasound was performed before study enrollment and sequentially to detect severe IVH (grade 3/4),

PVL, and ventriculomegaly. Thus, the trial aimed to initiate low-dose iNO therapy before significant lung injury occurred. The primary outcomes were death or BPD at 36 weeks of PMA and abnormal findings on chest radiography as assessed by a scoring system. There was no significant reduction in the primary outcome of death or BPD for the study subjects. Post hoc analysis showed that iNO reduced the risk for death or BPD in babies weighing more than 1000 g (16% of study patients) by 50% (RR = 0.60, 95% CI: 0.42–0.86, relative risk reduction (RRR) = 40%; *P* = .004). As in the study by Schreiber and colleagues,[71] there was a significant reduction in the incidence of brain injury (defined as severe IVH [grade 3/4]), PVL, and ventriculomegaly on brain imaging in the iNO-treated group (RR = 0.73, 95% CI: 0.55–0.98, NNT = 16; *P* = .03). Subgroup analysis suggested that this protective effect was confined to the 750- to 999-g birth weight group. Follow-up studies are needed to determine whether this short-term benefit translates into improved long-term neurodevelopmental outcomes. The incidence of BPD in the control group is relatively high and similar to that in the study by Schreiber and colleagues.[71]

EARLY RESCUE THERAPY TRIALS

Comparison of rescue therapy trials is complicated by variability among studies in respiratory disease severity at study entry along with blinding and timing of intervention.

Kinsella and Colleagues, 1999

This pilot double-blind multicenter trial enrolled 80 preterm neonates, with a gestational age (GA) of 34 weeks or less, 7 days of age or less, and severe hypoxemia (measured as an a/A ratio of 0.10 or less), who were on mechanical ventilation after surfactant treatment.[75] Enrollment was stratified by a GA of 28 weeks or less or 28 weeks or more, with randomization of babies to iNO at 5 ppm or placebo for 7 days, after which weaning was allowed. The primary outcome measure was survival to discharge. The incidence of BPD at 36 weeks of PMA, duration of ventilation, and incidence of severe IVH were secondary outcomes. Cranial ultrasound to detect the baseline IVH rate was performed before study enrollment. Even though oxygenation improved 1 hour after iNO treatment, the data showed only a trend toward a decrease in BPD (60% in iNO group versus 80% in placebo group; *P* = .30) and no differences in rates of severe IVH (37% versus 40%; *P* = .92). The lack of benefit could be attributable to the patient population in this trial, which was limited to critically ill preterm newborns (50% baseline mortality rate) with severe respiratory failure despite maximal intervention.

Van Meurs and Colleagues, 2005

This randomized multicenter trial enrolled 420 neonates, aged 34 weeks or less of gestation, with respiratory failure 4 hours or more after birth and surfactant treatment, with an OI of 10 or greater.[69] The neonates were randomized to receive iNO at 5 to 10 ppm or placebo gas, with weaning allowed more than 10 hours after starting treatment if Pa_{O_2} improved more than 10 mm Hg. If there was no response at 10 ppm, iNO was withdrawn. The primary outcome was incidence of death or BPD at 36 weeks of PMA. Room air challenge was offered to extubated infants and infants with 30% or less oxygen need at 36 weeks of PMA. Severe IVH and PVL were secondary outcomes. iNO did not reduce mortality or BPD, but post hoc analysis revealed that it reduced these rates in neonates weighing 1000 g or more (RR = 0.72, 95% CI: 0.54–0.96; *P* = .03). A cause for concern is the higher mortality these researchers observed in babies (<1 kg) treated with iNO compared with controls (RR = 1.28, 95%

CI: 1.06–1.54). They also observed a higher rate of severe IVH or PVL (RR = 1.40, 95% CI: 1.03–1.88) after controlling for antenatal or postnatal steroid use. Cranial ultrasound scans were not performed before study entry, and results of the examination were not available for 86 infants because of early death. Although smaller (47% of babies with a birth weight <750 g) and more critically ill (44% mortality in the control group, 17 babies with an OI <6.94 and a mean OI of 23) babies were enrolled, there was no significant impact of disease severity on the outcome measures. Follow-up of 92% of survivors in this cohort at 18 to 22 months of age showed no improvement in death or neurodevelopmental outcome in the iNO-treated group (RR = 1.07, 95% CI: 0.95–1.19). Moderate to severe cerebral palsy was higher in the iNO-treated group (RR = 2.41, 95% CI: 1.01–5.75).[76]

Other Unmasked Trials

The results of several unmasked randomized trials were published, with varying dosages and durations of iNO use, along with varying outcome measures.[77–80] The Franco-Belgium study group found that short-term oxygenation did not improve with iNO (10 ppm), but open-label use of iNO in the control group and outcome assessment after a short duration of treatment made interpretation difficult. The UK INNOVO (Neonatal Ventilation with Inhaled Nitric Oxide Versus Ventilatory support without Inhaled Nitric Oxide for preterm infants with Severe Respiratory Failure) trial enrolled newborns aged less than 34 weeks and less than 28 days with severe respiratory failure and used iNO at 5 to 40 ppm.[79] The investigators found no differences between treatment groups in long-term outcome at 1 year of corrected age. The study limitation was high crossover of the control group to the treatment group and also use of other pulmonary vasodilators, with a median OI of 32. A small single-center trial of babies aged less than 30 weeks who had severe RDS despite surfactant treatment at less than 7 days of age showed a significant reduction in death or BPD at 36 weeks of PMA in the iNO-treated group, but there was increased failure to respond to iNO in the neonates with a birth weight less than 750 g.[80] Another single-center study assessed severe IVH (grade 3/4) as the primary outcome measure in babies aged less than 34 weeks and treated with iNO at 20 ppm or with standard care for a maximum of 7 days and showed no statistically significant differences between the treatment groups.[81]

LATE THERAPY TRIALS

Subhedar and Colleagues, 1997

This was a single-center, non-blinded, randomized trial that investigated if two interventions (ie, postnatal dexamethasone and iNO) given together or alone reduce the incidence of BPD or death.[82] The investigators enrolled neonates at 32 weeks or less of GA, who were at risk for BPD based on a modified BPD prediction score and were randomized to iNO at a dose of 5–20 ppm or dexamethasone at a dose of 0.5–1 mg/kg for 6 days or to both or neither treatment. Cranial ultrasound scans were performed at baseline and weekly intervals to assess brain injury. No detectable difference in the incidence of BPD (RR = 1.05, 95% CI: 0.84–1.25) was noted, with 100% of survivors reported as having BPD. These researchers also observed a short-term increase in oxygenation in 20 preterm babies treated with iNO at 5 to 20 ppm and noted a 17% decrease in the OI after the initial 30 minutes. This transient effect did not translate into an improved BPD outcome, however.[83] Developmental assessment (95% follow-up of surviving infants) at 30 months of corrected age did not show differences in cerebral palsy or neurodevelopmental delay.[84]

Ballard and Colleagues, 2006

This recent multicenter trial measured the effect of iNO in improving survival without BPD in babies needing significant respiratory support at more than 1 week of age.[70] The researchers enrolled 582 neonates, 32 weeks or less of age, who were receiving respiratory support and also neonates weighing less than 800 g on CPAP because of high reintubation rates in this category (8%–9% of study patients). All neonates had cranial ultrasound scans for IVH surveillance before study entry. The babies received iNO at 20 ppm initially, with weekly weaning to 10, 5, and 2 ppm. The respiratory severity score (determined by multiplying the fraction of inspired oxygen by the mean airway pressure and equating a Pa_{O_2} of 40–70 mm Hg to an oxygen saturation goal of 88%–94%) of 3.5 was equal to an OI range of 5 to 9. Improved survival without BPD was noted in iNO group compared with controls (RR = 1.23, 95% CI: 1.01–1.51, NNT 14; *P* = .04). The benefit persisted at 40 and 44 weeks with decreased hospitalization and a decreased need for oxygen and ventilation. This effect was noted in infants in the 7- to 14-day-old age group (RR =1.81, 95% CI: 1.27–2.59, NNT = 5; *P* = .006) and was not present beyond 15 days of age. There was a modest 6% difference in BPD rates between the treatment groups. A study using a subcohort of this trial reported the effect of iNO on resistance and compliance of the respiratory system and observed no short- or medium-term benefit.[85] There was no evolution of neurologic findings on head ultrasound scans in the treatment group.

OUTCOME FROM CLINICAL TRIALS

A systematic review by Barrington and Finer[73] concluded that none of the previous individual trials showed any significant impact on mortality alone. In early prophylactic therapy trials, however, there was a favorable impact on mortality with iNO treatment (RR = 0.77, 95% CI: 0.60–0.98, NNT = 19; *P* = .03). No effect on the BPD rate was observed, however.

Effect on Bronchopulmonary Dysplasia or Death

The data on the combined outcome of death or BPD at 36 weeks of PMA in the early rescue therapy trials showed no benefit, although these trials vary considerably from one to another (**Fig. 3**). The preplanned subgroup analyses of the largest of the early rescue trials showed a reduced adverse outcome in iNO-treated neonates with a birth weight greater than 1 kg.[69] In the early prophylactic therapy trials, a marginal effect of improved outcome (RR = 0.91, 95% CI: 0.84–0.99; *P* = .03) with a NNT of 17 (95% CI: 8–100) was noted. The preplanned subgroup analyses of the larger trial showed that babies weighing more than 1 kg at birth experienced this benefit.[59] The late therapy trial showed a 21% increase in survival without BPD in neonates treated with iNO who were 7 to 14 days of age at randomization.[70]

Effect on Brain Injury

Although a trend for an increased incidence of severe IVH or PVL was noted in early rescue studies, there was no significant difference between control and iNO groups (RR = 1.16, 95% CI: 0.93–1.44; *P* = .20). The limitations to analysis of results are the varied entry criteria, lack of cranial ultrasound scans before study entry, short duration of iNO treatment, and more critically ill babies being enrolled in these trials. In contrast, the early prophylactic trials showed a reduction of this outcome (RR = 0.70, 95% CI: 0.53–0.91; *P* = .009) with a NNT of 14 (95% CI: 8–50). The late therapy trials showed no progression of neurologic injury (**Fig. 4**).

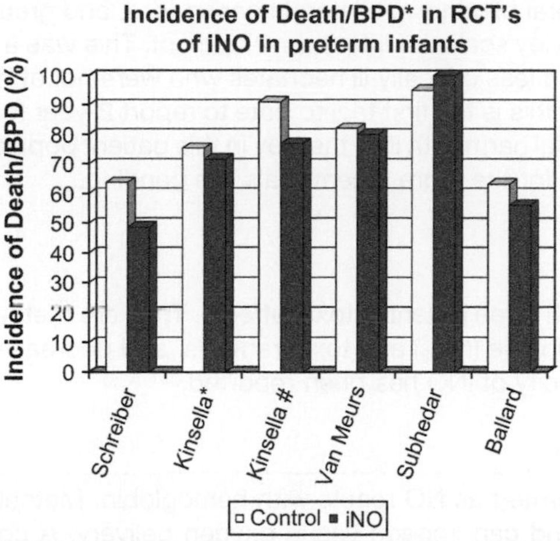

Fig. 3. Effect of inhaled NO on the incidence of death or BPD in RCTs. The trials show a modest benefit with a large number needed to treat (NNT) and pending confirmation from long-term outcome data. Kinsella * refers to the trial by Kinsella and colleagues in 2006.[59] Kinsella # refers to the trial by Kinsella and colleagues in 1999.[75]

Effect on Neurodevelopmental Outcome

Cochrane analysis of two studies reporting neurodevelopmental outcome did not show significant benefit.[79,84] The study by Mestan and colleagues[74] noted a significant reduction in the composite outcome of neurodevelopmental disability, defined as

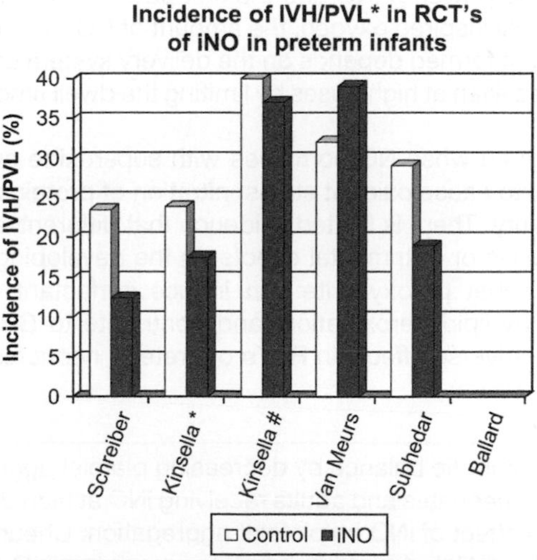

Fig. 4. Effect of inhaled NO on the incidence of severe neurologic injury in RCTs. IVH is defined as grade 3 or 4 intraventricular bleed. There seems to be decreased risk with early prophylactic therapy in comparison to rescue therapy trials because of the more critically ill study population in the latter group. Kinsella * refers to the trial by Kinsella and colleagues in 2006.[59] Kinsella # refers to the trial by Kinsella and colleagues in 1999.[75] (Data not available for study by Ballard).

cerebral palsy, bilateral blindness, bilateral hearing loss, and greater than 2 SD lower than the mean of Bayley scales of infant development. This was a single-center study with more mature and less critically ill neonates who were not at high risk for this outcome. Nevertheless, this is the first trial to date to report 2-year follow-up giving reassurance of no potential harm with iNO therapy in this patient population. The results on long-term outcomes for the more recent trials are pending.

POTENTIAL TOXICITIES

NO is associated with three potential toxic effects. They are methemoglobinemia, formation of nitrogen dioxide (NO_2) and toxic radicals, and decreased platelet aggregation. Little direct toxicity of iNO has been reported.

Methemoglobinemia

Methemoglobin is formed as NO reacts with hemoglobin. Methemoglobin has a low affinity for oxygen and can impede tissue oxygen delivery. A concentration greater than 5% to 10% has been associated with cyanosis and hypoxia. Preterm infants are more susceptible because of relatively low levels of the enzyme methemoglobin reductase.[86] Doses greater than 22 ppm are associated with higher levels of methemoglobin.[87] Hence, frequent monitoring of methemoglobin levels once treatment is commenced and until a stable dose is achieved is essential. None of the RCTs using doses of 20 ppm or less have reported any increase in the incidence of this adverse effect.

Nitrogen Dioxide and Peroxynitrite

On combining with oxygen, NO forms a toxic gas, NO_2, that has been implicated in oxidant stress injury to lungs and airways. The concentration of this toxic gas is proportional to the second power of iNO and the first power of inspired oxygen. For example, when using 90% inspired oxygen, the amount of NO_2 formed is 5 ppm over 20 seconds.[37] The amount formed depends on the delivery system used, and decreased levels can be achieved even at high doses by limiting the dwell time and vacuum-purging ambient air.[88]

Peroxynitrite is formed when NO combines with superoxide anion, a free radical, and has the potential to cause oxidant stress, nitration of proteins, lipid peroxidation, and, thereby, lung injury. There is limited evidence that different levels of this metabolite can have protective or detrimental effects on the developing lung.[37] Contradictory reports suggest that peroxynitrite can induce surfactant dysfunction, cause membrane damage by lipid peroxidation, and contribute to BPD.[89–92] There is no direct proof of these adverse effects in RCTs of preterm neonates, however.

Platelet Aggregation

NO also mediates thrombotic balance by decreasing platelet aggregation.[93] Bleeding times are prolonged in neonates and adults receiving iNO at high doses.[94,95] There are limited reports on the effect of iNO on platelet aggregation. Cheung and colleagues[96] studied mechanically ventilated preterm neonates receiving iNO and found that they had decreased platelet aggregation. This effect was not noted in a small study on term neonates.[97] This potential effect of iNO has caused concern for initiation of intracranial hemorrhage in preterm neonates at risk.[68] Although this was reported in early rescue trials,[69] there has been no evidence of this adverse outcome because of the confounding effect of illness severity.

PERSISTENT UNCERTAINTIES OF INHALED NITRIC OXIDE USE IN PRETERM INFANTS

Despite more than 2000 babies being enrolled in iNO trials, in preterm newborns, there are still questions to be answered, and the potential role of iNO needs to be further defined. The abundant laboratory evidence needs to be translated to beneficial clinical outcomes.

Dose and Duration of Treatment

The past decade has seen clinical trials of iNO using doses from 2 to 80 ppm, but toxicity concerns and lack of increased efficacy at high doses led most to gravitate to doses of 5 to 20 ppm. Van Meurs and colleagues[68] reported the dose response at 1, 5, 10, and 20 ppm in newborns aged 25 to 32 weeks of GA as a pilot study and found favorable changes in a/A ratio using doses of 5, 10, and 20 ppm. A study conducted as part of the INNOVO trial found no significant difference in dose response, defined as an increase in Pao_2 of at least 3 kPa for doses tested (5, 10, 20, and 40 ppm) in neonates aged less than 34 weeks and less than 28 days of postnatal age.[98] There is a minimum dose of 5 ppm and an equally effective safe increase to 20 ppm in preterm neonates.[67] There are large differences in the length of iNO treatment among clinical trials, with more recent trials using longer duration of treatment based on data that shows benefit in animal models.

Identification of Candidates who can Benefit from Treatment

This difficult question is partly answered by reviewing the clinical trials, which show that clinically relevant benefit seems to occur in babies weighing more than 1 kg with mild respiratory disease and neonates older than 7 days of age with established lung disease but who are at higher risk for adverse outcomes. Caution is needed in babies who weigh less than 1 kg and are critically ill because they are at higher risk for short- and long-term adverse outcomes regardless of iNO treatment. For example, the etiology for the new BPD is an aberration in alveolar and vascular development of the preterm lung.[99] Prematurity, along with multiple adverse stimuli like antenatal infection, lack of enteral nutrition, genetic differences, and mechanical ventilation, leads to growth arrest and BPD. This multifactorial causation of BPD and the lack of effect of iNO on many of the previously mentioned causes can diminish the effect of iNO in these sickest babies.

Future trials should investigate a specific subset of preterm neonates who have a lower inherent risk for neurologic injury but may benefit from iNO use. It seems reasonable to use iNO therapy in the critically ill very low birth weight baby with severe hypoxic respiratory failure who is unresponsive to conventional management.[72] It is important to recognize that the response to iNO depends on the disease, gestational age, timing, and dose of administration. The pathologic condition behind the clinical deterioration (ie, pulmonary hypoplasia, extrapulmonary shunt, sepsis, RDS) and its predicted response to iNO must be analyzed before attempting the use of iNO.

In centers with low BPD rates, the unknown long-term risks with iNO use in critically ill neonates weighing less than 1 kg probably outweigh the benefits offered by its use. In neonates weighing more than 1 kg, the modest benefits seen in trials so far, by treating a large number of babies at a high cost, do not seem to justify its routine use.

Long-Term Neurologic Outcome

Any assessment of the efficacy of iNO treatment should consider its effect on long-term outcomes. The surrogate markers of long-term outcome, such as BPD at 36 weeks of PMA, can cause global developmental delay, and a normal cranial ultrasound scan at the time of examination does not imply a normal neurodevelopmental outcome. Whether reduction of these surrogate markers improves long-term outcome still remains to be answered.

The long-term neurologic outcome data have not been reported for two of the recent large clinical trials. It should be interesting to see the differences in outcome between trials using iNO prophylactically versus with established lung disease and also to tease out the effect of low-dose prolonged duration of treatment. Future trials should address whether treatment with iNO before the occurrence of significant lung injury can improve neurologic outcome.

Assessment of Cost Benefit

It is difficult to define the subgroup of neonates who would have reduced adverse outcomes and also benefit from iNO treatment. The unknown risks, uncertain benefit, and significant expense of iNO therapy in this patient population require careful assessment and justification for its use.

SUMMARY

The available evidence for the use of iNO in the preterm neonate suggests that a beneficial effect of iNO depends on the patient population, duration of therapy, and underlying pathologic condition. The early and late use of iNO in preterm neonates cannot be recommended until long-term neurodevelopmental follow-up data from recently completed trials are available. The use of iNO as rescue therapy for babies weighing less than 1 kg is confounded by a patient population at high risk for an adverse neurologic outcome. Although endogenous NO is important for lung growth, there is little evidence that an exogenous supply of NO achieves that goal.

REFERENCES

1. Ignarro LJ, Buga GM, Wood KS, et al. Endothelium-derived relaxing factor produced and released from artery and vein is nitric oxide. Proc Natl Acad Sci U S A 1987;84:9265–9.
2. Palmer RM, Ferrige AG, Moncada S. Nitric oxide release accounts for the biological activity of endothelium-derived relaxing factor. Nature 1987;327:524–6.
3. Inhaled nitric oxide in full-term and nearly full-term infants with hypoxic respiratory failure. The Neonatal Inhaled Nitric Oxide Study Group. N Engl J Med 1997;336:597–604.
4. Clark RH, Kueser TJ, Walker MW, et al. Low-dose nitric oxide therapy for persistent pulmonary hypertension of the newborn. Clinical Inhaled Nitric Oxide Research Group. N Engl J Med 2000;342:469–74.
5. Mourani PM, Ivy DD, Gao D, et al. Pulmonary vascular effects of inhaled nitric oxide and oxygen tension in bronchopulmonary dysplasia. Am J Respir Crit Care Med 2004;170:1006–13.
6. Kinsella JP, Abman SH. Inhaled nitric oxide in the premature infant: animal models and clinical experience. Semin Perinatol 1997;21:418–25.
7. Kinsella JP, Parker TA, Galan H, et al. Effects of inhaled nitric oxide on pulmonary edema and lung neutrophil accumulation in severe experimental hyaline membrane disease. Pediatr Res 1997;41:457–63.
8. Moncada S, Palmer RM, Higgs EA. Nitric oxide: physiology, pathophysiology, and pharmacology. Pharmacol Rev 1991;43:109–42.
9. Mercier JC, Franco-Belgium Neonatal Study Group on Inhaled Nitric Oxide. Uncertainties about the use of inhaled nitric oxide in preterm infants. Acta Paediatr Suppl 2001;90:15–8.

10. Ignarro LJ. Biological actions and properties of endothelium-derived nitric oxide formed and released from artery and vein. Circ Res 1989;65:1–21.
11. Ignarro LJ, Cirino G, Casini A, et al. Nitric oxide as a signaling molecule in the vascular system: an overview. J Cardiovasc Pharmacol 1999;34:879–86.
12. Walter U. Physiological role of cGMP and cGMP-dependent protein kinase in the cardiovascular system. Rev Physiol Biochem Pharmacol 1989;113:41–88.
13. Frostell C, Fratacci MD, Wain JC, et al. Inhaled nitric oxide. A selective pulmonary vasodilator reversing hypoxic pulmonary vasoconstriction. Circulation 1991;83: 2038–47.
14. Coggins MP, Bloch KD. Nitric oxide in the pulmonary vasculature. Arterioscler Thromb Vasc Biol 2007;27:1877–85.
15. Hughes MN. Chemistry of nitric oxide and related species. Methods Enzymol. 2008;436:3–19.
16. Han RN, Stewart DJ. Defective lung vascular development in endothelial nitric oxide synthase-deficient mice. Trends Cardiovasc Med. 2006;16:29–34.
17. Parker TA, le Cras TD, Kinsella JP, et al. Developmental changes in endothelial nitric oxide synthase expression and activity in ovine fetal lung. Am J Physiol Lung Cell Mol Physiol 2000;278:L202–8.
18. Shaul PW, Afshar S, Gibson LL, et al. Developmental changes in nitric oxide synthase isoform expression and nitric oxide production in fetal baboon lung. Am J Physiol Lung Cell Mol Physiol 2002;283:L1192–9.
19. Shaul PW. Regulation of endothelial nitric oxide synthase: location, location, location. Annu Rev Physiol 2002;64:749–74.
20. Konduri GG, Bakhutashvili I, Eis A, et al. Oxidant stress from uncoupled nitric oxide synthase impairs vasodilation in fetal lambs with persistent pulmonary hypertension. Am J Physiol Heart Circ Physiol 2007;292:H1812–20.
21. Tristani-Firouzi M, Martin EB, Tolarova S, et al. Ventilation-induced pulmonary vasodilation at birth is modulated by potassium channel activity. Am J Physiol 1996; 271:H2353–9.
22. Shaul PW. Nitric oxide in the developing lung. Adv Pediatr 1995;42:367–414.
23. Young SL, Evans K, Eu JP. Nitric oxide modulates branching morphogenesis in fetal rat lung explants. Am J Physiol Lung Cell Mol Physiol 2002;282:L379–85.
24. Balasubramaniam V, Tang JR, Maxey A, et al. Mild hypoxia impairs alveolarization in the endothelial nitric oxide synthase-deficient mouse. Am J Physiol Lung Cell Mol Physiol 2003;284:L964–71.
25. Balasubramaniam V, Maxey A, Abman S. Inhaled nitric oxide reverses hypoxia induced lung hypoplasia in endothelial nitric oxide synthase-deficient mice. Chest 2005;128:613S–4S.
26. Balasubramaniam V, Maxey AM, Morgan DB, et al. Inhaled NO restores lung structure in eNOS-deficient mice recovering from neonatal hypoxia. Am J Physiol Lung Cell Mol Physiol 2006;291:L119–27.
27. Abman SH, Kinsella JP, Schaffer MS, et al. Inhaled nitric oxide in the management of a premature newborn with severe respiratory distress and pulmonary hypertension. Pediatrics 1993;92:606–9.
28. Kinsella JP, Ivy DD, Abman SH. Inhaled nitric oxide improves gas exchange and lowers pulmonary vascular resistance in severe experimental hyaline membrane disease. Pediatr Res 1994;36:402–8.
29. Stahlman M, Blankenship WJ, Shepard FM, et al. Circulatory studies in clinical hyaline membrane disease. Biol Neonate 1972;20:300–20.
30. Evans NJ, Archer LN. Doppler assessment of pulmonary artery pressure during recovery from hyaline membrane disease. Arch Dis Child 1991;66:802–4.

31. Skinner JR, Boys RJ, Hunter S, et al. Pulmonary and systemic arterial pressure in hyaline membrane disease. Arch Dis Child 1992;67:366–73.
32. Walther FJ, Benders MJ, Leighton JO. Persistent pulmonary hypertension in premature neonates with severe respiratory distress syndrome. Pediatrics 1992;90:899–904.
33. Halliday H, Hirschfeld S, Riggs T, et al. Respiratory distress syndrome: echocardiographic assessment of cardiovascular function and pulmonary vascular resistance. Pediatrics 1977;60:444–9.
34. Randala M, Eronen M, Andersson S, et al. Pulmonary artery pressure in term and preterm neonates. Acta Paediatr 1996;85:1344–7.
35. Golan A, Zalzstein E, Zmora E, et al. Pulmonary hypertension in respiratory distress syndrome. Pediatr Pulmonol 1995;19:221–5.
36. Kumar VH, Hutchison AA, Lakshminrusimha S, et al. Characteristics of pulmonary hypertension in preterm neonates. J Perinatol 2007;27:214–9.
37. Smyth RL. Inhaled nitric oxide treatment for preterm infants with hypoxic respiratory failure. Thorax 2000;55(Suppl 1):S51–5.
38. Rossaint R, Falke KJ, Lopez F, et al. Inhaled nitric oxide for the adult respiratory distress syndrome. N Engl J Med 1993;328:399–405.
39. Rossaint R, Pison U, Gerlach H, et al. Inhaled nitric oxide: its effects on pulmonary circulation and airway smooth muscle cells. Eur Heart J 1993;14(Suppl I):133–40.
40. Williams O, Rafferty GF, Hannam S, et al. Nasal and lower airway levels of nitric oxide in prematurely born infants. Early Hum Dev 2003;72:67–73.
41. Leipala JA, Williams O, Sreekumar S, et al. Exhaled nitric oxide levels in infants with chronic lung disease. Eur J Pediatr 2004;163:555–8.
42. Zimmerman JJ. Bronchoalveolar inflammatory pathophysiology of bronchopulmonary dysplasia. Clin Perinatol 1995;22:429–56.
43. Ogden BE, Murphy S, Saunders GC, et al. Lung lavage of newborns with respiratory distress syndrome. Prolonged neutrophil influx is associated with bronchopulmonary dysplasia. Chest 1983;83:31S–3S.
44. Kanwar S, Kubes P. Nitric oxide is an antiadhesive molecule for leukocytes. New Horiz 1995;3:93–104.
45. Gutierrez HH, Nieves B, Chumley P, et al. Nitric oxide regulation of superoxide-dependent lung injury: oxidant-protective actions of endogenously produced and exogenously administered nitric oxide. Free Radic Biol Med 1996;21:43–52.
46. Hamon I, Fresson J, Nicolas MB, et al. Early inhaled nitric oxide improves oxidative balance in very preterm infants. Pediatr Res 2005;57:637–43.
47. Afshar S, Gibson LL, Yuhanna IS, et al. Pulmonary NO synthase expression is attenuated in a fetal baboon model of chronic lung disease. Am J Physiol Lung Cell Mol Physiol 2003;284:L749–58.
48. MacRitchie AN, Albertine KH, Sun J, et al. Reduced endothelial nitric oxide synthase in lungs of chronically ventilated preterm lambs. Am J Physiol Lung Cell Mol Physiol 2001;281:L1011–20.
49. Bland RD, Albertine KH, Carlton DP, et al. Inhaled nitric oxide effects on lung structure and function in chronically ventilated preterm lambs. Am J Respir Crit Care Med 2005;172:899–906.
50. McCurnin DC, Pierce RA, Chang LY, et al. Inhaled NO improves early pulmonary function and modifies lung growth and elastin deposition in a baboon model of neonatal chronic lung disease. Am J Physiol Lung Cell Mol Physiol 2005;288:L450–9.
51. Tang JR, Markham NE, Lin YJ, et al. Inhaled nitric oxide attenuates pulmonary hypertension and improves lung growth in infant rats after neonatal treatment

with a VEGF receptor inhibitor. Am J Physiol Lung Cell Mol Physiol 2004;287: L344–51.
52. Martin RJ, Mhanna MJ, Haxhiu MA. The role of endogenous and exogenous nitric oxide on airway function. Semin Perinatol 2002;26:432–8.
53. Ballard PL, Gonzales LW, Godinez RI, et al. Surfactant composition and function in a primate model of infant chronic lung disease: effects of inhaled nitric oxide. Pediatr Res 2006;59:157–62.
54. Issa A, Lappalainen U, Kleinman M, et al. Inhaled nitric oxide decreases hyperoxia-induced surfactant abnormality in preterm rabbits. Pediatr Res 1999;45: 247–54.
55. Martin RJ, Walsh MC. Inhaled nitric oxide for preterm infants—who benefits? N Engl J Med 2005;353:82–4.
56. Cannon RO 3rd, Schechter AN, Panza JA, et al. Effects of inhaled nitric oxide on regional blood flow are consistent with intravascular nitric oxide delivery. J Clin Invest 2001;108:279–87.
57. Mayhan WG. Nitric oxide donor-induced increase in permeability of the blood-brain barrier. Brain Res 2000;866:101–8.
58. Martin RJ. Nitric oxide for preemies—not so fast. N Engl J Med 2003;349:2157–9.
59. Kinsella JP, Cutter GR, Walsh WF, et al. Early inhaled nitric oxide therapy in premature newborns with respiratory failure. N Engl J Med 2006;355:354–64.
60. Viscardi RM, Muhumuza CK, Rodriguez A, et al. Inflammatory markers in intrauterine and fetal blood and cerebrospinal fluid compartments are associated with adverse pulmonary and neurologic outcomes in preterm infants. Pediatr Res 2004;55:1009–17.
61. Haynes RL, Baud O, Li J, et al. Oxidative and nitrative injury in periventricular leukomalacia: a review. Brain Pathol 2005;15:225–33.
62. Aaltonen M, Soukka H, Halkola L, et al. Inhaled nitric oxide treatment inhibits neuronal injury after meconium aspiration in piglets. Early Hum Dev 2007;83:77–85.
63. Kinsella JP, Abman SH. Inhaled nitric oxide in the premature newborn. J Pediatr 2007;151:10–5.
64. Pawloski JR, Hess DT, Stamler JS. Export by red blood cells of nitric oxide bioactivity. Nature 2001;409:622–6.
65. Steinhorn RH, Porta NF. Use of inhaled nitric oxide in the preterm infant. Curr Opin Pediatr 2007;19:137–41.
66. Peliowski A, Finer NN, Etches PC, et al. Inhaled nitric oxide for premature infants after prolonged rupture of the membranes. J Pediatr 1995;126:450–3.
67. Skimming JW, Bender KA, Hutchison AA, et al. Nitric oxide inhalation in infants with respiratory distress syndrome. J Pediatr 1997;130:225–30.
68. Van Meurs KP, Rhine WD, Asselin JM, et al. Response of premature infants with severe respiratory failure to inhaled nitric oxide. Preemie NO Collaborative Group. Pediatr Pulmonol 1997;24:319–23.
69. Van Meurs KP, Wright LL, Ehrenkranz RA, et al. Inhaled nitric oxide for premature infants with severe respiratory failure. N Engl J Med 2005;353:13–22.
70. Ballard RA, Truog WE, Cnaan A, et al. Inhaled nitric oxide in preterm infants undergoing mechanical ventilation. N Engl J Med 2006;355:343–53.
71. Schreiber MD, Gin-Mestan K, Marks JD, et al. Inhaled nitric oxide in premature infants with the respiratory distress syndrome. N Engl J Med 2003;349:2099–107.
72. Subhedar N, Dewhurst C. Is nitric oxide effective in preterm infants? Arch Dis Child Fetal Neonatal Ed 2007;92:F337–41.
73. Barrington KJ, Finer NN. Inhaled nitric oxide for preterm infants: a systematic review. Pediatrics 2007;120:1088–99.

74. Mestan KK, Marks JD, Hecox K, et al. Neurodevelopmental outcomes of premature infants treated with inhaled nitric oxide. N Engl J Med 2005;353:23–32.
75. Kinsella JP, Walsh WF, Bose CL, et al. Inhaled nitric oxide in premature neonates with severe hypoxaemic respiratory failure: a randomised controlled trial. Lancet 1999;354:1061–5.
76. Hintz SR, Van Meurs KP, Perritt R, et al. Neurodevelopmental outcomes of premature infants with severe respiratory failure enrolled in a randomized controlled trial of inhaled nitric oxide. J Pediatr 2007;151:16–22, 22.e1–3.
77. Early compared with delayed inhaled nitric oxide in moderately hypoxaemic neonates with respiratory failure: a randomised controlled trial. The Franco-Belgium Collaborative NO Trial Group. Lancet 1999;354:1066–71.
78. Hascoet JM, Fresson J, Claris O, et al. The safety and efficacy of nitric oxide therapy in premature infants. J Pediatr 2005;146:318–23.
79. Field D, Elbourne D, Truesdale A, et al. Neonatal ventilation with inhaled nitric oxide versus ventilatory support without inhaled nitric oxide for preterm infants with severe respiratory failure: the INNOVO multicentre randomised controlled trial (ISRCTN 17821339). Pediatrics 2005;115:926–36.
80. Dani C, Bertini G, Pezzati M, et al. Inhaled nitric oxide in very preterm infants with severe respiratory distress syndrome. Acta Paediatr 2006;95:1116–23.
81. Srisuparp P, Heitschmidt M, Schreiber MD. Inhaled nitric oxide therapy in premature infants with mild to moderate respiratory distress syndrome. J Med Assoc Thai 2002;85(Suppl 2):S469–78.
82. Subhedar NV, Ryan SW, Shaw NJ. Open randomised controlled trial of inhaled nitric oxide and early dexamethasone in high risk preterm infants. Arch Dis Child Fetal Neonatal Ed 1997;77:F185–90.
83. Subhedar NV, Shaw NJ. Changes in oxygenation and pulmonary haemodynamics in preterm infants treated with inhaled nitric oxide. Arch Dis Child Fetal Neonatal Ed 1997;77:F191–7.
84. Bennett AJ, Shaw NJ, Gregg JE, et al. Neurodevelopmental outcome in high-risk preterm infants treated with inhaled nitric oxide. Acta Paediatr 2001;90:573–6.
85. Di Fiore JM, Hibbs AM, Zadell AE, et al. The effect of inhaled nitric oxide on pulmonary function in preterm infants. J Perinatol 2007;27:766–71.
86. Kravitz H, Elegant LD, Kaiser E, et al. Methemoglobin values in premature and mature infants and children. AMA J Dis Child 1956;91:1–5.
87. Guthrie SO, Walsh WF, Auten K, et al. Initial dosing of inhaled nitric oxide in infants with hypoxic respiratory failure. J Perinatol 2004;24:290–4.
88. Sokol GM, Van Meurs KP, Wright LL, et al. Nitrogen dioxide formation during inhaled nitric oxide therapy. Clin Chem 1999;45:382–7.
89. Drury JA, Nycyk JA, Subhedar NV, et al. Inhaled nitric oxide does not increase lipid peroxidation in preterm infants. Eur J Pediatr 1998;157:1033.
90. Haddad IY, Ischiropoulos H, Holm BA, et al. Mechanisms of peroxynitrite-induced injury to pulmonary surfactants. Am J Physiol 1993;265:L555–64.
91. Radi R, Beckman JS, Bush KM, et al. Peroxynitrite-induced membrane lipid peroxidation: the cytotoxic potential of superoxide and nitric oxide. Arch Biochem Biophys 1991;288:481–7.
92. Hallman M, Waffarn F, Bry K, et al. Surfactant dysfunction after inhalation of nitric oxide. J Appl Physiol 1996;80:2026–34.
93. Radomski MW, Palmer RM, Moncada S. Endogenous nitric oxide inhibits human platelet adhesion to vascular endothelium. Lancet 1987;2:1057–8.
94. George TN, Johnson KJ, Bates JN, et al. The effect of inhaled nitric oxide therapy on bleeding time and platelet aggregation in neonates. J Pediatr 1998;132:731–4.

95. Hogman M, Frostell C, Arnberg H, et al. Bleeding time prolongation and NO inhalation. Lancet 1993;341:1664–5.
96. Cheung PY, Salas E, Etches PC, et al. Inhaled nitric oxide and inhibition of platelet aggregation in critically ill neonates. Lancet 1998;351:1181–2.
97. Christou H, Magnani B, Morse DS, et al. Inhaled nitric oxide does not affect adenosine 5′-diphosphate-dependent platelet activation in infants with persistent pulmonary hypertension of the newborn. Pediatrics 1998;102:1390–3.
98. Ahluwalia J, Tooley J, Cheema I, et al. A dose response study of inhaled nitric oxide in hypoxic respiratory failure in preterm infants. Early Hum Dev 2006;82:477–83.
99. Jobe AJ. The new BPD: an arrest of lung development. Pediatr Res 1999;46:641–3.

Racial Disparity in Low Birth Weight and Infant Mortality

James W. Collins, Jr., MD, MPH[a,*], Richard J. David, MD[b]

KEYWORDS

- African-American • Low birth weight • Infant mortality
- Racial discrimination • Racial disparities • Poverty

The infant mortality rate (IMR) is more than the discrete number of infant deaths that occur in the first year of life per 1000 live births; it is a symbolic benchmark of how a nation cares for its future generations. By this standard, infant mortality in the United States has two glaring characteristics: it is high compared with other developed nations, and African-American infants have a 2.4-fold greater mortality rate than non-Latino white infants.[1] Despite an advanced and expensive health care system, the United States' ranking among industrialized countries has plummeted from sixth to twenty-seventh during the past 50 years.[1,2] The IMR of African Americans has increased from 1.6 to 2.4 times that of whites from the 1950s through 2005.[2,3] In 2005, the IMR of African-American infants equaled 13.6 per 1000 live births compared with 5.7 per 1000 live births for white infants.[3] Deterioration of the US white infant mortality ranking internationally has paralleled the widening racial disparity over the past half century.[2] Reflecting the public health importance of these phenomena, *Healthy People 2010* calls for a decrease in the US overall IMR to 4.5 per 1000 live births and an elimination of the racial disparity in IMRs.[4]

The five leading causes of infant mortality for African Americans and whites[5] are listed in the **Table 1**. Disorders related to short gestation (<37 weeks) are the leading cause of death for African-American infants, whereas congenital malformations are the leading cause of death for white infants. The African American/white mortality rate ratios ranged from only 1.2 for congenital malformations to 3.9 for disorders of short gestation.

Funding support to Dr. Collins was provided by the Centers for Disease Control and Prevention (grant TS-356-15/15), Chicago Community Trust, and March of Dimes (grant 12-FY04-45).

[a] Department of Pediatrics, Northwestern University's Feinberg School of Medicine, Children's Memorial Hospital, 2300 Children's Plaza, Division of Neonatology, Box 45, Chicago, IL 60614, USA

[b] Department of Pediatrics, University of Illinois at Chicago, John Stroger Cook Hospital, 1901 W. Harrisson Street, Chicago, IL 60612, USA

* Corresponding author.

E-mail address: jcollins@northwestern.edu (J.W. Collins).

Clin Perinatol 36 (2009) 63–73
doi:10.1016/j.clp.2008.09.004 perinatology.theclinics.com
0095-5108/08/$ – see front matter

Table 1
Cause-specific infant death rates: United States, 2000

Causes of Infant Death	African American	White	Rate Ratio (African American to White)
All causes	14.0	5.7	2.4
Congenital malformations (Q00–Q99)	1.7	1.4	1.2
Disorders related to short gestation (P07)	3.0	0.8	3.9
Sudden infant death syndrome (R95)	1.2	0.6	2.4
Maternal pregnancy complications (P01)	0.9	0.3	3.1
Complications of placenta, cord, membranes (P02)	0.5	0.2	2.0

Death rates are expressed as deaths per 1000 live births.
Data from Infant deaths and mortality rates for the five leading causes of infant death by race and Hispanic origin of mother: United States. 2000 linked file. In: National vital statistics reports 2002;50:21. Codes (in parentheses) are from the *International Classification of Diseases, 10th Revision*.

Short gestation is tightly linked with low birth weight (LBW; <2500 g) and, particularly, with very low birth weight (VLBW; <1500 g). Moreover, LBW is a leading determinant of first-year mortality risk and the primary factor underlying the racial disparity in IMRs.[6] It is closely linked to serious long-term physical, mental, and emotional disabilities. An expanding body of published literature shows that LBW is also a major risk factor for several chronic diseases of adulthood, including coronary artery disease and type II diabetes.[7–9] In contrast to the marked improvements in birth weight–specific mortality among African Americans and whites during the past 50 years, race-specific LBW rates have stagnated.[10] In 2006, African Americans had a LBW rate of 14.0% compared 7.3% for whites.[3]

Most pertinent, the approximately 1% of births occurring at a VLBW account for more than half of infant deaths and nearly two thirds of the racial gap in infant mortality.[6] Since 1950, VLBW rates have steadily increased among African Americans. Reflecting the increased prevalence of pregnancies conceived with assistant reproductive technology, VLBW rates have begun to increase among whites.[10,11] In 2005, African Americans had a VLBW rate of 3.3% compared with 1.2% for whites.[3]

Although the underlying causes of these persistent racial inequalities have not been empirically established, progress has been made in understanding the complicated issue of race and infant outcome. The challenge is to identify and eliminate the effects of lifelong underserved minority status on women's health. In this review, the authors look beyond traditional risk factors and explore the social context of race in this country in an effort to understand African-American women's long-standing pregnancy outcome disadvantage. In the process, new insights are highlighted concerning likely causes for the poor birth outcomes of white infants in this country compared with infants in most other industrialized nations.

RACE, TRADITIONAL RISK FACTORS, AND INFANT BIRTH WEIGHT

For the last part of the twentieth century, the emphasis in epidemiologic studies of LBW incidence was to identify a set of social individual characteristics that differed in quantity between the races but that exerted qualitatively similar effects on African-American and white women. Young maternal age, low education attainment, low income, unmarried marital status, short interpregnancy interval, health-eroding personal behaviors (cigarette smoking, alcohol intake, and illicit drug use), and inadequate prenatal care use are well-documented risk factors for LBW.[12–15] Numerous studies have found that the disparities in the incidence of LBW and VLBW infants are not only persistent but actually widen as women's sociodemographic status, medical status, and behavioral status decline, however.[13,14,16,17] College-graduated African-American women who receive adequate prenatal care still have more than a twofold greater LBW rate than college-educated white women who receive adequate prenatal care.[13,18]

GEOGRAPHIC ANCESTRY AND BIRTH WEIGHT

Some investigators have viewed race as a proxy for geographic ancestry. They assumed that because "controlling for socioeconomic factors" did not eliminate racial disparities in infant mortality, these disparities in birth outcomes must result from genetic differences between African-American and white women.[18,19] The authors have argued against this, based on the weight of evidence from population genetics and the clear relation of genetic arguments to social and political trends at this moment in scientific history.[20] The scientific evidence accumulated against the existence of genetic "race" has become overwhelming. Protein and DNA evidence demonstrates that more than 90% of human genetic variation is found within the population of any continent, with only an additional 5% to 10% accounted for by differences in gene frequencies among continental populations.[21,22]

One compelling line of evidence against the hypothesized linkage of continent of ancestry and birth weight was the authors' comparison of birth weights in three groups of women delivering in Illinois over a 15-year period: US-born white women, US-born black women, and sub-Saharan African–born black women.[23] If there were specific alleles responsible for preterm birth and they were more frequent in African populations, thus contributing to the racial differential in infant birth weight observed in the North America, one would expect African-born black women, possessing the purest African ancestry, to deliver the smallest infants of the three groups. US-born black women, given their high percentage of European ancestry, would be expected to have intermediate birth weights between African-born black women and US-born white women. The authors found the complete opposite. The overall birth weight distributions for infants of African-born black women and US-born white women were essentially identical; however, infants born to US-born black women comprised a distinctly different population weighing hundreds of grams less (**Fig. 1**). Moreover, infants of US-born black women had higher rates of LBW and VLBW than infants of US-born white women or infants of sub-Saharan African–born black women when appropriate confounders were controlled.[23] Confirming the earlier study, we found that Caribbean-born black women gave birth to infants hundreds of grams heavier and had a lower LBW rate than US-born black women[24] A study by Fang and colleagues[25] of births in New York City found that within poor neighborhoods, immigrant black mothers had lower LBW rates than US-born black mothers.

The possibility that the phenomenon observed in women immigrating to the United States from Africa and the Caribbean reflected a "healthy immigrant effect" seems remote. We examined the birth weight patterns of US-born female descendents of foreign-born African-American and European-American women.[26] Our findings strongly contradicted predictions based on continent geography or race. Recent European

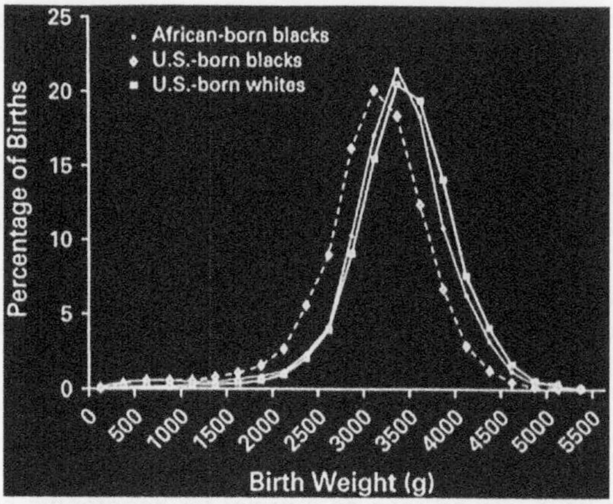

Fig. 1. Birth weight distribution of three Illinois subpopulations, 1980–1995. (*From* David R, Collins J. Differing birth weight among infants of US-born blacks, African-born blacks, and US-born whites. N Engl J Med 1997;337:1211; with permission. Copyright © 1997, Massachusetts Medical Society.)

immigrants to the United States gave birth to female babies of similar birth weight to the female babies born to established white families. Furthermore, when these girls of recent European immigrants subsequently grew up in the United States, their daughters' birth weights were higher than their own. In stark contrast, African-born and Caribbean-born African-American immigrants gave birth to girls who were heavier than established African-American families. Most striking, these first-generation African-American girls grew up in the United States and gave birth to daughters whose own birth weights were less than their own birth weights and approximated those in established African-American families. This intergenerational trend was the opposite of that found in the nonimmigrant population and opposite of the trend in European immigrant families.[25]

Because Mexican Americans are the second largest and fastest growing minority group in the United States, the pregnancy outcome of Mexican-American women is of particular public health significance. Interestingly, their LBW rate is actually less than that of non-Latino white women. Nevertheless, it has been well documented that US-born Mexican-American women have a greater LBW rate than Mexican-born women.[26,27] Acculturation to a US lifestyle has been identified as a major postulated factor that explains the nativity differential in pregnancy outcome among Mexican-American women.[28–30]

Of course, neither putative genetic differences nor social disadvantage associated with ethnic minority status explains the poor outcomes of US white infants compared with infants of other countries. An adequate disease model to deal with the public health problem of adverse birth outcomes in the United States requires a broader perspective. It must explain the dramatically poor outcomes for African Americans and the less flagrant but more widespread problem of poor infant health for the majority population.

Life-Course Conceptual Model

Lu and Halfon[31] proposed a life-course conceptual model to explain the discordant pregnancy outcome of white and African-American women in the United States. In their conceptual model, the racial disparity in LBW rates reflects a greater prevalence of prepregnancy contextual risk factors and a lower prevalence of prepregnancy protective variables among African Americans compared with whites. Life-course factors influence pregnancy outcome through two proposed mechanisms: early life (fetal) programming of reproductive potential and cumulative wear and tear (weathering). For both pathways, a key underlying mechanism is stress and the body's response to it. The social and biologic processes evident in racial comparisons offer promise in understanding adverse outcomes for US whites once the concept of stress related to social class is incorporated into the analytic framework.

Fetal programming

There has been a rapid outpouring of studies that describe what is programmed during fetal life with regard to the health status of that fetus as an adult.[8–10,32–35] Emanuel[36] hypothesized that the early in utero conditions of a woman's life are important determinants of later pregnancy outcome.

It has been shown that when women experience stress during their pregnancies, their brain and placenta secrete a stress hormone: corticotropin-releasing hormone (CRH).[37–39] This hormone passes into the fetal circulation during critical periods of neuroendocrine and hypothalamic-pituitary-adrenal axis (HPA) development. This could lead to a female infant with higher stress reactivity later in life (ie, they secrete an increased amount of CRH and cortisol when exposed to stress) and place that woman at greater risk for preterm labor when she becomes pregnant 20 or 30 years later.[40] This may be related to feedback resistance as a consequence of altered expression of glucocorticoid receptors in the developing female fetal brain.[37–39,41]

One aspect of heightened stress reactivity is inefficient termination of the cortisol stress response after the stress has passed, resulting in chronic exposure of body systems to elevated stress hormones. This has been referred to as allostatic load.[31] Increased allostatic load, with all the associated health risks, has been shown to correlate with lower social class and with being African American, even in the absence of poverty.[42]

Fetal programming acts at the level of the DNA in a phenomenon called epigenetics, which is basically volume control for genes. Gene expression can be turned up or down and switched on or off simply by methylating or demethylating DNA. Two individuals with the same genetic code can end up with extremely different levels of stress reactivity for life based on whether a segment of their DNA is methylated or demethylated.[43] This epigenetic process, in turn, has a lot to do with whether or not their mothers were stressed during pregnancy.[39]

Although the mechanisms underlying gene-environment interactions are incompletely understood, the biologic pathways are beginning to get mapped in animal models. There are two areas of the fetal brain that are particularly vulnerable to the cytotoxic effect of stress hormones: the hippocampus and the amygdala. The hippocampus acts as the brake on the HPA axis, whereas the amygdala accentuates the action of the HPA axis. Prenatal stress increases the release of glucocorticoids from fetal adrenal glands, which can down-regulate glucocorticoid receptors in the hippocampus and, at the same time, up-regulate glucocorticoid receptors in the amygdala. As a result, the hippocampus is made less sensitive to negative feedback and the amygdala is made more sensitive to positive feedback. One ends up with a female fetus with a hyperreactive HPA axis that may predispose her to preterm birth.[31,37]

African-American and white women's aberrant fetal growth as measured by LBW is an important risk factor for LBW in their offspring. We found that women who were themselves of LBW have greater rates of delivering infants that have a LBW, are intrauterine growth retarded, and are preterm than women who were themselves not of LBW, regardless of the adequacy of prenatal care use.[44,45] Reflecting the high prevalence of LBW among African-American mothers, a greater percentage of LBW, growth retarded, and preterm African-American infants were attributable to maternal LBW compared with white infants.[44,45]

Residential environment

Residential segregation is a distinguishing organizational characteristic of American life.[46] Not surprisingly, we found that African-American and white women in the Chicago metropolitan area were exposed to the extremes of residential environment during their life course.[47] In Cook County, Illinois, most African-American, but not white, women have a lifelong residence in a poor neighborhood.[47]

An extensive body of literature shows that neighborhood poverty during adulthood is an independent risk factor for the delivery of a LBW infant.[12,13,48–52] In 1950, Yankauer[50] published the seminal study on infant mortality, race, and urban segregation. He found that the percentage of white and nonwhite infant deaths in New York City neighborhoods rose as the percentage of nonwhite residents increased. The education levels and occupations of nonwhites were similar, suggesting that the ghetto environment was an independent risk factor for infant mortality. Rauh and colleagues[53] and Pearl and colleagues[48] independently found that for African-American (but not white) women, residence in impoverished neighborhoods had a significant negative effect on infant birth weight independent of individual poverty. Using vital record data and US census data from eight geographic areas (in Maryland, Michigan, North Carolina, and Pennsylvania), O'Campo and colleagues[51] found a significant association between neighborhood deprivation and the risk for preterm birth among non-Latino white and African-American women.

Using median family income of census tract residence to measure ecologic risk, the authors found the same enduring racial disparities, especially among low-risk African-American mothers.[13] African-American women who lived in higher income neighborhoods still had LBW rates that exceeded those of white women who resided in low-income neighborhoods. Furthermore, in affluent Chicago neighborhoods, African-American women still had a twofold greater infant VLBW rate than white women regardless of age, education, and marital status.[52]

To the extent that life-course factors associated with direct exposure to neighborhood poverty singularly explain the racial disparity in infant outcome, one would expect the gap to abate among women who never resided in impoverished neighborhoods. Our exploratory data showed that African-American women unexposed to the health-eroding consequences of early life and cumulative exposures to neighborhood poverty had a fivefold greater VLBW rate than their white peers.[54] When differences in adult sociodemographic and medical risk status were taken into account, however, the racial gap narrowed, giving African-American women a twofold greater VLBW rate than whites.[54]

Weathering Hypothesis

Young and advanced maternal age are well-described risk factors for LBW infants among white women. Instead of the U- or J-shaped age curve for infant LBW among white women, the risk for infant LBW for African-American women grows monotonically with advancing age.[13,14,55,56] Most striking, infant LBW rates start to increase among African-American women in their late twenties and early thirties.[55,56] Geronimus[56] termed the deterioration in reproductive health status over the childbearing years among African-American women as *weathering*.

The weathering hypothesis conceptualizes the physical consequences of social inequality on female reproductive outcome. Geronimus[56] found that the rates of moderately low birth weight (MLBW; 1500–2499 g) and VLBW infants among African-American women who resided in low-income Michigan neighborhoods increased as age rose from 20 to 34 years. Rauh and colleagues[53] reported that among African Americans in New York City, neighborhood poverty exacerbated the effect of maternal aging on infant MLBW risk but not on VLBW risk. The authors found that the increase in MLBW rates associated with advancing maternal age was accelerated in extremely impoverished compared with nonimpoverished urban neighborhoods.[55]

Neighborhood poverty drives the weathering phenomenon among urban African-American women and contributes to the racial disparity in infant birth weight. In a recent study, the authors found that the weathering pattern of maternal age and infant birth weight was limited to African-American women with lifelong residence in low-income urban neighborhoods.[47] Interestingly, infant LBW rates did not increase with maternal age among African-American women with lifelong residence in high-income neighborhoods. Moreover, African-American women in their early thirties with lifelong residence in high-income neighborhoods had an infant LBW rate one-half that of African-American women in their early thirties with a lifelong residence in low-income neighborhoods.[47]

LIFELONG EXPOSURE TO INTERPERSONAL RACIAL DISCRIMINATION

The conventional investigative approach to the racial disparity in the rates of preterm birth has been based on the implicit assumption that there is a set of risk factors differing in quantity between the races but exerting similar effects on black and white women. This conceptualization does not take into account the nonrandom, pervasive, and multifaceted inequality that is bound up in the historical context of race, nor does it capture its effect on human beings over time.[2] Racial discrimination is an example of this sort of factor.[2] Even quantitative measures, such as neighborhood income, may differ so widely over the life course of white and African-American women that their lives are qualitatively different, as pointed out previously.

The authors used an interviewer-administered closed-ended questionnaire to capture the variability of perceived lifetime exposure to racial discrimination and described its association with infant birth weight.[57] **Table 2** shows that African-American mothers who delivered preterm VLBW infants were more likely to experience interpersonal racial discrimination during their lifetime than African-American mothers who delivered term non-LBW infants.[57] The adverse effect of perceived discrimination was strongest among women aged 20 to 29 years, generally considered the optimal childbearing decade, whereas it was reduced or absent among teenaged women and those older than 30 years of age. Similarly, the association between maternal exposure to interpersonal racial discrimination and VLBW was strongest among women with more than 12 years of formal education. The adjusted odds ratio of VLBW for maternal lifetime exposure to interpersonal racism in one or more and in three or more domains equaled 1.7 (95% confidence interval: 1.0–9.2) and 2.6 (95% confidence interval: 1.2–5.3), respectively.

Stress and Adverse Outcomes for White Women

Although white women of childbearing age are not subject to the double jeopardy of race and class that characterizes the experience of most African-American women, they are nevertheless subject to adverse health effects brought on by stress related to their social situation. Given the nature of work life for US women of childbearing age, with the highest workforce participation in history and longer work hours on average than in any other industrialized country, the argument for unhealthy life stress for

Table 2
Maternal lifetime exposure to interpersonal racial discrimination and infant birth weight by selected characteristics

	Reported Racial Discrimination in One or More Domains Very Low Birth Weight (n = 104) Percentage (n)	Reported Racial Discrimination in One or More Domains Non-Low Birth Weight (n = 208) Percentage (n)	Odds Ratio (95% Confidence Interval)
Maternal age (years)			
<20	50 (14)	44 (27)	1.3 (0.5–3.2)
20–24	62 (16)	32 (20)	3.4 (1.3–8.9)
25–29	60 (12)	40 (17)	2.2 (0.7–6.5)
≥30	52 (15)	49 (17)	1.1 (0.4–3.0)
Maternal education (years)			
<12	39 (12)	34 (26)	1.2 (0.5–2.9)
12	53 (18)	39 (30)	1.8 (0.8–4.0)
>12	75 (27)	52 (24)	2.8 (1.1–7.1)
Prenatal care			
Early[a]	52 (37)	42 (53)	1.5 (0.8–2.7)
Late or none	63 (20)	37 (30)	2.8 (1.2–6.6)
Cigarette smoking			
Yes	52 (16)	30 (13)	2.5 (0.9–6.4)
No	57 (41)	43 (70)	1.8 (1.0–3.1)

[a] Initiation in the first trimester.

From Collins J, David R, Handler A, et al. Very low birth weight in African-American infants: the role of maternal exposure to interpersonal racial discrimination. Am J Public Health 2004;94:2126; with permission.

nonaffluent white women seems quite plausible.[58] Indeed, job strain, defined as the combination of high demand and low control, has been shown to be associated with lower birth weight and an increased rate of preterm birth among white women.[59]

SUMMARY

In the United States, African-American infants have significantly worse outcomes than white infants. An extensive body of literature strongly suggests that closing the racial gap in prenatal care use cannot singularly lead to closure of the gap in the incidence of LBW. An expanding literature shows that aberrant early life (ie, fetal) programming and cumulative wear and tear (ie, weathering) underlie African-American women's reproductive outcome disadvantage. Eliminating the racial gap in birth outcomes takes a life-course approach, addressing early life disadvantages in addition to lifelong exposure to neighborhood poverty, interpersonal racial discrimination, and job strain.

REFERENCES

1. Guyer B, Hoyert J, Freedman M, et al. Annual summary of vital statistics—trends in the health of Americans during the 20th century. Pediatrics 2000;106:1307–17.
2. David R, Collins J. Bad outcomes in black babies: race or racism? Ethn Dis 1991;1:236–44.
3. Martin J, Kung H, Matthews T, et al. Annual summary of vital statistics: 2006. Pediatrics 2008;121:788–801.

4. Healthy People 2010. US Department of Health and Human Services. Available at: http://www.healthypeople.gov/about/goals.htm. Accessed June 19, 2008.
5. Infant deaths and mortality rates for the five leading causes of infant death by race and Hispanic origin of mother: United States. 2000 linked file. In: National vital statistics reports. 2002;50:21. Available at: http://www.cdc.gov/nchs/data/nvrs/nvser50/50-12t7.pdf. Accessed March 18, 2005.
6. Matthews T, MacDorman F. Infant mortality statistics from the 2004 period linked birth/infant death dataset. National Vital Statistics Reports 2007;55:1–13.
7. Barker D, Osmond C, Simmonds S. Fetal and placenta size and risk of hypertension in adult life. BMJ 1990;301:259–62.
8. Rich-Edwards J, Stampfer M, Manson J, et al. Birth weight and risk of cardiovascular disease in a cohort of women followed up since 1976. BMJ 1997;315:396–400.
9. Rich-Edwards J, Colditz G, Stampfer M, et al. Birthweight and the risk for type 2 diabetes in adult women. Ann Intern Med 1999;130:278–84.
10. Coutinho R, David R, Collins J. Relation of parental birth weight to infant birth weight among African-Americans and whites in Illinois: a transgenerational study. Am J Epidemiol 1997;146:810–9.
11. Centers for Disease Control and Prevention. Infant mortality and low birth weight among black and white infants—US, 1980–2000. MMWR 2002;51:499–592.
12. Collins J, David R. The differential effect of traditional risk factors on infant birthweight among blacks and whites in Chicago. Am J Public Health 1990;80:679–81.
13. Collins J, Wall S, David R. Adequacy of prenatal care utilization, maternal ethnicity, and infant birthweight in Chicago. J Natl Med Assoc 1997;89:198–203.
14. Berg C, Wilcox L, Almanda P. The prevalence of socioeconomic status and behavorial characteristics and their impact on very low birth weight in black and white infants in Georgia. Matern Child Health J 2001;5:75–84.
15. Kleinman J, Kessal S. Racial differences in low birth weight. N Engl J Med 1987;317:744–53.
16. Foster H, Wu L, Bracken M, et al. Intergenerational effects of high socioeconomic status and low birth weight and preterm birth among African-Americans. J Natl Med Assoc 2000;92:213–21.
17. Schoendorf K, Hogue C, Kleinman J, et al. Mortality among infants of black as compared to white college-educated parents. N Engl J Med 1992;326:1522–6.
18. Dizon-Townson DS. Preterm labour and delivery: a genetic predisposition. Paediatr Perinat Epidemiol 2001;15(suppl):57–62.
19. van den Oord E. Ethnic differences in birth weight: maternal effects emerge from an analysis involving mixed race US couples. Ethn Dis 2006;16:706–11.
20. David R, Collins J. Disparities in infant mortality: what's genetics got to do with it? Am J Public Health 2007;97:1191–7.
21. Race, Ethnicity and Genetics Working Group of the National Human Genome Research Institute. The use of racial, ethnic and ancestral categories in human genetics research. Am J Hum Genet 2005;77:519–32.
22. Goodman AH. Why genes don't count (for racial differences in health). Am J Public Health 2000;90:1699–702.
23. David R, Collins J. Differing birth weight among infants of US-born blacks, African-born blacks, and US-born whites. N Engl J Med 1997;337:1209–14.
24. Pollotto E, Collins J, David R. Enigma of maternal race and infant birth weight: a population-based study of US-born black and Caribbean-born black women. Am J Epidemiol 2000;151:1080–5.

25. Fang J, Madhavan S, Alderman M. Low birth weight: race and maternal nativity: the impact of community income. Pediatrics 1999;103:1–6.
26. Collins J, Wu S, David R. Differing intergenerational birth weights among the descendants of US-born and foreign-born Whites and African-Americans in Illinois. Am J Epidemiol 2002;155:210–6.
27. Collins JW, David RJ. Pregnancy outcome of Mexican-American women: the effect of generational residence in the United States. Ethn Dis 2004;14:312–21.
28. Fuentes-Afflick E, Hessol N, Perez-Stable E. Maternal birthplace, ethnicity, and low birth weight in California. Arch Pediatr Adolesc Med 1998;152:1105–12.
29. Cobas J, Balcazar H, Benin H, et al. Acculturation and low birth weight among Latino women: a reanalysis of HHANES data with structural equation models. Am J Public Health 1996;86:394–6.
30. Gundelman S, English P. Effect of United States residence on birth outcomes among Mexican-American immigrants: an exploratory study. Am J Epidemiol 1995;142:S30–8.
31. Lu M, Halfon N. Racial and ethnic disparities in birth outcomes: a life-course perspective. Matern Child Health J 2003;7:13–30.
32. Godfrey K, Robinson S. Maternal nutrition, placental growth, and fetal programming. Proc Nutr Soc 1998;57:105–11.
33. Barker D, Winter P, Osmond C, et al. Weight in infancy and death from ischemic heart disease. Lancet 1989;2:577–80.
34. Ness R, Catov J. Invited commentary: timing and the types of cardiovascular risk factors in relation to offspring birth weight. Am J Epidemiol 2007;166:1365–7.
35. Law C, Shiell A. Is blood pressure inversely related to birth weight? The strength of evidence from systematic review of the literature. J Hypertens 1996;94: 3246–50.
36. Emanuel I. Maternal health during childhood and later reproductive performance. Ann N Y Acad Sci 1986;477:27–39.
37. Wadhwa PD. Psychoneuroendocrine processes in human pregnancy influence fetal development and health. Psychoneuroendocrinology 2005;30:724–43.
38. Wadhwa P, Garite TJ, Porto M, et al. Placental corticotropin-releasing hormone (CRH), spontaneous preterm birth, and fetal growth restriction: a prospective investigation. Am J Obstet Gynecol 2004;191:1063–9.
39. Seckl J, Meaney M. Glucocorticoid "programming" and PTSD risk. Ann N Y Acad Sci 2006;1071:351–78.
40. Mulder E, Robles de Medina PG, Huizink AC, et al. Prenatal maternal stress: effects on pregnancy and the (unborn) child. Early Hum Dev 2002;70:3–14.
41. Merlot E, Couret D, Otten W. Prenatal stress, fetal imprinting and immunity. Brain Behav Immun 2008;22:42–51.
42. Geronimus A, Hicken M, Keene D, et al. "Weathering" and age patterns of allostatic load scores among Blacks and Whites in the United States. Am J Public Health 2006;96:826–33.
43. Weaver ICG, Cervoni N, Champagne FA, et al. Epigenetic programming by maternal behavior. Nat Neurosci 2004;7:847–54.
44. Collins J, Pierce M, Prachand N, et al. Low birth weight across generations. Matern Child Health J 2003;7:229–39.
45. Simon D, Vyas S, Prachand N, et al. Relation of maternal low birth weight to infant growth retardation and prematurity. Matern Child Health J 2006;10:321–7.
46. National Research Council. A common destiny. Blacks and American society. Washington, DC: National Academy Press; 1989.

47. Collins J, Wambach, David J, Rankin R. Women's lifelong exposure to neighborhood poverty and low birth weight: a population-based study. Mat Child Health J, in press.
48. Pearl M, Braveman P, Abrams B. The relationship between neighborhood socioeconomic characteristics to birth weight among 5 ethnic groups in California. Am J Public Health 2001;91:1804–14.
49. Pickett K, Collins J, Masi C, et al. The effects of racial density and income incongruity on pregnancy outcome. Soc Sci Med 2005;60:2229–38.
50. Yankauer A. The relationship of fetal and infant mortality to residential segregation. An inquiry into social epidemiology. Am Sociol Rev 1950;15:644–8.
51. O'Campo P, Burke J, Culhane J, et al. Neighborhood deprivation and preterm birth among non-Hispanic Blacks and Whites in eight geographic areas in the US. Am J Epidemiol. 2008;167:155–67.
52. Collins J, Herman A, David R. Prevalence of very low birth weight in relation to income-incongruity among African-American and white parents in Chicago. Am J Public Health 1997;87:414–7.
53. Rauh V, Andrews H, Garfinkel R. The contribution of maternal age to racial disparities in birth weight: a multilevel perspective. Am J Public Health 2001;91: 1815–24.
54. Collins J, David R, Simon D, et al. The relation of race to preterm birth among women with a lifelong residence in high-income Chicago neighborhoods: an exploratory study. Ethn Dis 2007;17:113–7.
55. Collins JW, Simon DM, Jackson TA, et al. Advancing maternal age and infant birth weight among urban African-Americans: the effect of neighborhood poverty. Ethn Dis 2006;16:180–6.
56. Geronimus A. Black/White differences in the relationship of maternal age to birth weight: a population-based test of the weathering hypothesis. Soc Sci Med 1996; 42:589–97.
57. Collins J, David R, Handler A, et al. Very low birth weight in African-American infants: the role of maternal exposure to interpersonal racial discrimination. Am J Public Health 2004;94:2132–8.
58. Evans J, Lippoldt C, Marianna P. Trends in working hours in OECD countries, OECD. Labour market and social policy occasional papers. 2001, No. 45, Paris, France, OECD Publishing. 10.1787/674061356827.
59. Oths K, Dunn L, Palmer N. A prospective study of psychosocial job strain and birth outcomes. Epidemiology 2001;12:744–6.

Evaluation and Treatment of Hypotension in the Preterm Infant

E.M. Dempsey, MBBCh, FRCPI[a], K.J. Barrington, MBChB, MRCP, FRCP[b,*]

KEYWORDS

- Blood pressure • Shock • Volume expansion
- Inotropes • Glucocorticoids

Despite our limited understanding of the pathophysiology of hypotension and the benefits of therapeutic intervention in the preterm infant, a significant number of preterm newborns receive cardiovascular support.[1] The proportion of extremely preterm infants receiving intervention varies greatly among neonatal intensive care units (NICUs), ranging from 29% to 98% in a recent study.[2] Although some of this variation may reflect different population characteristics, much is solely related to differing patterns of practice.[1] The current review addresses issues regarding cardiovascular support in this unique population of patients: (1) definition of hypotension and shock in the preterm infant, (2) clinical assessment of hypotension and shock, (3) the short- and long-term consequences of hypotension, and (4) the therapeutic options available.

DEFINITION OF HYPOTENSION AND SHOCK IN THE PRETERM INFANT

The definition of hypotension in the preterm infant is contentious. Hypotension could be defined as a "statistically low blood pressure." This assumes that normative data have been derived from a population of patients and that if the value decreases lower than a certain percentile (eg, third, fifth, tenth percentile), the patient is deemed to be hypotensive. Many normative blood pressure reference ranges exist based on birth weight, gestational age, and postnatal age criteria.[3–8] Considerable variation exists among these reference ranges because of frequent methodologic flaws: retrospective data collection, small numbers of patients, collection of only a few data points and averaging over wide time ranges, combined invasive and noninvasive measurements, and inclusion of small for dates and appropriate for gestational age infants. Many

[a] Department of Neonatology, Cork University Maternity Hospital, Cork, Ireland
[b] Department of Pediatrics, CHU-Ste Justine, Ste-Justine Hospital, University of Montreal, 3175 Côte Sainte-Catherine, Montréal, Quebec, PQ, Canada
* Corresponding author.
E-mail address: keith.barrington@mcgill.ca (K. Barrington).

Clin Perinatol 36 (2009) 75–85
doi:10.1016/j.clp.2008.09.003 perinatology.theclinics.com

studies have a priori excluded infants who were thought to require treatment with pressor agents, have included data obtained while they were receiving such agents, or have excluded data from those with poor outcomes, which tends to exclude the most immature infants and sometimes leads to tiny sample sizes.[6] Other normal ranges have been generated that, although demonstrating the postnatal increases in blood pressure, have lumped all preterm infants together.[7]

Other normal values have been generated and widely applied without any empiric validation. The most popular criterion for diagnosing hypotension[9] seems to be the Joint Working Group of the British Association of Perinatal Medicine[10] recommendation that the mean arterial blood pressure in millimeters of mercury should be maintained at or greater than the mean gestational age in weeks. Despite a complete lack of published evidence to support this recommendation, it has been used as the primary entry criterion by several recent randomized therapeutic intervention trials.[11,12] It is essential that any statistical definition of hypotension that is based on empiric observation integrates the known increases with increasing postnatal and gestational age and is preferably derived from a population of preterm infants with minimal exclusions apart from treatments designed to change the blood pressure.

The question of how to define what is a "normal" blood pressure is difficult. It may be preferable to define hypotension by a blood pressure value lower than which there is a statistically increased risk for adverse outcome (ie, "unsafe blood pressure") if such a threshold exists and can be defined. The authors attempted to answer this question in a large database from very low birth weight (VLBW) infants and identified a statistically worse outcome with decreasing mean blood pressure thresholds. The incidence of adverse outcome (defined as grade 3 or 4 intraventricular hemorrhage [IVH]) increased from 21% to 31% when the definition of hypotension was reduced from 20 to 15 mm Hg in all patients less than 28 weeks of age. These definitions (20 and 15 mm Hg) accounted for only 7.1% and 1.2%, respectively, of the overall population of infants less than 28 weeks of age, however.[13] When less extreme definitions of hypotension were applied, the increase in risk for severe IVH associated with hypotension was small. Even if we could define a threshold lower than which there is an increased chance of adverse outcome, this does not necessarily mean that intervention is going to result in improved outcome at such a value.

The ideal definition would be a threshold blood pressure lower than which intervention results in improved outcome (ie, operational threshold). This value is unlikely to be a single value; it would have to be patient specific and would depend on several factors, including gestation, birth weight, and postnatal age, and perhaps the cause of the hypotension. Such a threshold currently remains elusive.

Hypotension and Shock

Shock is a pathologic state characterized by inadequate tissue oxygen delivery to meet demand. There is little or no correlation between systemic blood flow and blood pressure in the preterm infant;[14] extremely low systemic perfusion, shock, can occur with normal blood pressure. Conversely, preterm infants with blood pressure lower than average often have no biochemical or clinical signs of shock, presumably have adequate tissue oxygen delivery, and probably do not require treatment. We have called this approach "permissive hypotension."

When systemic oxygen delivery decreases, there are several initial compensatory responses that occur to maintain perfusion and oxygen delivery to the most vital organs, including peripheral vasoconstriction, which maintains blood pressure (ie, shock without hypotension). Progression to the uncompensated phase is characterized by signs of poor perfusion accompanied by low blood pressure (ie, shock with hypotension), ultimately leading to the irreversible stage if appropriate therapy is not instituted. In contrast to the permissive hypotension approach mentioned previously, intervention to improve perfusion may be warranted in infants with shock despite normal blood pressure.

RECOGNITION OF HYPOTENSION AND SHOCK IN THE PRETERM INFANT

Clinical Signs

Currently, there is no validated clinical scoring system available to diagnose shock, and the assessment of adequate end organ blood flow in the preterm infant is subjective. Bedside evaluation includes assessment of capillary refill time, color, heart rate, blood pressure, and urine output. None of these parameters in isolation is specific in identifying poor perfusion. Capillary refill time values exist for the term neonate,[15,16] but there are limited data on capillary refill times in the preterm neonate.[14,17] Osborn and colleagues[14] showed a weak association between capillary refill time and systemic blood flow. Wodey and colleagues[17] have shown a significant relation between cardiac index and capillary refill time in preterm neonates. The authors recently confirmed a limited relation between capillary refill values obtained in the forehead, sternum, and foot and simultaneously obtained superior vena cava (SVC) flow measurements.[18]

The relation between skin color and illness severity in the newborn has been evaluated using an objective measurement tool.[19] Colorimeter values were found to be significantly different in the high-illness severity group, particularly in the blue-yellow axis; however, no data on blood pressure or cardiac function were given. Further investigations of whether an objective measurement of when an infant is "off color" might help with diagnosis of shock are warranted.

Heart rates are extremely variable, vary with gestational[20] and postnatal age, and correlate with oxygen consumption; however, neither absolute heart rate nor trend analysis of heart rate is validated as a way to assess cardiac function. Urine output is low and variable in the first 24 hours; however, good urine output is somewhat reassuring. Although the positive predictive value (PPV) of each of these individual measures for identifying poor perfusion is unknown and likely to be low, it does seem that clinical assessment using a combination of signs allows one to identify patients with poor outcomes.[21]

Central venous pressure (CVP) monitoring is commonly performed in adult and pediatric intensive care, in which it is often used to guide fluid management.[22,23] Normal values for CVP in preterm infants have a wide range (2.8–13.9 mm Hg),[24] and there are numerous technical difficulties in obtaining CVP measurements. It is unclear if CVP correlates with circulating blood volume in the preterm infant; in any case, most preterm infants with lower blood pressure in the first few days are not hypovolemic. Thus, CVP monitoring is of limited use in the NICU.[25] Mixed venous saturation monitoring is frequently used in adult and pediatric intensive care units, but its role in the preterm neonate is limited by the interatrial shunting and technical difficulties encountered in safely obtaining a value.

Serum Lactate Values

Serial lactate measurements are useful in critically ill adults as a manifestation of poor tissue oxygen delivery.[26] Lactate values have been analyzed in several clinical situations in the preterm infant,[27] including sepsis[28] and necrotizing enterocolitis.[29] Values obtained during the first day of postnatal life can predict outcome.[30,31] Deshpande and Platt[31] showed a worse outcome when lactate concentrations remained persistently elevated in sick ventilated newborns (23–40 weeks of gestation). Mortality was 57% if two lactate values were greater than 5.6 mmol/L, highlighting the importance of serial lactate assessments. Groenendaal and colleagues[30] estimated the PPV and negative predictive value (NPV) of arterial lactate within 3 hours after birth in a cohort of preterm babies and found that with a cutoff value of 5.7 mmol/L, the PPV was 0.47 and NPV was 0.92 for a combined adverse outcome (death or poor neurodevelopmental outcome).

Data are limited on the use of serum lactate values specifically in hypotensive newborns. Only one previous study has evaluated the role of lactate in assessment of perfusion. Wardle and colleagues,[32] in an assessment of peripheral oxygenation, found no difference in lactate levels between normotensive and hypotensive preterm infants. In the authors' cohort of VLBW infants, they identified a weak negative correlation between lactate values and SVC flow. A combined lactate value of more than 4 mmol and prolonged capillary refill times of more than 4 seconds in the foot resulted in a PPV of 80% and a NPV of 88% for identifying low SVC flow, highlighting the value of combining clinical and biochemical parameters.[33]

Objective Assessment of Flow

The peripheral perfusion index (PPI) is readily obtained from some bedside pulse oximeter devices. It is essentially a relative measure of the pulse strength and may permit a continuous noninvasive estimate of peripheral perfusion. Its role has recently been reviewed in the adult intensive care unit.[34] In the neonatal acute care setting, a low PPI has been shown to correlate with illness severity[35] and may be useful to detect left obstructive heart lesions in term newborns.[36] PPI monitoring warrants further evaluation in the assessment of perfusion in the preterm infant.

Functional echocardiography may have an important role to play in assessing the adequacy of circulatory status in the preterm infant. It provides an objective assessment of cardiac function and output and permits assessment of response to therapeutic interventions.[37] In the preterm infant, circulatory shunting complicates the measurement of systemic blood flow: left ventricular output is equal to pulmonary blood flow minus any left-to-right shunting across a foramen ovale, and right ventricular output is equal to systemic blood flow plus left-to-right foraminal shunting.[38,39] In comparison, SVC flow provides a shunt-independent assessment of blood flow to the upper body.[40] Low SVC blood flow has been associated with adverse short- and long-term outcomes.[33,41] Functional echocardiography is rational and noninvasive. It gives useful information about hemodynamics; however, the PPV of low SVC flow measurement for adverse outcome is low,[42] and therapy aimed at preventing low flow has not yet been shown to be beneficial.[43]

Near-infrared spectroscopy (NIRS) has been used to assess the adequacy of peripheral oxygenation and cerebral oxygenation[44] in the preterm infant. Wardle and colleagues[32] evaluated oxygen delivery and consumption in the forearm of 30 preterm babies, 15 of whom were hypotensive by Watkins' criteria.[5] They identified lower oxygen delivery and oxygen consumption in the hypotensive babies, with no difference in fractional oxygen extraction (FOE). There was no difference in NIRS-measured variables (oxygen delivery, oxygen consumption, and FOE) in patients who had an adverse outcome compared with those who had a normal outcome. NIRS has yet to demonstrate that its use results in improved outcome in the preterm infant, and its use in the NICU as a clinical monitor has recently been questioned.[45] Future randomized trials of cardiovascular support could incorporate functional echocardiography and NIRS to identify patients who may benefit from cardiovascular support.

Intramucosal pH or P_{CO_2}

Using gastric tonometry, the intramucosal pH or P_{CO_2} of the stomach can be calculated and used as an index of local perfusion.[46] Because splanchnic blood flow decreases early during compensated shock states, it can be used as an index of adequate overall oxygen delivery.[47] Its use in the neonatal population is limited to a study of 38 VLBW infants in whom recurrent low intramucosal pH was significantly associated with an increase in gastrointestinal complications.[48] There was no statistically significant association between intramucosal pH and death. Its role has yet to be evaluated in assessment of cardiovascular stability in the preterm infant.

SHOULD WE WORRY ABOUT HYPOTENSION?

The authors recently performed a systematic review to determine if there was a blood pressure threshold that accurately discriminated between preterm infants with a good outcome and those with an adverse outcome.[49] They identified 18 studies in total, none of which were methodologically robust. The overall assessment of the data was that there is some association between having a lower blood pressure and having a worse outcome; however, there are several potential confounding factors that preclude the elucidation of strong inferences from this association. The definition of hypotension varied substantially across the studies. One definition that has been used is a single mean blood pressure value less than 30 mm Hg.[50] Such a definition may result in an artifactual association between hypotension and adverse outcome because the more immature babies, at greatest risk for IVH, are much more likely to be hypotensive by this rule.

The authors identified four studies that met the greatest proportion of their inclusion criteria.[5,13,50–52] Using continuous invasive blood pressure monitoring, Miall-Allen and colleagues[52] identified an excess of IVH in preterm newborns with a mean blood pressure less than 30 mm Hg. Bada and colleagues[50] showed that infants who developed moderate to severe IVH had lower blood pressure values for their postnatal ages than matched control infants who did not develop IVH. Watkins and colleagues,[5] having taken postnatal age and birth weight into account, identified an association between a lower blood pressure (less than tenth percentile from self-constructed tables) and the frequency of severe IVH. The exact timing and duration of hypotension were not taken into account. Each of these studies was confounded by the fact that pressors were used and not accounted for in the analyses. More recently, Cunningham and colleagues[51] found no association between the development of severe IVH and a prolonged period with a mean blood pressure less than gestational age in weeks. Data collected from the Canadian Neonatal Network[13] have shown that those infants who had a lowest blood pressure less than their gestational age, or a blood pressure less than the tenth percentile using Watkins' criteria, were statistically slightly more likely to have severe IVH. This minor increase in risk was no longer apparent when pressor use was accounted for, however. Infants in the database who were not hypotensive and yet received inotropes were more likely to have a worse outcome than hypotensive patients who had not received such treatment. This finding could be interpreted in many different ways, one of which is that the adverse outcomes attributed in the past to hypotension are actually caused by the treatment of hypotension. An alternative explanation is as follows: physicians sometimes give cardiovascular support to infants who are unwell and poorly perfused despite an acceptable blood pressure (compensated shock), and such infants do poorly despite treatment. In contrast, the authors sometimes do not treat infants who have a statistically lower blood pressure but who appear to be well perfused, and such infants do well. Either of these explanations calls into question the common practice of routinely treating infants according to simplistic blood pressure thresholds.

CURRENT THERAPIES

Many different therapeutic algorithms exist for treatment of hypotension.[53,54] These typically consist of volume expansion, followed by inotropic support (often dopamine as a first line) and, more recently, corticosteroids. The authors recently surveyed Canadian neonatologists concerning their approach to the diagnosis and treatment of hypotension in the VLBW infant.[9] Three predominant regimens currently exist in practice; each consists of volume, followed by dopamine (91%), with the subsequent addition of steroid, epinephrine, or dobutamine. There is little evidence to support this current approach.

Volume

The initial approach by most clinicians to hypotension in the preterm infant is volume replacement. There is no physiologic rationale for this approach and no reliable evidence to support it; most infants who are hypotensive have normal circulating blood volumes.[55–57] Furthermore, an increasing volume of fluid administered during the first few days of life is associated with an increasing prevalence of bronchopulmonary dysplasia (BPD).[58,59] This correlation was confirmed by a prospective controlled trial that demonstrated improved survival and decreased BPD rates in preterm babies who were randomized to low fluid intakes versus those given a more liberal fluid intake.[60] Goldberg and colleagues[61] found an increase in the incidence of IVH in preterm infants receiving rapid volume expansion, and adverse neurologic outcome[62] has been reported in VLBW infants who had received colloid boluses. The relative lack of response to volume administration is also evidence that hypotensive preterm infants are rarely hypovolemic.[63–65] There is therefore no empiric evidence to support the use of fluid boluses as therapy of hypotension, with observational data supporting adverse cardiovascular, pulmonary, and neurologic outcomes.

Inotropes

There are several randomized controlled trials[66–70] comparing the effects of various different catecholamine agents in systemic hypotension. Dopamine reliably increases blood pressure but seems to do so largely by increasing vascular resistance[71] and often leads to a decrease in systemic perfusion. Dobutamine does not reliably increase blood pressure but usually is associated with an increase in left ventricular output[69] and SVC flow.[72] Epinephrine increases blood pressure[11] and may increase systemic flows, but limited data are available.[73,74] The greatest concern remains the paucity of evidence that clinically important outcomes are improved by the use of any of these catecholamine pressor agents.

Glucocorticoids

There are a several prospective randomized trials addressing corticosteroid use for prevention[75,76] and treatment of hypotension[12,77–80] in the newborn. In one of the prophylactic studies, a reduction in the amount of inotrope required was noted, and in the second, there was no difference in inotrope use. No data are provided on long-term follow-up in either of these studies. There was an increase in the number of adverse effects, however, including hyperglycemia necessitating insulin infusion and gastric perforation in the treated group. In the treatment of hypotension trials, there was variation across the studies with respect to increase in blood pressure and reduction in inotrope use. No advantage of steroids has been documented for any clinically relevant outcomes (death or IVH rate), and no long-term outcome data are provided in any of the trials. The use of glucocorticoids for the prevention and treatment of hypotension cannot be recommended until clinically important benefits are demonstrated in future trials.

SUMMARY

The definition and subsequent appropriate treatment of hypotension and the clinical diagnosis of shock remain elusive, as evidenced by the continued wide variation in practices across NICUs.[2] Currently, many infants receive potentially toxic therapies based solely on simplistic criteria, such as a mean blood pressure less than the gestational age in weeks, in the absence of any evidence that such an approach is beneficial. An approach to treatment that includes blood pressure values but also clinical signs and biochemical values before deciding to initiate therapy markedly reduces the number of infants who receive therapy and is associated with good outcomes.[21,81] Good clinical practice requires a careful assessment of the risks and benefits of an intervention before starting it. The available evidence suggests that an infant who is clinically well perfused despite a numerically low blood pressure is at low risk and may not benefit from intervention. The frequency of treatment can be reduced by a clinically selective approach to as few as 11% of VLBW infants[21] with no evidence of adverse results. It is incumbent on those promoting a more interventionist approach to perform the requisite randomized controlled trials to prove that clinical outcomes are improved.

REFERENCES

1. Al-Aweel I, Pursley DM, Rubin LP, et al. Variations in prevalence of hypotension, hypertension, and vasopressor use in NICUs. J Perinatol 2001;21(5):272–8.
2. Laughon M, Bose C, Allred E, et al. Factors associated with treatment for hypotension in extremely low gestational age newborns during the first postnatal week. Pediatrics 2007;119(2):273–80.
3. Lee J, Rajadurai VS, Tan KW, et al. Blood pressure standards for very low birthweight infants during the first day of life. Arch Dis Child Fetal Neonatal Ed 1999;81(3):F168–70.
4. Spinazzola RM, Harper RG, de Soler M, et al. Blood pressure values in 500- to 750-gram birthweight infants in the first week of life. J Perinatol 1991;11(2): 147–51.
5. Watkins AM, West CR, Cooke RW, et al. Blood pressure and cerebral haemorrhage and ischaemia in very low birthweight infants. Early Hum Dev 1989; 19(2):103–10.
6. Versmold HT, Kitterman JA, Phibbs RH, et al. Aortic blood pressure during the first 12 hours of life in infants with birth weight 610 to 4,220 grams. Pediatrics 1981;67(5):607–13.
7. Hegyi T, Anwar M, Carbone MT, et al. Blood pressure ranges in premature infants: II. The first week of life. Pediatrics 1996;97(3):336–42.
8. Hegyi T, Carbone MT, Anwar M, et al. Blood pressure ranges in premature infants. I. The first hours of life. J Pediatr 1994;124(4):627–33.
9. Dempsey EM, Barrington KJ. Diagnostic criteria and therapeutic interventions for the hypotensive very low birth weight infant. J Perinatol 2006;26(11):677–81.

10. Report of Working Group of the British Association of Perinatal Medicine and Neonatal Nurses Association on categories of babies requiring neonatal care. Arch Dis Child 1992;67(7 Spec No):868–9.
11. Pellicer A, Valverde E, Elorza MD, et al. Cardiovascular support for low birth weight infants and cerebral hemodynamics: a randomized, blinded, clinical trial. Pediatrics 2005;115(6):1501–12.
12. Ng PC, Lee CH, Bnur FL, et al. A double-blind, randomized, controlled study of a "stress dose" of hydrocortisone for rescue treatment of refractory hypotension in preterm infants. Pediatrics 2006;117(2):367–75.
13. Barrington KJ, Stewart S, Lee S, et al. Differing blood pressure thresholds in preterm infants, effects on frequency of diagnosis of hypotension and intraventricular haemorrhage. Pediatric Academic Societies Annual Meeting 2002, abstract. Baltimore, Maryland, May 4–7, 2002.
14. Osborn D, Evans N, Klucklow M. Clinical detection of upper body blood flow in very premature infants using blood pressure, capillary refill time and central-peripheral temperature difference. Arch Dis Child Fetal Neonatal Ed 2004; 2(89):F168–73.
15. Raju NV, Maisels MJ, Kring E, et al. Capillary refill time in the hands and feet of normal newborn infants. Clin Pediatr (Phila) 1999;38(3):139–44.
16. Strozik KS, Pieper CH, Roller J, et al. Capillary refilling time in newborn babies: normal values. Arch Dis Child Fetal Neonatal Ed 1997;76(3):F193–6.
17. Wodey E, Pladys P, Betremieux P, et al. Capillary refilling time and hemodynamics in neonates: a Doppler echocardiographic evaluation. Crit Care Med 1998;26(8): 1437–40.
18. Miletin J, Pichova K, Dempsey EM. Bedside detection of low systemic flow in the very low birth weight infant on day 1 of life. Eur J Pediatr 2008, Epub ahead of print.
19. De Felice C, Flori ML, Pellegrino M, et al. Predictive value of skin color for illness severity in the high-risk newborn. Pediatr Res 2002;51(1):100–5.
20. Giussani DA, Forhead AJ, Fowden AL. Development of cardiovascular function in the horse fetus. J Physiol 2005;565(Pt 3):1019–30.
21. Dempsey EM, Al-Hazzani F, Barrington KJ, et al. Permissive hypotension in the ELBW. Pediatric Academic Societies Annual Meeting 2005, abstract 560. Washington DC, May 14–17, 2005.
22. Peron JM, Bureau C, Gonzalez L, et al. Treatment of hepatorenal syndrome as defined by the International Ascites Club by albumin and furosemide infusion according to the central venous pressure: a prospective pilot study. Am J Gastroenterol 2005;100(12):2702–7.
23. Pittman JA, Ping JS, Mark JB, et al. Arterial and central venous pressure monitoring. Int Anesthesiol Clin 2004;42(1):13–30.
24. Trevor Inglis GD, Dunster KR, Davies MW, et al. Establishing normal values of central venous pressure in very low birth weight infants. Physiol Meas 2007; 28(10):1283–91.
25. Skinner JR, Milligan DW, Hunter S, et al. Central venous pressure in the ventilated neonate. Arch Dis Child 1992;67(4 Spec No):374–7.
26. Nguyen HB, Rivers EP, Knoblich BP, et al. Early lactate clearance is associated with improved outcome in severe sepsis and septic shock. Crit Care Med 2004;32(8):1637–42.
27. Izraeli S, Ben-Sira L, Harell D, et al. Lactic acid as a predictor for erythrocyte transfusion in healthy preterm infants with anemia of prematurity. J Pediatr 1993;122(4):629–31.

28. Fitzgerald MJ, Goto M, Myers TF, et al. Early metabolic effects of sepsis in the preterm infant: lactic acidosis and increased glucose requirement. J Pediatr 1992;121(6):951–5.
29. Abubacker M, Yoxall CW, Lamont G, et al. Peri-operative blood lactate concentrations in pre-term babies with necrotising enterocolitis. Eur J Pediatr Surg 2003; 13(1):35–9.
30. Groenendaal F, Lindemans C, Uiterwaal CS, et al. Early arterial lactate and prediction of outcome in preterm neonates admitted to a neonatal intensive care unit. Biol Neonate 2003;83(3):171–6.
31. Deshpande SA, Platt MP. Association between blood lactate and acid-base status and mortality in ventilated babies. Arch Dis Child Fetal Neonatal Ed 1997; 76(1):F15–20.
32. Wardle SP, Yoxall CW, Weindling AM, et al. Peripheral oxygenation in hypotensive preterm babies. Pediatr Res 1999;45(3):343–9.
33. Miletin J, Dempsey EM. Low superior vena cava flow on day one and adverse outcome in the very low birth weight infant. Arch Dis Child Fetal Neonatal Ed 2008;F368–71.
34. Bendjelid K. The pulse oximetry plethysmographic curve revisited. Curr Opin Crit Care 2008;14(3):348–53.
35. De Felice C, Latini G, Vacca P, et al. The pulse oximeter perfusion index as a predictor for high illness severity in neonates. Eur J Pediatr 2002;161(10):561–2.
36. Granelli AW, Ostman-Smith I. Noninvasive peripheral perfusion index as a possible tool for screening for critical left heart obstruction. Acta Paediatr 2007;96(10): 1455–9.
37. Kluckow M, Seri I, Evans N, et al. Functional echocardiography: an emerging clinical tool for the neonatologist. J Pediatr 2007;150(2):125–30.
38. Evans N, Iyer P. Assessment of ductus arteriosus shunt in preterm infants supported by mechanical ventilation: effect of interatrial shunting. J Pediatr 1994; 125(5 Pt 1):778–85.
39. Evans N, Iyer P. Incompetence of the foramen ovale in preterm infants supported by mechanical ventilation. J Pediatr 1994;125(5 Pt 1):786–92.
40. Kluckow M, Evans N. Superior vena cava flow in newborn infants: a novel marker of systemic blood flow. Arch Dis Child Fetal Neonatal Ed 2000;82(3):F182–7.
41. Osborn DA, Evans N, Kluckow M, et al. Low superior vena cava flow and effect of inotropes on neurodevelopment to 3 years in preterm infants. Pediatrics 2007; 120(2):372–80.
42. Barrington KJ, Dempsey EM. Cardiovascular support in the preterm: treatments in search of indications. J Pediatr 2006;148(3):289–91.
43. Paradisis M. Randomised trial of milrinone versus placebo for prevention of low systemic blood flow in very preterm infants. Pediatric Academic Societies Annual Meeting 2007. Toronto, Canada, May 5–8, 2007.
44. Naulaers G, Morren G, Van Huffel S, et al. Measurement of tissue oxygenation index during the first three days in premature born infants. Adv Exp Med Biol 2003; 510:379–83.
45. Nicklin SE, Hassan IA, Wickramasinghe YA, et al. The light still shines, but not that brightly? The current status of perinatal near infrared spectroscopy. Arch Dis Child Fetal Neonatal Ed 2003;88(4):F263–8.
46. Heard SO. Gastric tonometry: the hemodynamic monitor of choice (Pro). Chest 2003;123(5 Suppl):469S–74S.
47. Silva E, De Backer D, Creteur J, et al. Effects of fluid challenge on gastric mucosal PCO2 in septic patients. Intensive Care Med 2004;30(3):423–9.

48. Campbell ME, Costeloe KL. Measuring intramucosal pH in very low birth weight infants. Pediatr Res 2001;50(3):398–404.
49. Dempsey EM, Barrington KJ. Treating hypotension in the preterm infant: when and with what: a critical and systematic review. J Perinatol 2007;27(8):469–78.
50. Bada HS, Korones SB, Perry EH, et al. Mean arterial blood pressure changes in premature infants and those at risk for intraventricular hemorrhage. J Pediatr 1990;117(4):607–14.
51. Cunningham S, Symon AG, Elton RA, et al. Intra-arterial blood pressure reference ranges, death and morbidity in very low birthweight infants during the first seven days of life. Early Hum Dev 1999;56(2–3):151–65.
52. Miall-Allen VM, de Vries LS, Whitelaw AG, et al. Mean arterial blood pressure and neonatal cerebral lesions. Arch Dis Child 1987;62(10):1068–9.
53. Dasgupta SJ, Gill AB. Hypotension in the very low birthweight infant: the old, the new, and the uncertain. Arch Dis Child Fetal Neonatal Ed 2003;88(6):F450–4.
54. Subhedar NV. Treatment of hypotension in newborns. Semin Neonatol 2003;8(6): 413–23.
55. Kluckow M, Evans N. Relationship between blood pressure and cardiac output in preterm infants requiring mechanical ventilation. J Pediatr 1996;129(4):506–12.
56. Bauer K, Linderkamp O, Versmold HT. Systolic blood pressure and blood volume in preterm infants. Arch Dis Child 1993;69(5 Spec No):521–2.
57. Wright IM, Goodall SR. Blood pressure and blood volume in preterm infants. Arch Dis Child Fetal Neonatal Ed 1994;70(3):F230–1.
58. Van Marter LJ, Pagano M, Allred EN, et al. Rate of bronchopulmonary dysplasia as a function of neonatal intensive care practices. J Pediatr 1992;120(6):938–46.
59. Van Marter LJ, Leviton A, Allred EN, et al. Hydration during the first days of life and the risk of bronchopulmonary dysplasia in low birth weight infants. J Pediatr 1990;116(6):942–9.
60. Tammela OK. Appropriate fluid regimens to prevent bronchopulmonary dysplasia. Eur J Pediatr 1995;154(8 Suppl 3):S15–8.
61. Goldberg RN, Chung D, Goldman SL, et al. The association of rapid volume expansion and intraventricular hemorrhage in the preterm infant. J Pediatr 1980; 96(6):1060–3.
62. Greenough A, Cheeseman P, Kavvadia V, et al. Colloid infusion in the perinatal period and abnormal neurodevelopmental outcome in very low birth weight infants. Eur J Pediatr 2002;161(6):319–23.
63. Rennie JM. Cerebral blood flow velocity variability after cardiovascular support in premature babies. Arch Dis Child 1989;64(7 Spec No):897–901.
64. Barr PA, Bailey PE, Sumners J, et al. Relation between arterial blood pressure and blood volume and effect of infused albumin in sick preterm infants. Pediatrics 1977;60(3):282–9.
65. Pladys P, Wodey E, Betremieux P, et al. Effects of volume expansion on cardiac output in the preterm infant. Acta Paediatr 1997;86(11):1241–5.
66. Hentschel R, Hensel D, Brune T, et al. Impact on blood pressure and intestinal perfusion of dobutamine or dopamine in hypotensive preterm infants. Biol Neonate 1995;68(5):318–24.
67. Greenough A, Emery EF. Randomized trial comparing dopamine and dobutamine in preterm infants. Eur J Pediatr 1993;152(11):925–7.
68. Klarr JM, Faix RG, Pryce CJ, et al. Randomized, blind trial of dopamine versus dobutamine for treatment of hypotension in preterm infants with respiratory distress syndrome. J Pediatr 1994;125(1):117–22.

69. Roze JC, Tohier C, Maingueneau C, et al. Response to dobutamine and dopamine in the hypotensive very preterm infant. Arch Dis Child 1993;69(1 Spec No):59–63.
70. Ruelas-Orozco G, Vargas-Origel A. Assessment of therapy for arterial hypotension in critically ill preterm infants. Am J Perinatol 2000;17(2):95–9.
71. Zhang J, Penny DJ, Kim NS, et al. Mechanisms of blood pressure increase induced by dopamine in hypotensive preterm neonates. Arch Dis Child Fetal Neonatal Ed 1999;81(2):F99–104.
72. Osborn D, Evans N, Kluckow M, et al. Randomized trial of dobutamine versus dopamine in preterm infants with low systemic blood flow. J Pediatr 2002;140(2): 183–91.
73. Phillipos EZ, Barrington K, Robertson M. Dopamine versus epinephrine for inotropic support in the neonate: a randomised blinded trial. Pediatr Res 1996;39:A238.
74. Chatterjee A, Bussey M, Leuschen MP, et al. The pharmacodynamics of inotropic drugs in premature neonates. Pediatr Res 1993;33:206A.
75. Kopelman AE, Moise AA, Holbert D, et al. A single very early dexamethasone dose improves respiratory and cardiovascular adaptation in preterm infants. J Pediatr 1999;135(3):345–50.
76. Efird MM, Heerens AT, Gordon PV, et al. A randomized-controlled trial of prophylactic hydrocortisone supplementation for the prevention of hypotension in extremely low birth weight infants. J Perinatol 2005;25(2):119–24.
77. Bourchier D, Weston PJ. Randomised trial of dopamine compared with hydrocortisone for the treatment of hypotensive very low birthweight infants. Arch Dis Child Fetal Neonatal Ed 1997;76(3):F174–8.
78. Krediet T, van der Ent K. Rapid increase of blood pressure after low dose hydrocortisone in low birth weight neonates with hypotension refractory to high doses of cardiac inotropes. Pediatr Res 1998;38(210A).
79. Osiovich HPE, Lemke P. A short course of hydrocortisone in hypotensive neonates: a randomised double blind control trial. Pediatr Res 2000;43:A422.
80. Gaissmaier RE, Pohlandt F. Single-dose dexamethasone treatment of hypotension in preterm infants. J Pediatr 1999;134(6):701–5.
81. Batton B, Batton D, Riggs T, et al. Blood pressure during the first 7 days in premature infants born at postmenstrual age 23 to 25 weeks. Am J Perinatol 2007; 24(2):107–15.

Indications for Home Apnea Monitoring (or Not)

Jean M. Silvestri, MD[a,b,*]

KEYWORDS

- Apnea of prematurity • Apparent life-threatening event
- Apnea • Home monitoring • Prematurity

There is widespread use of cardiorespiratory monitoring for preterm infants in the neonatal ICU (NICU). The clinician often struggles with decisions regarding discontinuing cardiorespiratory monitoring before discharge or prescribing home monitoring. For very low birth weight infants, one of the key determinants for hospital discharge is the maturation of cardiorespiratory control with resolution of apnea and bradycardia. In addition, monitors may be part of the diagnostic and therapeutic plan for infants who have experienced an apparent life-threatening event (ALTE). This article focuses on issues that affect decision making regarding home monitor use in two groups of patients: infants who have apnea of prematurity (AOP) and infants who experience an ALTE.

Although there is a large body of literature describing AOP and ALTEs, there is no consensus on the use of home monitoring. The "*Summary Proceedings From the Apnea-of-Prematurity Group*"[1] published in 2005 identified a number of key treatment issues to be resolved. One of the crucial issues is there is no standard definition of what duration of apnea, degree of bradycardia, or drop in oxygen saturation is clinically significant. Definitions vary by geographic location. From a study of 14,532 neonates of less than 34 weeks' gestation cared for across the United States, 1588 (11%) were discharged on home apnea monitors. The most important variables determining discharge on a home apnea monitor were the medical preference at the site of care and a diagnosis of apnea. This article reviews existing data to guide a decision to discontinue monitoring at hospital discharge or to prescribe monitoring in the home.

[a] Department of Pediatrics, Rush University Medical Center, 1653 West Congress Parkway, Chicago, IL 60612, USA
[b] Neonatal Intensive Care Unit, Rush Children's Hospital, Chicago, IL, USA
* Department of Pediatrics, Rush University Medical Center, 1653 West Congress Parkway, Chicago, IL 60612, USA.
E-mail address: jean_m_silvestri@rsh.net

Clin Perinatol 36 (2009) 87–99
doi:10.1016/j.clp.2008.09.012 perinatology.theclinics.com

APNEA OF PREMATURITY

Despite the American Academy of Pediatrics' definition of AOP (cessation of breathing that lasts for 20 seconds or is associated with bradycardia, oxygen desaturation, cyanosis in an infant younger than 37 weeks' gestational age),[2] management is variable, depending on the NICU of birth.[3,4] Local practice preferences may result in controversy regarding discharge planning of the convalescing preterm infant who has a history of apnea. This section examines a number of factors relevant to the timing of discharge of an infant who has a history of apnea and to whether home apnea monitoring is indicated.

Natural History

AOP typically is not a clinical problem for infants born at 35 to 36 weeks' gestational age but occurs in up to 85% of infants of less than 34 weeks' gestational age.[5] AOP increases in frequency with decreasing maturity and resolves with increasing maturity. In an early study of 231 preterm infants 26 to 36 6/7 weeks' gestational age who had apnea, apnea resolved in 92% of infants by 37 weeks' postconceptional age (PCA), and more than 98% of these infants were without apnea by 40 weeks' PCA.[6] This sample was limited at the lower gestational ages, only 19 infants were less than 28 weeks' gestational age. A later study demonstrated that among 226 extremely premature infants born at 24 to 28 weeks' gestational age apnea persisted beyond 36 weeks' PCA in all gestational age groups.[7] There was a higher incidence of persistent apnea beyond 40 weeks PCA among infants born at 24 weeks' gestation than in infants born at 28 weeks' gestation. In addition, among infants born at 24 to 28 weeks' gestation, bronchopulmonary dysplasia was associated with a later resolution of apnea.

The large longitudinal Collaborative Home Infant Monitoring Evaluation (CHIME) reinforced the observations of resolution of apnea with increasing PCA.[8] The CHIME study, however, used respiratory inductance plethysmography (RIP) rather than impedance monitors. Because RIP detects obstruction as well as central apnea, the dissimilar definition of events does not allow a direct comparison with prior studies. The risk of conventional events, defined as (1) apnea lasting 20 seconds or longer; (2) in infants of less than 44 weeks' PCA, a heart rate lower than 60 beats per minute (bpm) for at least 5 seconds or lower than 80 bpm for at least 15 seconds; or (3) in infants of 44 weeks' PCA or more, a heart rate lower than 50 bpm for at least 5 seconds or lower than 60 bpm for at least 15 seconds, was present for all infants but was higher among the preterm groups than for term infants and declined with advancing PCA. The risk of an extreme event, defined as (1) apnea lasting 30 seconds or longer, (2) in infants of less than 44 weeks' PCA, a heart rate lower than 60 bpm for at least 10 seconds; or (3) in infants of 44 weeks' or more PCA, a heart rate lower than50 bpm for 10 seconds or more, was higher among preterm infants until 43 weeks' PCA.

In addition, a pattern of resolution of apnea and bradycardia has been observed.[7] Clinically evident apnea and bradycardia requiring stimulation and intervention typically resolve first, followed by self-resolving apnea and bradycardia, followed by transient episodes of bradycardia without observed apnea. Although these studies demonstrate a pattern of improvement with advancing maturity and can help determine when to discontinue respiratory stimulants and monitoring, resolution cannot be predicted precisely for an individual infant.

Determination of Cardiorespiratory Stability

What is the normal respiratory pattern of a preterm infant who is ready for discharge? A number of monitoring studies have been performed in an attempt to determine a convalescing preterm infant's cardiorespiratory stability (or instability) before discharge. An early study performed in-hospital recordings in 83 infants (mean gestational age at birth, 30 weeks) who had a history of cyanosis, apnea, and bradycardia and who were ready for discharge at 36 to 44 weeks' PCA.[9] Stability was defined as having needed no nursing intervention for the past week. Rare episodes of brief bradycardia lasting several seconds (not defined further) not associated with color change or intervention did not exclude discharge. In-hospital recordings demonstrated abnormalities of apnea lasting 20 seconds or longer, excessive periodic breathing, or bradycardia lower than 80 bpm in 92% of these so-called "asymptomatic" infants. Recorded events did not correlate with subsequent clinical events.

Another study also identified abnormal findings by predischarge multichannel recordings among 187 infants at a mean PCA of 37.4 weeks (mean gestational age at birth, 27 weeks) who were thought to be ready for discharge.[10] Apnea lasting 12 seconds or longer (usually between 12 and 19 seconds and often obstructive and mixed) or apnea associated with a 10% fall in heart rate or a 10-point drop in hemoglobin saturation were demonstrated in 91% of recordings. In 12 healthy, asymptomatic infants the findings were so severe, frequent, or prolonged that their discharge was delayed. No relationship was found between predischarge recordings and clinical outcomes.

In contrast, predischarge recordings among 106 infants considered stable for discharge on caffeine therapy (31 weeks' mean gestational age at birth) were performed at a younger mean PCA of 35 weeks.[11] These studies demonstrated abnormalities of apnea lasting 20 seconds or longer or bradycardia lower than 80 bpm for longer than 5 seconds in 30% of infants. This subset of infants was discharged on home recording monitors and had more postdischarge complications and pathologic apnea recorded. The infants without predischarge abnormalities were discharged on caffeine without home monitoring.

A study of 12-hour in-hospital recordings of heart rate, hemoglobin saturation, and RIP instead of impedance compared 35 infants who had persistent bedside apnea and bradycardia alarms and 33 infants who had not had alarms for 2 days before the study and who were being prepared for discharge.[12] The referral infants with alarms were of significantly younger mean gestational age at birth (29.1 versus 30.6 weeks) but of significantly older mean PCA at time of study (36.1 versus 35.3 weeks). Although both groups had recorded apnea, bradycardia, and desaturation, apneas lasting longer than 20 seconds were infrequent in either group. The referral infants had more frequent episodes of desaturation and bradycardia preceded by brief apnea that was significantly shorter in referral infants than in controls. The referral infants also had lower baseline oxygen saturation, which may have contributed to their underlying vulnerability.

Outpatient home monitoring studies also demonstrate that apnea, bradycardia, and desaturation continue in convalescing preterm infants after discharge. The use of conventional impedance home cardiorespiratory monitors showed that 79% of 29 preterm infants who had persistent apnea and bradycardia at the time of discharge continued to demonstrate significant events, defined as apnea lasting 20 seconds or longer or age-related bradycardia, after discharge.[13] Most events occurred in the first month after discharge. Bradycardia, with and without central apnea, was the most prevalent event recorded.

The CHIME study enrolled 443 preterm infants of less than 34 weeks' gestation, a birth weight less than 1750 g, and age less than 120 days at the time of discharge into two groups: 76 (17%) symptomatic preterm infants and 367 (83%) asymptomatic preterm infants. "Symptomatic" was defined as clinically observed apnea and bradycardia associated with cyanosis in the NICU within 5 days of discharge.[8] Both symptomatic and asymptomatic preterm infants continued to have conventional and extreme events (as defined previously) that declined over time. The rate of extreme events was higher in both preterm groups than in healthy term infants through 43 weeks PCA. A key finding of the CHIME study is that after discharge asymptomatic preterm infants continued to have events, with 20% of asymptomatic preterm infants experiencing at least one extreme event. With the use of RIP monitors, a high frequency of obstructed breathing was noted, with at least three obstructed breaths found in 50% of conventional events of apnea lasting at least 20 seconds and in 70% of extreme events of apnea lasting longer than 30 seconds.

In summary, both in-hospital and at-home studies demonstrate that convalescing preterm infants continue to have cardiorespiratory patterns with both central and obstructive apnea, heart rate decelerations, and bradycardia and episodes of desaturation. These episodes continue to occur even though the infants have achieved a period of cardiorespiratory stability and clinically seem to be asymptomatic and ready for discharge.

Defining Symptomatic Versus Asymptomatic Preterm Infants

The clinical finding that an infant is "asymptomatic" and the comfort level of the discharging physician are critical in determining which infants will be discharged on home monitoring. An asymptomatic infant may be identified by clinical bedside observation of apnea, bradycardia, and cyanosis, as commonly done in every NICU; however, observation may be complicated by a number of factors. Most hospital monitors as well as currently available home monitors rely on impedance and thus do not detect obstruction. Convalescing preterm infants who are being prepared for discharge typically are swaddled in open cribs to maintain body temperature. Because swaddling limits direct observation of chest wall movements, bradycardia and drops in hemoglobin saturation are recorded, rather than apnea, and central or obstructive apnea is difficult to identify.

No standard thresholds exist for apnea or bradycardia alarms. With increased vigilance in oxygen monitoring, standard protocols for hemoglobin saturation thresholds have been instituted. When oximetry is not used, prolonged episodes of hypoxemia and cyanosis may not be recognized,[14] raising the issue of how long oximetry should continue in healthy, convalescing preterm infants. One study demonstrated that the time to resolution of clinically apparent apnea was longer in centers in which the duration of pulse oximetry use was longer.[4]

In any NICU there are frequent alarms that do not precede a life-threatening event, raising the question of whether the alarm was a false alarm or whether, instead, there was intervention before a life-threatening event could occur. Alarms and responses to alarms have not been examined in a rigorous fashion. Hospitals also vary in their response and documentation of events. It is well known that the number and duration of episodes of apnea and bradycardia are underdocumented.[15–17] In a study comparing nursing documentation with computer recording of apnea, nurses identified only 54% of 1266 apneas recorded in 27 infants, with apnea detection improving as apnea duration increased.[16] Documentation also was evaluated in predischarge recordings of 44 infants.[17] Nursing documentation identified approximately one third of the recorded episodes of apnea and bradycardia. Episodes also were misclassified. Of the 100 apneas documented by nurses, only 20% were true apnea. Bradycardia was less likely to be misclassified; of the 190 instances documented by nurses, 80% were true bradycardia.

Distinguishing between symptomatic and asymptomatic infants is a problem both for the skilled medical community caring for multiple infants and for the concerned parents or caretakers of an individual infant at home on a monitor. There may be considerable error in reporting apnea when relying on parental reports.[18] Also, more than 60% of documented significant events may not be associated with any reported clinical symptoms,[13] raising the question of what episodes of apnea and bradycardia are significant.

What is a Significant Episode of Apnea and Bradycardia?

Studies demonstrate most preterm infants have apnea. The problem lies in determining what duration of apnea is a problem. This question was one of the issues addressed in the CHIME study,[8] because multiple investigators from five clinical sites and four other institutions had to agree on definitions. The definition of an extreme event was set at a level where all investigators thought there would be physiologic compromise; however, the extent of abnormality necessary to cause injury has yet to be determined definitively.

In the NICU the concern for the preterm infant arises not from the apnea itself but the from the consequences of apnea: a drop in heart rate, blood pressure, or oxygenation.[19,20] As a result, one authority has suggested disabling the respiratory channel while monitoring in the NICU, because one is never monitoring only respiratory movements.[20] Studies of hospitalized very low birth weight infants[21] and of discharged symptomatic and asymptomatic preterm infants[8] demonstrated that increasing duration of apnea and bradycardia was associated with greater drop in hemoglobin saturation.

The clinician also struggles with the definition of "clinically significant" bradycardia. In one study, brief episodes of bradycardia lasting several seconds that were not associated with color change and did not require intervention were recognized and did not exclude infants from discharge.[9] These episodes were not defined further, however. Subsequent studies have identified transient episodes of bradycardia, defined as a drop in heart rate below 90 bpm.[22,23] These episodes were common: they occurred in 68% of 66 infants of 32 to 36 weeks' PCA, and 68% of these events were not associated with apnea lasting 15 seconds or longer.[22] In a much smaller study of 19 healthy preterm infants, transient episodes of bradycardia were found in about half of infants at 40, 44, and 52 weeks' PCA.[23] No infant had a heart rate nadir below 50 bpm, and only one infant had a nadir to below 60 bpm. Nadirs below 70 were uncommon. With the preterm infant's higher heart rate, one would expect that the transient bradycardia would be less common.

Is There Harm?

Every preterm infant experiences apnea, bradycardia, and drops in hemoglobin saturation. These events vary in frequency, duration, and severity. Because events are common and improve with maturation, one could argue that they are without consequence. On the other hand, a study of 15 preterm infants (mean gestational age at birth, 28 ± 3 weeks) found cerebral perfusion decreased dramatically during apnea and bradycardia with heart rates lower than 80 bpm and remained constant with heart rates higher than 80 bpm.[24] These infants had variable clinical courses and were studied at a mean of 19.9 ± 13 days. Although this study was small and lacked longitudinal data, one could infer that altered cerebral perfusion may effect neurodevelopmental outcome.

The relationship between neurodevelopmental outcome at 3 years of age and the number of days with any documented apnea in hospital was assessed in 175 preterm infants (mean gestational age at birth, 27.6 ± 2.2 weeks).[25] Investigators acknowledged the uncertainty of categorizing the frequency/severity of the events and used the number of days a nurse recorded any apnea. Analysis revealed that 23% of infants had impairment. An increasing number of apnea days recorded in hospital was associated with poor outcome. In contrast to in-hospital recording of apnea, data from the CHIME study have begun to assess the severity of events recorded after discharge that may alter neurodevelopmental outcome.[26] Among the 118 preterm infants evaluated at 1 year of age, a dose effect was suggested, in that having no, one to four, or more than five conventional events was associated with unadjusted mean Mental Developmental Index (MDI) values of 100.4 ± 10.3, 96.8 ± 11.5, and 95.8 ± 10.6, respectively. The adjusted mean MDI for preterm infants who had five or more conventional events was 4.9 points lower than in preterm infants who had no events. Whether these findings result directly from the events or combinations of the events during hospitalization or at home or from some underlying cause in the infant requires further study.

Whom to Monitor or Not

The caveats noted in the previous sections show why there is controversy about which infants should be monitored and why there are regional differences in monitoring practice. Most centers are able to identify preterm infants who have persistent apnea and bradycardia who are candidates for discharge on home cardiorespiratory monitoring. When infants continue to have events, and monitoring is chosen, there must be a period before discharge of cardiorespiratory stability without episodes requiring vigorous or frequent stimulation. The PCA at discharge often is higher for infants discharged on a home monitor than for infants not discharged on a monitor.[7]

The challenge is to identify which infant does not need a home monitor at discharge. Much discussion and considerable controversy have centered around this topic; decisions typically are made on the basis of regional customary practice.[3,4] Completion of an apnea and bradycardia–free period is the typical criterion for discharge without a home cardiorespiratory monitor. A survey preformed at a Hot Topics in Neonatology conference in 1996 found that 67% of the 252 neonatologists questioned used an apnea-free interval of 5 to 7 days as a criterion for discharge without a monitor.[27] Methodology for published studies has used the clinical guideline of a minimum of 5 days "spell-free" without methylxanthines before discharge.[7] A retrospective study of a select group of 91 infants (29.7 ± 0.3 weeks' mean gestation age at birth) demonstrated that no apnea occurred more than 8 days after an apnea-free interval unless there was a specific cause such as sepsis.[27] There is controversy about how to define "apnea free." The author's standard is for a monitored infant to complete 5 to 7 days without episodes of apnea and bradycardia before discharge. The apnea-free period (being asymptomatic) is defined by clinical criteria and bedside observation. Low heart rate limits in the Rush Hospital NICU are set at 100 bpm for infants under 34 weeks' gestation and at 80 bpm for infants over 34 weeks' gestation. The authors and colleagues do not to perform predischarge recordings; most infants will have recorded episodes, and the recordings do not have predictive value.

Oximetry typically is discontinued when an infant has been stable in room air for more than 48 hours. The author's view of transient episodes of bradycardia is that an occasional transient, self-relieved episode of bradycardia in the range of 70 to 80 bpm lasting less than 5 to 10 seconds does not by itself delay an infant's discharge. If infant has multiple episodes or require stimulation, however, the infant is reassessed, and the "countdown" to achieve an apnea and bradycardia–free interval is restarted.

Bradycardia awake with feeding is considered a different phenomenon and by itself is not considered an impediment to discharge. Methylxanthines used to achieve cardiorespiratory stability add another dimension to the decision making. Methylxanthines decrease the frequency of apnea and thus are effective treatment for AOP.[28] There have been no systematic trials examining the timing of discontinuation of respiratory stimulants and discharge criteria. Clinical practice has been to discontinue methylxanthines after a period without apnea and bradycardia or at the time when apnea begins to decrease in frequency at 34 to 36 weeks' PCA. Only a small proportion of infants require reinstitution of stimulants and discharge on medication. Some investigators do not discharge infants receiving methylxanthines without a home monitor.[7,13]

At the Hot Topics meeting in 1996, 27% of 266 neonatologists almost never used xanthines at discharge, and 66% used them occasionally.[27] A retrospective study has demonstrated that infants who had abnormal predischarge event recordings on caffeine were discharged on home monitors and caffeine and that those who had normal recordings were discharged on caffeine alone.[11] Larger prospective studies are needed to validate these findings and to inform clinical practice. The author's approach has been to discontinue caffeine in hospital and observe. If an infant is without apnea and bradycardia for 7 days without caffeine, the infant is discharged without a monitor. If episodes recur and are mild, the author observes to achieve a 5 to 7 day period without apnea and bradycardia. If an infant is receiving caffeine at discharge, monitoring is ordered. Typically caffeine is discontinued at term gestation, and monitoring continues to document resolution of apnea. The author's hesitancy to prescribe caffeine at discharge arises from concerns about compliance with medication administration, cost, and added responsibility for the parent.

APPARENT LIFE-THREATENING EVENTS

The term "apparent life-threatening event" was defined in 1986 by the National Institutes of Health Conference on Infantile Apnea and Home Monitoring as "an episode that is frightening to the observer that is characterized by some combination of apnea (central or occasionally obstructive), color change (usually cyanotic or pallid but occasionally erythematous or plethoric), marked change in muscle tone (usually marked limpness), choking or gagging. In some cases, the observer fears that the infant has died."[29] A difficulty in reviewing the ALTE literature is that an ALTE typically is a chief complaint and not a specific diagnosis and thus has not always been well defined. In addition, as with the literature on AOP, one must decide which events are normal or abnormal. An episode of lifelessness primarily associated with apnea and color change has been reported in 3% to 5.3% of healthy infants.[30,31] Also, by definition, the diagnosis of an ALTE is subjective and is based on the observations of a frightened, often medically naïve, observer. This section provides a brief overview of the heterogeneity of diagnoses and management and of the risk of recurrence, examines monitoring studies in infants who have experienced an ALTE, and discusses decision making regarding home monitoring.

Overview

A careful, thorough, and detailed history and physical examination are keys in directing a focused diagnostic work-up and determining underlying causes for an ALITE. Identifying a cause for the ALTE is especially difficult because infants often appear well at the time of presentation and represent diverse pathophysiology. Possible diagnoses include gastrointestinal problems (typically gastroesophageal reflux), seizures, respiratory and infectious problems, prematurity, upper airway obstruction, breath holding, inborn errors of metabolism, and child abuse. The cause remains unknown in up to 50% of infants who experience an ALTE. If no cause is determined, the ALTE is considered idiopathic.

After a significant ALTE or an inconclusive history or physical examination, most infants are hospitalized for observation and diagnostic studies.[32,33] The challenge is to identify the infants who may be at risk for recurrent events and significant morbidity and death. There is no standardized approach to testing, and, as seen with AOP, there is significant regional variation. A retrospective study of hospital admissions for ALTE for 12,067 patients from 36 children's hospitals across the United States highlighted the variability in length of stay, diagnostic testing, and treatment. Infants with a history of prematurity were excluded from the study.[34] During hospitalization, the infant typically undergoes continuous cardiorespiratory monitoring with oximetry. Diagnostic testing may include memory monitoring, multichannel recordings, or polysomnography to direct further work-up and to identify any underlying cardiorespiratory instability.

Mortality and Morbidity: Risk of Rehospitalization, Recurrent Events, and Neurodevelopmental Sequelae

Evidence is lacking regarding the true risk of subsequent events and death, in part because of the heterogeneity of diagnoses and groups at risk. In most instances, the infant experiences a single event and recovers and survives. When a serious underlying condition is identified, that diagnosis dictates the outcome. Infants who have required vigorous or repeated stimulation or resuscitation are at higher risk of death.[35,36]

In the large study of 12,067 term infants who experienced an ALTE the rate of rehospitalization was 2.5% and was associated with a discharge diagnosis of cardiovascular disorders and gastroesophageal reflux.[34] A study of 59 infants found that a history of multiple ALTEs before admission and an age of 1 month or less identified infants at higher risk.[37] Prematurity was an additional factor predictive of subsequent events.

From one case series of 73 infants (88% of whom experienced an idiopathic ALTE), apnea and bradycardia documented during the initial hospital investigation predicted subsequent events recorded at home.[13] An attempt to identify infants at high risk for subsequent ALTEs using predischarge polysomnography has failed to demonstrate convincing results.[38,39]

Data from the CHIME study has begun to assess the severity of events recorded after discharge that may alter neurodevelopmental outcome.[26] The CHIME study included 138 monitored term infants (26% had experienced idiopathic ALTE, 37% were healthy term infants, and 37% were siblings of a infant who had suffered sudden infant death) who underwent neurodevelopmental evaluations at 1 year of age. A dose effect was suggested in that having no, one to four, and five or more conventional events (as defined earlier) was associated with unadjusted mean MDI values of 103.6 ± 10.6, 104.2 ± 10.7, and 97.7 ± 10.9, respectively. The adjusted mean MDI for term infants having five or more conventional events was 5.6 points lower than that of infants who had no events. As noted for AOP, it is not known whether these findings result from the events themselves or from some underlying pathology in the infant.

Home Monitoring Studies of Infants who Experience an Idiopathic Apparent Life-Threatening Event

When no cause is determined, home monitoring may be prescribed for an infant who has experienced an idiopathic ALTE. A number of early studies were performed in patients who experienced idiopathic ALTE using home monitoring without event-recording capability, thus making clinical correlation tenuous. Studies using home monitoring with memory capability have proved useful in establishing a diagnosis in infants who experience recurrent idiopathic ALTEs when the initial evaluation was unremarkable.[40,41] In two case series of infants who experienced recurrent severe ALTEs, cardiorespiratory monitoring as well as monitoring of oxygenation allowed the diagnosis of seizures, suffocation, and Munchausen's syndrome by proxy. Home monitoring with memory capability can describe underlying mechanisms better and clarify the natural history and frequency of recurrence of ALTE in infants.

In a program using monitors with memory capability, subsequent significant events occurred in 33% of the 73 infants who experienced an ALTE.[13] Most of the significant events were recorded in the first month of monitoring. Sixty percent of 134 documented significant events were not associated with any reported clinical symptoms; conversely, only 61% of the 144 reported clinical events had significant documented apnea and/or bradycardia. As with AOP, these findings raise the question of the threshold of significance for apnea and bradycardia and highlight the difficulty in correlating recorded significant events with clinical events observed by the caregivers.

Term (n = 107) and preterm (n = 45) infants who had experienced an idiopathic ALTE were enrolled as two groups in the CHIME study that enrolled 1079 infants overall.[8] Although all infants being monitored for an idiopathic ALTE had an increased risk for repeated extreme events (as described earlier), the difference was statistically significant only for the preterm infants who experienced an ALTE. Of the 116 term and preterm infants who had at least one extreme event, 51.7% had a second event; 57.3% of the infants who experienced a second event had a third event; and 80% of the infants who had a third event experienced a fourth event. Most subsequent events occurred within 6 weeks of the prior event.

Prescribing Home Monitoring for Apparent Life-Threatening Events

The goals in the evaluation of an infant who experiences ALTE are to identify a treatable cause and to initiate treatment. Home monitoring is useful in infants who are at increased risk of recurrent events[2] because the infant is still immature or because the ALTE required vigorous stimulation or resuscitation and the true risk of morbidity cannot be determined.

In infants who have experienced an idiopathic ALTE the decision to use home monitoring should be individualized. In certain infants home monitoring with memory capability may be useful in helping the infants make the transition to home. Monitoring with memory capability helps identify underlying mechanisms and accurately records the frequency, severity, and resolution of events.

When maturing cardiorespiratory patterns and resolving AOP have contributed to an ALTE, monitoring through age 43 weeks documenting resolution of apnea and bradycardia usually is sufficient.[8] Subsequent events, if they occur, typically occur within 6 weeks of the initial ALTE. This experience supports monitoring for up to 6 weeks or until the resolution of events has been documented. It is of interest is that almost half the parents of infants who had experienced an ALTE, were followed in a monitoring program, and had met the criteria for discontinuing monitoring were unwilling to discontinue monitoring.[13]

CONSEQUENCES OF PRESCRIBING A HOME MONITOR FOR APNEA OF PREMATURITY OR AN APPARENT LIFE-THREATENING EVENT

When a home monitor is prescribed, the parents become partners in care and must understand the indications for and the limitations and duration of monitoring for their infant. No study has demonstrated that monitors save lives and prevent sudden, unexpected death.[2] Indeed, infants have died while on home monitors.[42–44] Monitors, whether in the NICU or at home, are there to alert the caretaker to a potentially life-threatening event. Because monitored infants have numerous false alarms, families should be counseled that these events occur and that they should observe the infant before intervening. All caregivers should be trained to administer appropriate intervention; such training includes training in cardiopulmonary resuscitation highlighting appropriate stimulation for resuscitation and the need to avoid shaking the infant. All monitors should have event-recording (memory) capability to document events, to distinguish true apnea and bradycardia from false alarms, and to document compliance.[2] A support system for the family should be in place and should provide appropriate teaching and directions for monitor use and appropriate technical and medical support and follow-up. Because most events occur in the early weeks of monitoring,[13] appropriate support is important to encourage compliance with monitor use.

One also must consider the impact of home monitoring on the family and on post-discharge care. Caring for an infant or newborn, and especially a preterm infant on an apnea home monitor, is challenging. Studies have shown that caregivers of monitored infants experience stress and fatigue, with a variable impact on family life.[45,46] In addition, the use of an apnea monitor placed an infant at significantly increased risk of rehospitalizaton.[47]

A plan for duration of monitoring should be in place when the monitor is prescribed. In addition, all caregivers should be instructed in safe infant sleep practices, which should include supine sleeping with the face uncovered and avoiding overheating. A safe sleep environment also requires a firm sleeping surface, no loose bedding or soft crib toys in the crib, and a smoke-free environment.

Monitoring and Sudden Infant Death

Since the National Institutes of Health Consensus Statement on Infantile Home Apnea Monitoring in 1986, the controversial association of apnea and sudden infant death syndrome (SIDS) and intervention with home monitoring has been debated. A large, prospective monitoring study published in 1983 of 6914 term infants and 2337 preterm infants was unable to identify cardiorespiratory patterns that were predictive of SIDS in 24-hour recordings performed in the first 6 weeks of life.[48]

In a large, retrospective series of 3406 infants followed for 5 years in monitoring programs in California, mortality was not greater in infants for whom monitoring was not recommended than in those for whom monitoring was recommended.[42] More recent data from the CHIME study demonstrated that many infants experience apnea and bradycardia and do not die.[8] In addition, the resolution of extreme events occurred before the age of the peak incidence of SIDS, suggesting that extreme events are not a precursor to SIDS.

The perceived association between apnea and SIDS allowed home monitoring to flourish. There are limited indications for home monitoring, and home monitoring in its current form is not a strategy to reduce sudden infant death. A monitor is a tool to capture and identify events and has not been shown to reduce the number or severity of events or to prevent these events or death. Novel strategies examining recordings preceding events[49] may provide insights into alternative monitoring or identification of a subset of the infants at highest risk. Further insights into best practices and predicting adverse outcomes will come with well-structured multicenter prospective studies.

ACKNOWLEDGEMENT

The author acknowledges the editorial assistance of Jill and William J. Malan in preparing this article.

REFERENCES

1. Finer NN, Higgins R, Kattwinkel J, et al. Summary proceedings from the apnea-of-prematurity group. Pediatrics 2006;117:S47–51.
2. Committee on Fetus and Newborn. Apnea, sudden infant death syndrome, and home monitoring. Pediatrics 2003;111:914–7.
3. Sychowski SP, Dodd E, Thomas P, et al. for the Pediatrix-Obstetrix Center for Research and Education. Home apnea monitor use in preterm infants discharged from newborn intensive care units. J Pediatr 2001;139:245–8.
4. Eichenwald EC, Blackwell M, Lloyd JS, et al. Inter-neonatal intensive care unit variation in discharge timing: influence of apnea ad feeding management. Pediatrics 2001;108:928–33.
5. Barrington K, Finer N. The natural history of the appearance of apnea of prematurity. Pediatr Res 1991;29:372–5.
6. Henderson-Smart DJ. The effect of gestational age on the incidence and duration of recurrent apnoea in newborn babies. Aust Paediatr J 1981;17:273–6.
7. Eichenwald EC, Aina A, Stark AR. Apnea frequently persists beyond term gestation infants delivered at 24–28 weeks. Pediatrics 1997;100:354–9.
8. Ramanathan R, Corwin MJ, Hunt CE, et al. Cardiorespiratory events recorded on home monitors. Comparison of healthy infants with those at increased risk for SIDS. J Am Med Assoc 2001;285:2199–207.
9. Rosen CL, Glaze DG, Frost JD Jr. Home monitor follow-up of persistent apnea and bradycardia in preterm infants. Am J Dis Child 1986;140:547–50.
10. Barrington KJ, Finer N, Li D. Predischarge respiratory recordings in very low birth weight newborn infants. J Pediatr 1996;129:934–40.
11. Subhani M, Katz S, DeCristofaro JD. Prediction of postdischarge complications by predischarge event recordings in infants with apnea of prematurity. J Perinatol 2000;2:92–5.
12. DiFiore JM, Arko MK, Miller MJ, et al. Cardiorespiratory events in preterm infants referred for apnea monitoring studies. Pediatrics 2001;108:1304–8.
13. Côté A, Hum C, Brouillette RT, et al. Frequency and timing of recurrent events in infants using home cardiorespiratory monitors. J Pediatr 1998;312:783–9.
14. Poets CF, Stebbens VA, Richard D, et al. Prolonged episodes of hypoxemia in preterm infants undetectable by cardiorespiratory monitors. Pediatrics 1995;95:860–3.
15. Southall DP, Levitt GA, Richards JM, et al. Undetected episodes of prolonged apnea and severe bradycardia in preterm infants. Pediatrics 1983;72:541–51.
16. Muttitt SC, Finer NN, Tierney AJ, et al. Neonatal apnea: diagnosis by nurse versus computer. Pediatrics 1988;82:713–20.
17. Razi NM, Humphreys J, Pandit PB, et al. Predischarge monitoring of preterm infants. Pediatr Pulmonol 1999;27:113–6.
18. Steinschneider A, Santos V. Parental reports of apnea and bradycardia: temporal characteristics and accuracy. Pediatrics 1991;88:1100–5.
19. Upton CJ, Milner AD, Stokes GM. Apnoea, bradycardia, and oxygen saturation in preterm infants. Arch Dis Child 1991;66:381–5.
20. Poets CF. Monitoring in the NICU. In: Mathew OP, editor. Respiratory control disorders. New York: Marcel Dekker, Inc.; 2003. p. 217–35.

21. Finer NN, Barrington KJ, Hayes BJ, et al. Obstructive, mixed and central apnea in the neonate: physiologic correlates. J Pediatr 1992;121:943–50.
22. Hodgman JE, Gonzalez F, Hoppenbrouwers T, et al. Apnea, transient episodes of bradycardia, and periodic breathing in preterm infants. Am J Dis Child 1990;144:54–7.
23. Hodgman JE, Hoppenbrouwers T, Cabal LA. Episodes of bradycardia during early infancy in the term and preterm infant. Am J Dis Child 1993;147:960–4.
24. Perlman JM, Volpe JJ. Episodes of apnea and bradycardia in the preterm newborn: impact on cerebral circulation. Pediatrics 1985;76:333–8.
25. Janvier A, Khairy M, Kokkotis A, et al. Apnea is associated with neurodevelopmental impairment in very low birth weight infants. J Perinatol 2004;24:763–8.
26. Hunt CE, Corwin MJ, Baird T, et al. Cardiorespiratory events detected by home memory monitoring and one-year neurodevelopmental outcome. J Pediatr 2004;145:465–71.
27. Darnall RA, Kattwinkel J, Nattie C, et al. Margin of safety for discharge after apnea in preterm infants. Pediatrics 1997;100:795–801.
28. Henderson-Smart DJ, Steer P. Methylxanthine treatment for apnea in preterm infants. Cochrane Database Syst Rev 2001;(3):CD000140.
29. National Institutes of Health Consensus Development Conference on Infantile Apnea and Home Monitoring, Sept 29 to Oct 1, 1986. Pediatrics 1987;79:292–9.
30. Mitchell EA, Thompson JMD. Parental reported apnoea, admissions to hospital and sudden infant death syndrome. Acta Paediatr 2001;90:417–22.
31. Fleming P, Blair P, Platt MW, et al. The case control study: results and discussion. In: Fleming P, Bacon C, Blair P, editors. Sudden unexpected deaths in infancy. The CESDI SUDI studies 1993–1996. London: The Stationary Office; 2000. p. 13–96.
32. Brand DA, Altman RL, Purtill K, et al. Yield of diagnostic testing in infants who have had an apparent life-threatening event. Pediatrics 2005;115:885–93.
33. Kahn A. Recommended clinical evaluation of infants with an apparent life-threatening event. Consensus document of the European society for the study and prevention of infant death, 2003. Eur J Pediatr 2004;163:108–15.
34. Tieder JS, Cowan CA, Garrison MM, et al. Variation in inpatient resource utilization and management of apparent life-threatening events. J Pediatr 2008;152:629–35.
35. Samuels MP. Apparent life-threatening events: pathogenesis and management. In: Marcus CL, Carroll JL, Donnelly DF, editors. Sleep and breathing in children. 2nd edition. New York: Informa Healthcare USA, Inc.; 2008. p. 229–54.
36. Oren J, Kelly D, Shannon DC. Identification of a high-risk group for sudden infant death syndrome among infants who were resuscitated for sleep apnea. Pediatrics 1986;77:495–9.
37. Claudius I, Keens T. Do all infants with apparent life-threatening events need to be admitted? Pediatrics 2007;119:679–83.
38. Rosen CL, Frost JD, Harrison GM. Infant apnea: polygraphic studies and follow-up monitoring. Pediatrics 1983;71:731–6.
39. Daniëls H, Naulaers G, Deroost F, et al. Polysomnography and home documented monitoring of cardiorespiratory pattern. Arch Dis Child 1999;81:434–6.
40. Samuels MP, Poets CF, Noyes JP, et al. Diagnosis and management after life threatening events in infants and young children who received cardiopulmonary resuscitation. BMJ 1993;306:489–92.

41. Poets CF, Samuels MP, Noyes JP, et al. Home event recordings of oxygenation, breathing movements, and heart rate and rhythm in infants with recurrent life-threatening events. J Pediatr 1993;123:693–701.
42. Davidson Ward SL, Keens TG, Chan LS, et al. Sudden infant death syndrome in infants evaluated by apnea programs in California. Pediatrics 1986;77:451–5.
43. Meny RG, Carroll JL, Carbone T, et al. Cardiorespiratory recordings from infants dying suddenly and unexpectedly at home. Pediatrics 1994;93:44–9.
44. Poets CF, Meny RG, Chobanian MR, et al. Gasping and other cardiorespiratory patterns during sudden infant deaths. Pediatr Res 1999;45:350–4.
45. Ahmann E, Wulff L, Meny RG. Home apnea monitoring and disruptions in family life: a multidimensional controlled study. Am J Public Health 1992;82:719–22.
46. Williams PD, Press A, Williams AR, et al. Fatigue in mothers of infants discharged to the home on apnea monitors. Appl Nurs Res 1999;12:69–77.
47. Malloy MH, Graubard B. Access to home apnea monitoring and its impact on rehospitalization among very low birth weight infants. Arch Pediatr Adolesc Med 1995;149:326–32.
48. Southall DP, Richards JM, Swiet M, et al. Identification of infants destined to die unexpectedly during infancy: evaluation of predictive importance of prolonged apnoea and disorders of cardiac rhythm. BMJ 1983;286:1092–6.
49. Hunt C, Corwin MJ, Lister G, et al. Precursors of cardiorespiratory events in infants detected by home memory monitor. Pediatr Pulmonol 2008;43:87–8.

Short Bowel Syndrome: How Short is Too Short?

Praveen S. Goday, MBBS, CNSP

KEYWORDS

- Short bowel syndrome • Intestinal failure • Prognosis
- Enteral feeding • Neonate

Intestinal failure is characterized by the inability to maintain energy, fluid, electrolyte, or micronutrient balance and can result from surgical resection, obstruction, dysmotility, congenital defect, or disease-associated loss of absorption.[1] The most common condition resulting in intestinal failure is short bowel syndrome (SBS), which occurs after massive resection of small bowel.[2,3] In infants, necrotizing enterocolitis and intestinal anomalies are most frequently responsible for SBS. The intestinal anomalies responsible for SBS include intestinal atresias, gastroschisis, and volvulus.

Any definition of SBS must include two important concepts: a shortened length of intestine and a need for parenteral nutrition (PN). The Canadian Association of Pediatric Surgeons defines SBS as the need for PN greater than 42 days after bowel resection or a residual small bowel length of less than 25% expected for gestational age.[4] This definition leads us to the question that is the subject of this article, which is addressed in the next section.

Wessel and Kocoshis[5] make an important distinction between intestinal failure and SBS. The implied difference between the two entities is that SBS is associated with significant loss of absorptive surface area, whereas intestinal failure is a lack of satisfactory absorption despite an apparently adequate intestinal surface area.[5] So, patients who have SBS may have intestinal failure, whereas patients who have intestinal failure may not have SBS. This article focuses only on SBS with associated intestinal failure and attempts to elucidate the prognostic factors that ultimately predict successful weaning from PN.

Intestinal adaptation is defined as the ability to maintain normal growth and fluid and electrolyte balance without the need for PN support. It is a compensatory response that follows an abrupt decrease in mucosal surface area after an extensive small bowel resection and includes a variety of anatomic and physiologic changes that increase the gut's digestive and absorptive capacity. It begins shortly after intestinal resection and is complete within 36 to 48 months.[6,7]

Division of Pediatric Gastroenterology and Nutrition, Department of Pediatrics, Medical College of Wisconsin, 8701 Watertown Plank Road, Milwaukee, WI 53045, USA
E-mail address: pgoday@mcw.edu

Clin Perinatol 36 (2009) 101–110
doi:10.1016/j.clp.2008.09.006 perinatology.theclinics.com
0095-5108/08/$ – see front matter

HOW SHORT IS TOO SHORT?

Neonates, especially premature neonates, are at a distinct advantage with regard to intestinal adaptation. The small bowel length beyond 35 weeks of gestation is double that of an infant between 19 and 27 weeks of gestation,[8] suggesting that the residual intestine may have greater potential for increase in length in a preterm infant than in a full-term baby.[9,10] Median small bowel length increases from 114.8 cm between 19 and 27 weeks of gestation through 172.1 cm between 27 and 35 weeks of gestation to a length of 248.0 cm in neonates greater than 35 weeks of gestation.[8] At 1 year of age, small bowel length is approximately 380 cm.[11]

Intestinal resections can be divided into three categories based on the residual length of the small intestine along the antimesenteric border. Resections can be short (residual small intestine: 100–150 cm), large (residual small intestine: 40–100 cm), or massive (residual small intestine: <40 cm).[7] From a prognostic perspective, however, this approach is simplistic; we also need to consider the gestational age of the patient at the time of surgery, the portion of bowel resected, and the functional integrity of the remaining small intestine.[7]

All our knowledge about prognostic factors that determine survival and weaning from PN comes from retrospective studies. One early study suggested that the presence of 15 cm of small bowel with an ileocecal valve (ICV) or 40 cm of small bowel in the absence of an ICV was associated with survival.[12] These data have been partially improved on by several studies published in the past decade (**Table 1**). The newer data, too, should be interpreted carefully because all these studies included patients over several years; the shortest study studied patients over a 12-year span, whereas the longest studied patients over 27 years. Two studies have shown that infants born in more recent years have better outcomes than infants born earlier.[13,14]

FACTORS PREDICTING MORTALITY

In a large population-based study, the overall incidence of SBS was 22.1 per 1000 neonatal intensive care unit (NICU) admissions and 24.5 per 100,000 live births, with a much greater incidence in premature infants.[15] The SBS case fatality rate was 37.5%.[15] In the retrospective studies detailed in this article, mortality has ranged from 10.3% to 27.5%. In general, studies have found increased mortality with decreased small bowel length (<15 cm[16] or <10% of a given infant's length for gestational age[17]) and with persistent cholestasis (defined as a direct bilirubin measurement $\geq$2 mg/dL[16] or $\geq$2.5 mg/dL[17]).

ANATOMIC PREDICTORS OF ADAPTATION

All the newer retrospective studies have found that small bowel length is an important prognostic factor.[6,7,14,16,17] Two studies identified children with residual small bowel length greater than 15 cm[16] and greater than 40 cm[7] as more likely to be weaned off PN. Spencer and colleagues[17] found that small bowel length $\geq$10% of expected length for gestational age was a significant predictor of adaptation.

Absolute residual length measurements should no longer be used as a predictor of adaptation. Infants who have SBS today span a much wider gestational age range than their counterparts in the late 1970s (three of the "newer" studies date back to patients from that era). If one were to prognosticate purely on the basis of residual small bowel length, the most accurate method of prediction would be to use the percentage of small bowel length for gestational age. These data also suggest that surgeons should report the remaining length of small bowel accurately. If surgeons report

Table 1
Factors predicting successful weaning from total parenteral nutrition that have been identified by five retrospective studies

	Sondheimer and colleagues[6]	Andorsky and colleagues[14]	Quiros-Tejeira and colleagues[16]	Goulet and colleagues[7]	Spencer and colleagues[17]
No. children	44	30	78	87	80
Study period	1985–1996	1985–1998	1975–2000	1975–1991	1977–2003
Surgical factors					
Small bowel length	Yes	Yes	>15 cm	>40 cm	≥10% of expected length for gestational age
Presence of ICV	No	No	Yes	Yes	Yes
Intact colon	—	No	Yes	—	—
<50% of colon resected	—	No	Yes	—	—
Primary anastomosis	—	No	Yes	—	—
More recent year of surgery	—	Yes	—	No	—
Enteral intake					
Percentage of daily kilocalories through the enteral route at 6 weeks	—	Yes	—	—	—
Percentage of daily kilocalories through the enteral route at 12 and 24 weeks	Yes	—	—	—	—
Potentially modifiable factors					
Intake of breast milk	—	Yes	—	—	—
Intake of amino acid–based formula	—	Yes	—	—	—

Data from Refs.[6,7,14,16,17]

only the resected length, the estimated residual small bowel length can be calculated from the known small bowel length for the child's gestational age.[8]

Although the length of the resected specimen is important, it is also important to know the portion of small bowel that was resected (ie, jejunum versus ileum) because the area of small bowel that is resected also influences the degree of adaptation that is possible. The ileum has a much greater capacity for adaptation than the more proximal portions of the bowel.[18] In addition to intrinsic differences between these two small bowel segments, chyme moves less rapidly through the ileum than through the jejunum because of less vigorous motility. This increases the opportunity for nutrient absorption during adaptation.[19] Also, ileal resection causes the rate of gastric emptying to hasten as a result of the loss of the ileogastric reflex that normally slows it down, diminishing the opportunity for nutrient absorption.[20]

Because the ileum is contiguous with the ICV, which, in turn, is contiguous with the colon, these three elements have to be considered together. The ICV slows the transit time of intestinal contents and prevents reflux of colonic contents and bacteria into the ileum. Resection of the ICV can cause bacterial reflux into the small bowel. The ensuing bacterial overgrowth can deconjugate bile salts, reduce bile salt absorption, and impair gut function.[5] An intact colon or remnant of colon may contribute to adaptation after small bowel loss.[21,22] In colonic resections, the usual colonic functions of water, electrolyte, and short-chain fatty acid (SCFA) absorption and slowing of intestinal transit are lost.[23] Thus, colonic resection may also diminish adaptation.

Most studies have identified preservation of the ICV as a favorable indicator of long-term adaptation. Whether this actually reflects the ICV itself or the terminal ileum that is contiguous with it is unclear. Spencer and colleagues[17] found it difficult to separate the influence of ICV resection from colonic resection and decided to use only ICV resection in their analysis. Quiros-Tejeira and colleagues[16] were able to show that apart from patients with a preserved ICV, patients with an intact colon or with at least greater than 50% of colon length remaining were more likely to adapt. However, these researchers also showed that primary anastomosis rather than an ostomy or ostomies was associated with a greater degree of adaptation.[16] The benefits of maintaining intestinal continuity can be physiologically explained by the fact that all portions of the gut are exposed to enteral nutrients and biliary and pancreatic secretions, leading to a greater degree of adaptation.

Apart from the length of bowel remaining after a resection, the condition, area, and motility of the bowel may affect the ability of the infant or child to tolerate enteral feedings. These factors can be indirectly assessed by the enteral tolerance to breast milk or formula at specific intervals after the initial resection. Sondheimer and colleagues[6] assessed the percent of daily energy intake through the enteral route at 12 weeks after surgery. In infants obtaining 75% of their calories enterally by 12 weeks, the likelihood of weaning off PN is 90%, whereas those tolerating 50% of their calories enterally have only a 75% likelihood of being weaned off PN. In children who tolerate only 25% enterally, the likelihood of weaning is only 50%.[6] These investigators also extended their observations to 24 weeks after surgery, whereas Andorsky and colleagues[14] confirmed that this is generally true even 6 weeks after the initial surgery.

Most of the anatomic predictors are not modifiable, with the possible exception of restoring intestinal continuity at the time of intestinal surgery. Only one of these studies[14] has shown that use of breast milk and amino acid–based formulas is associated with a shorter duration of PN. The effect of these and other nutrients is discussed further in the section on nutritional modifiers of adaptation.

From a clinical perspective, these data lead us to the following conclusions. We should use the percentage of residual small bowel length for gestational age as the prime anatomic predictor of adaptation—the greater the percentage, the better is the likelihood of adaptation. Other anatomic factors should then be added into the prognostic mix: presence of the ICV, presence of an intact colon or most of the colon, and presence of an ostomy. Because these infants usually spend at least 3 to 6 weeks in the NICU after surgery, the percentage of enteral calories tolerated by these infants at specific time intervals can be used to refine the prognosis.

NUTRITIONAL MODIFIERS OF ADAPTATION

In rodent models, sole use of PN without enteral feeding causes small bowel atrophy.[24] The use of enteral feeding contributes greatly to intestinal adaptation. After massive small bowel resection, only limited adaptation can occur in the absence of enteral nutrition.[24] In protracted diarrhea of infancy, the combination of PN and enteral nutrition is superior to PN alone in stimulating intestinal regeneration of disaccharidases.[25] The same is considered to be true of intestinal adaptation in SBS.

Specific enteral nutrients stimulate epithelial cell proliferation through a complex process. These nutrients probably work through trophic paracrine hormones that are secreted in the intestinal epithelium to stimulate epithelial cell proliferation and reduce apoptosis.[26] Among digestible carbohydrates, it has been shown that disaccharides are more trophic to the rat small bowel than monosaccharides.[27] This has led to the "functional workload" hypothesis.[28] This hypothesis states that it is the workload induced in the epithelium—the need for digestion and absorption of nutrients within the lumen—that serves as an important trophic stimulus for adaptation.[28] Certain enteral nutrients may be more effective stimulants than others, probably because they confer a greater workload while being digested and absorbed or because they result in enhanced release of trophic factors. They probably orchestrate these changes through afferent sensory neurons that detect changes in the chemical contents of the gut lumen and then set off the subsequent neural, hormonal, and immune signals supporting nutrient digestion and absorption.[29–31] This "functional workload" premise should also apply during the consumption of a mixed diet.

Evaluation of specific macronutrients reveals that hydrolyzed protein is more trophic to the gut than intact protein.[32] Similarly, long-chain fats stimulate small bowel adaptation better than medium-chain fats.[32] Free fatty acids are more trophic than long-chain triglycerides (LCTs), protein, starch, or medium-chain triglycerides (MCTs) in enhancing intestinal adaptation.[33] LCTs seem to be potentially more trophic than MCTs; LCTs also stimulate biliary and pancreatic secretions, which, in turn, are also trophic factors.[34] Among long-chain fatty acids, eicosapentanoic and docosahexanoic acids are more effective in inducing structural changes associated with adaptation than less highly unsaturated fats.[35] Despite their inability to stimulate adaptation to the extent of LCTs, MCTs are considered to be beneficial in SBS for several reasons. MCTs are hydrolyzed more rapidly than LCTs by pancreatic lipase into free fatty acids and glycerol. They can also be absorbed intact into the portal circulation even in the absence of lipase and bile.[36] MCTs can be absorbed to a certain extent from the stomach and duodenum; the unabsorbed fraction is then absorbed in the proximal jejunum.

Biliary and pancreatic secretions can also serve as potent stimuli for small bowel adaptation. Surgical manipulations in rodents, such as transplantation of the ampulla of Vater into the distal small intestine[37] or diversion of pancreatic and biliary secretions into self-emptying ileal loops, induce villus hyperplasia in the ileum.[38]

Gut adaptation involves hormonal mediators, such as enteroglucagon, glucagon-like peptides, neurotensin, peptide YY, growth hormone, and insulin-like growth factor. A detailed review of these hormones and their role in gut adaptation is outside the scope of this article and can be found elsewhere.[39–41] Other factors in the intestinal lumen that potentially contribute to intestinal adaptation include polyamines (spermine and spermidine), epidermal growth factor (EGF), and trefoil peptides.[18,42] Glutamine, an enterocyte fuel, and SCFAs, a fuel for colonocytes produced by bacterial fermentation of dietary fiber, also play roles in intestinal adaptation.[42,43]

ENTERAL FEEDING IN SHORT BOWEL SYNDROME: WHAT TO FEED AND HOW TO FEED

There are no prospective or randomized data to guide the choice of enteral feeds in SBS. Only one of the retrospective studies addressed this question.[14] In this study, breast milk feeding was shown to be an important factor in gut adaptation.[14] Breast milk, surprisingly, fulfills many of the needs of infants who have SBS. Its chemical complexity is a double-edged sword. Although it is a complex food that definitely increases functional overload, the presence of lactose, complex fats, and proteins can lead to feeding intolerance in infants who have SBS. From a trophic perspective, however, lactose is a disaccharide, and although breast milk lacks hydrolyzed protein, it has LCTs, glutamine,[44] and growth factors like growth hormone[45,46] and EGF.[47,48] As is discussed elsewhere in this article, breast milk is also less likely to provoke an allergy in the neonate.

Amino acid–based formulas were also found to be associated with a shorter duration of PN in the study by Andorsky and colleagues.[14] Even before this study, Bines and colleagues[49] reported on four patients who had SBS and feeding intolerance, who were all weaned off PN within 15 months of being started on an amino acid–based formula. Physiologic data fail to lend significant support to an amino acid–based formula in SBS. Such a formula does not increase functional workload significantly because of its elemental nature. The carbohydrates are glucose polymers, and the protein is in the form of amino acids. A factor that could favor amino acid–based formulas, however, is that the formula used in the study by Bines and colleagues[49] had a large proportion of LCTs. Second, allergic sensitization[50] and allergic colitis have been described in infants who have SBS.[51,52]

Although there are no clinical data to support them, semielemental formulas containing hydrolyzed protein and MCTs are used widely and are generally well tolerated.

A practical approach to infant feeding in SBS is outlined here. Breast milk becomes the feed of choice when it is available. When it is unavailable or poorly tolerated, it may be appropriate to consider a protein hydrolysate formula initially, especially in children with good anatomic prognostic factors who are likely to adapt successfully. In children with poor prognostic factors, an elemental formula may be considered initially in the absence of breast milk. In any child in whom there is persistent feeding intolerance, an amino acid–based formula must be considered.

How to Feed

In all children who have SBS requiring PN, a continuous enteral infusion of breast milk or formula must be considered. The sole exception may be children with practically no small bowel, such as after surgery for extensive midgut volvulus. As soon as postoperative ileus resolves, feeds are administered in a continuous fashion through a nasogastric or a gastrostomy tube. Children who seem to have a poorer prognosis may benefit from early gastrostomy tube placement. Continuous feeds optimize absorption (and probably adaptation) by permitting total saturation of the transporters in the gut

24 hours a day. Enteral nutrition is usually started slowly and advanced based on stool or ostomy output and other abdominal symptoms and signs.

When there is an ostomy and an accompanying mucus fistula, the ostomy output can be infused into the mucus fistula with the aim of providing nutrients for absorption and luminal secretions, both of which should encourage adaptation of the distal bowel. A review on this topic concluded that mucus fistula refeeding is safe, improves weight gain, and potentially reduces total PN–related complications in infants who have SBS.[53] However, skin breakdown, bag leakage, and difficulties in performing this at home may make this difficult.[54,55]

OTHER FACTORS THAT MAY INFLUENCE ADAPTATION

In an effort to provide SCFAs as an energy source to an intact colon, dietary fiber in the form of pectin, a soluble fiber,[56] or green beans[56] has been used. SCFAs are meant to stimulate sodium and water absorption, and patients can be expected to have decreased stool output while receiving supplemental fiber. This approach does not always decrease stool output and may cause abdominal distention from the fermentation of fiber. In patients without a colon or with a short colon and no ICV, dietary fiber would not be expected to work and should be avoided. There are no controlled studies on the use of these materials, and more study is needed.

Children who have SBS with small bowel bacterial overgrowth are more difficult to wean off PN.[57] This suggests that in children who have SBS, bacterial overgrowth should be aggressively managed.

SUMMARY

SBS is the most common cause of intestinal failure in infants and is often caused by necrotizing enterocolitis and intestinal anomalies. Several anatomic factors can be used to predict patients with a poor prognosis. These prognostic factors can be used to guide various therapies and to counsel parents. The few modifiable factors, such as the use of continuous enteral feeding along with PN, should be used to optimize outcome.

REFERENCES

1. O'Keefe SJ, Buchman AL, Fishbein TM, et al. Short bowel syndrome and intestinal failure: consensus definitions and overview. Clin Gastroenterol Hepatol 2006;4(1): 6–10.
2. Buchman AL, Scolapio J, Fryer J. AGA technical review on short bowel syndrome and intestinal transplantation. Gastroenterology 2003;124(4):1111–34.
3. Vanderhoof JA, Langnas AN. Short-bowel syndrome in children and adults. Gastroenterology 1997;113(5):1767–78.
4. Grant D. Intestinal transplantation: 1997 report of the international registry. Intestinal Transplant Registry. Transplantation 1999;67(7):1061–4.
5. Wessel JJ, Kocoshis SA. Nutritional management of infants with short bowel syndrome. Semin Perinatol 2007;31(2):104–11.
6. Sondheimer JM, Cadnapaphornchai M, Sontag M, et al. Predicting the duration of dependence on parenteral nutrition after neonatal intestinal resection. J Pediatr 1998;132(1):80–4.
7. Goulet O, Baglin-Gobet S, Talbotec C, et al. Outcome and long-term growth after extensive small bowel resection in the neonatal period: a survey of 87 children. Eur J Pediatr Surg 2005;15(2):95–101.

8. Touloukian RJ, Smith GJ. Normal intestinal length in preterm infants. J Pediatr Surg 1983;18(6):720–3.
9. Siebert JR. Small-intestine length in infants and children. Am J Dis Child 1980; 134(6):593–5.
10. Sukhotnik I, Siplovich L, Shiloni E, et al. Intestinal adaptation in short-bowel syndrome in infants and children: a collective review. Pediatr Surg Int 2002;18(4): 258–63.
11. Weaver LT, Austin S, Cole TJ. Small intestinal length: a factor essential for gut adaptation. Gut 1991;32(11):1321–3.
12. Wilmore DW. Factors correlating with a successful outcome following extensive intestinal resection in newborn infants. J Pediatr 1972;80(1):88–95.
13. Kubota A, Yonekura T, Hoki M, et al. Total parenteral nutrition-associated intrahepatic cholestasis in infants: 25 years' experience. J Pediatr Surg 2000;35(7): 1049–51.
14. Andorsky DJ, Lund DP, Lillehei CW, et al. Nutritional and other postoperative management of neonates with short bowel syndrome correlates with clinical outcomes. J Pediatr 2001;139(1):27–33.
15. Wales PW, de Silva N, Kim J, et al. Neonatal short bowel syndrome: population-based estimates of incidence and mortality rates. J Pediatr Surg 2004;39(5): 690–5.
16. Quiros-Tejeira RE, Ament ME, Reyen L, et al. Long-term parenteral nutritional support and intestinal adaptation in children with short bowel syndrome: a 25-year experience. J Pediatr 2004;145(2):157–63.
17. Spencer AU, Neaga A, West B, et al. Pediatric short bowel syndrome: redefining predictors of success. Ann Surg 2005;242(3):403–9.
18. Wilmore DW. Growth factors and nutrients in the short bowel syndrome. JPEN J Parenter Enteral Nutr 1999;23(5 Suppl):S117–20.
19. Summers RW, Kent TH, Osborne JW. Effects of drugs, ileal obstruction, and irradiation on rat gastrointestinal propulsion. Gastroenterology 1970;59(5):731–9.
20. Dorney SF, Ament ME, Berquist WE, et al. Improved survival in very short small bowel of infancy with use of long-term parenteral nutrition. J Pediatr 1985; 107(4):521–5.
21. Nightingale JM, Lennard-Jones JE, Gertner DJ, et al. Colonic preservation reduces need for parenteral therapy, increases incidence of renal stones, but does not change high prevalence of gall stones in patients with a short bowel. Gut 1992;33(11):1493–7.
22. Jeppesen PB, Mortensen PB. The influence of a preserved colon on the absorption of medium chain fat in patients with small bowel resection. Gut 1998;43(4): 478–83.
23. DiBaise JK, Young RJ, Vanderhoof JA. Intestinal rehabilitation and the short bowel syndrome: part 1. Am J Gastroenterol 2004;99(7):1386–95.
24. Johnson LR, Copeland EM, Dudrick SJ, et al. Structural and hormonal alterations in the gastrointestinal tract of parenterally fed rats. Gastroenterology 1975;68(5 Pt 1): 1177–83.
25. Greene HL, McCabe DR, Merenstein GB. Protracted diarrhea and malnutrition in infancy: changes in intestinal morphology and disaccharidase activities during treatment with total intravenous nutrition or oral elemental diets. J Pediatr 1975; 87(5):695–704.
26. Stern LE, Huang F, Kemp CJ, et al. Bax is required for increased enterocyte apoptosis after massive small bowel resection. Surgery 2000; 128(2):165–70.

27. Weser E, Babbitt J, Hoban M, et al. Intestinal adaptation. Different growth responses to disaccharides compared with monosaccharides in rat small bowel. Gastroenterology 1986;91(6):1521–7.
28. Tappenden KA. Mechanisms of enteral nutrient-enhanced intestinal adaptation. Gastroenterology 2006;130(2 Suppl. 1):S93–9.
29. Buchan AM. Nutrient tasting and signaling mechanisms in the gut. III. Endocrine cell recognition of luminal nutrients. Am J Physiol 1999;277(6 Pt 1): G1103–7.
30. Furness JB, Kunze WA, Clerc N. Nutrient tasting and signaling mechanisms in the gut. II. The intestine as a sensory organ: neural, endocrine, and immune responses. Am J Physiol 1999;277(5 Pt 1):G922–8.
31. Raybould HE, Cooke HJ, Christofi FL. Sensory mechanisms: transmitters, modulators and reflexes. Neurogastroenterol Motil 2004;16(Suppl 1):60–3.
32. Vanderhoof JA, Grandjean CJ, Burkley KT, et al. Effect of casein versus casein hydrolysate on mucosal adaptation following massive bowel resection in infant rats. J Pediatr Gastroenterol Nutr 1984;3(2):262–7.
33. Grey VL, Garofalo C, Greenberg GR, et al. The adaptation of the small intestine after resection in response to free fatty acids. Am J Clin Nutr 1984;40(6): 1235–42.
34. Goulet O, Ruemmele F, Lacaille F, et al. Irreversible intestinal failure. J Pediatr Gastroenterol Nutr 2004;38(3):250–69.
35. Vanderhoof JA, Park JH, Herrington MK, et al. Effects of dietary menhaden oil on mucosal adaptation after small bowel resection in rats. Gastroenterology 1994; 106(1):94–9.
36. Bach AC, Babayan VK. Medium-chain triglycerides: an update. Am J Clin Nutr 1982;36(5):950–62.
37. Altmann GG. Influence of bile and pancreatic secretions on the size of the intestinal villi in the rat. Am J Anat 1971;132(2):167–77.
38. Weser E, Hernandez MH. Studies of small bowel adaptation after intestinal resection in the rat. Gastroenterology 1971;60(1):69–75.
39. Williamson RC. Intestinal adaptation (second of two parts). Mechanisms of control. N Engl J Med 1978;298(26):1444–50.
40. Booth IW, Lander AD. Short bowel syndrome. Baillieres Clin Gastroenterol 1998; 12(4):739–73.
41. Drucker DJ. Biological actions and therapeutic potential of the glucagon-like peptides. Gastroenterology 2002;122(2):531–44.
42. Jeppesen PB, Mortensen PB. Enhancing bowel adaptation in short bowel syndrome. Curr Gastroenterol Rep 2002;4(4):338–47.
43. Briet F, Flourie B, Achour L, et al. Bacterial adaptation in patients with short bowel and colon in continuity. Gastroenterology 1995;109(5):1446–53.
44. Rhoads JM, Argenzio RA, Chen W, et al. L-glutamine stimulates intestinal cell proliferation and activates mitogen-activated protein kinases. Am J Physiol 1997; 272(5 Pt 1):G943–53.
45. Byrne TA, Morrissey TB, Nattakom TV, et al. Growth hormone, glutamine, and a modified diet enhance nutrient absorption in patients with severe short bowel syndrome. JPEN J Parenter Enteral Nutr 1995;19(4):296–302.
46. Shulman DI, Hu CS, Duckett G, et al. Effects of short-term growth hormone therapy in rats undergoing 75% small intestinal resection. J Pediatr Gastroenterol Nutr 1992;14(1):3–11.
47. Hodin RA, Meng S, Nguyen D. Immediate-early gene expression in EGF-stimulated intestinal epithelial cells. J Surg Res 1994;56(6):500–4.

48. Stern LE, Falcone RA Jr, Huang F, et al. Epidermal growth factor alters the bax:bcl-w ratio following massive small bowel resection. J Surg Res 2000; 91(1):38–42.
49. Bines J, Francis D, Hill D. Reducing parenteral requirement in children with short bowel syndrome: impact of an amino acid-based complete infant formula. J Pediatr Gastroenterol Nutr 1998;26(2):123–8.
50. Mazon A, Solera E, Alentado N, et al. Frequent IgE sensitization to latex, cow's milk, and egg in children with short bowel syndrome. Pediatr Allergy Immunol 2008;19(2):180–3.
51. Powell GK. Enterocolitis in low-birth-weight infants associated with milk and soy protein intolerance. J Pediatr 1976;88(5):840–4.
52. Taylor SF, Sondheimer JM, Sokol RJ, et al. Noninfectious colitis associated with short gut syndrome in infants. J Pediatr 1991;119(1 (Pt 1)):24–8.
53. Richardson L, Banerjee S, Rabe H. What is the evidence on the practice of mucous fistula refeeding in neonates with short bowel syndrome? J Pediatr Gastroenterol Nutr 2006;43(2):267–70.
54. Wong KK, Lan LC, Lin SC, et al. Mucous fistula refeeding in premature neonates with enterostomies. J Pediatr Gastroenterol Nutr 2004;39(1):43–5.
55. Al-Harbi K, Walton JM, Gardner V, et al. Mucous fistula refeeding in neonates with short bowel syndrome. J Pediatr Surg 1999;34(7):1100–3.
56. Finkel Y, Brown G, Smith HL, et al. The effects of a pectin-supplemented elemental diet in a boy with short gut syndrome. Acta Paediatr Scand 1990;79(10): 983–6.
57. Kaufman SS, Loseke CA, Lupo JV, et al. Influence of bacterial overgrowth and intestinal inflammation on duration of parenteral nutrition in children with short bowel syndrome. J Pediatr 1997;131(3):356–61.

Anemia in the Preterm Infant: Erythropoietin Versus Erythrocyte Transfusion—It's not that Simple

Isabelle Von Kohorn, MD, Richard A. Ehrenkranz, MD*

KEYWORDS

- Erythropoietin • Transfusion • Very low birth weight
- Infant • Premature

Since the late 1980s recombinant human erythropoietin (r-EPO) has been studied as an alternative to packed red blood cell (RBC) transfusion in the treatment of anemia of prematurity (AOP). Two decades later hematologists and neonatologists have not reached consensus on when r-EPO should be used in very low birth weight (VLBW, <1500 g) infants. Initial trials and reports focused on the use of r-EPO to prevent or treat AOP with the goal of eliminating RBC transfusion. Later studies found response to r-EPO was influenced by (1) significant volumes of blood loss, especially in the smallest, sickest infants, (2) the physiology of r-EPO, which requires days to weeks to increase hematocrit, and (3) the need for supplementation with protein, iron, folate, and vitamin E. In addition, recent reports have warned of undesirable side effects, including a possible increase in retinopathy of prematurity (ROP) with early administration of r-EPO.

This article reviews the history of AOP treatment, starting with the physiology of AOP and the development of specialized transfusion techniques for the VLBW population. It then describes the initial trials of r-EPO to prevent or treat AOP and the implementation of restrictive RBC transfusion criteria. Finally, it discusses recent concerns about the side effects of r-EPO administration and outlines therapies that may limit the need for r-EPO administration, shifting the cost–benefit balance away from treatment with r-EPO to prevent or treat AOP.

Dr. Von Kohorn was supported by National Institute of Child Health and Human Development Training Grant T32HD07094.
Division of Perinatal Medicine, Department of Pediatrics, Yale University School of Medicine, 333 Cedar Street, New Haven, CT 06520-8064, USA
* Corresponding author.
E-mail address: richard.ehrenkranz@yale.edu (R.A. Ehrenkranz).

Clin Perinatol 36 (2009) 111–123
doi:10.1016/j.clp.2008.09.009 perinatology.theclinics.com

PHYSIOLOGY OF ANEMIA OF PREMATURITY

During the third trimester of gestation, fetal RBC production transitions from hepatic to marrow erythropoiesis. The glycoprotein hormone EPO is the driving force behind RBC production, and fetal hematocrit rises in conjunction with fetal levels of EPO.[1] EPO production switches near term from liver to kidney; the "hypoxia sensor" of the liver is much less sensitive than the kidney. Nonetheless, fetal EPO production is responsive to decreased RBC mass and rises appropriately in response to pathologic conditions, for example, in the setting of erythroblastosis faetalis.[2]

After birth, infants display a physiologic drop in hematocrit accompanied by a fall in blood EPO levels. Although cord blood levels of EPO are high, little EPO is found in full-term neonatal blood from the second day of life until 6 to 8 weeks of age.[3] This decrease in EPO and subsequent lack of erythropoiesis after birth leads to the "physiologic nadir" of hematocrit around 3 months of life in the term infant. Oxygen delivery to tissues seems to be preserved in full-term infants at the physiologic nadir, and symptoms of anemia are rarely seen without exacerbating factors.

Premature infants experience a lower nadir of hematocrit than full-term infants, resulting in a normocytic, normochromic anemia coincident with a low reticulocyte count and low EPO level. The nadir is inversely related to gestational age. This condition is termed "anemia of prematurity."[4] Some premature infants tolerate AOP well. Others, especially the smallest, sickest infants, develop signs and symptoms such as tachycardia, tachypnea, apnea and bradycardia, poor weight gain, oxygen requirement, diminished activity, pallor, and elevated serum lactate.[4,5] These symptoms can lead to increased length of stay in the hospital and infectious complications if in-dwelling lines are needed for nutritional support and hydration.

Physiologic studies of the preterm infant indicate that stimulation of endogenous EPO is governed by hypoxia and anemia, as it is in the adult population; compared with adults, however, preterm infants have been shown to have a relatively low EPO level for a given hematocrit.[6] Further investigation demonstrated the importance of factors other than hematocrit governing RBC production in the preterm infant. In 1977 Stockman and colleagues[7] determined that oxygen unloading capacity influences erythropoiesis. They reported that hemoglobin levels in premature infants with a right-shifted oxyhemoglobin dissociation curve, because of a lower proportion of fetal hemoglobin (HbF < 30%), fell 2 to 3 g/dL lower than those infants with a left-shifted dissociation curve (HbF > 60%) before endogenous EPO production resumed. In 1984 Stockman and colleagues[8] published data showing that endogenous EPO also is sensitive to dissolved oxygen; central venous oxygen tension varies inversely with EPO level in the premature infant. Still, the most premature infants seem to display a much lower mean EPO level in the face of similar "available oxygen" than seen in adults.[9] Interestingly, these data about the physiology of AOP indicate that RBC transfusion, which increases the proportion of hemoglobin A in the preterm neonate, may contribute to a lower nadir of hematocrit by improving oxygen availability to the tissues and lowering the stimulus for EPO production.[5]

The natural history of AOP often is exacerbated by iatrogenic factors such as low hematocrit at birth and postnatal phlebotomy as well as by endogenous factors such as rapid infant growth, shortened RBC lifespan, and expansion of blood volume. Technological advances have decreased the volume of blood needed for neonatal laboratory studies. Despite these improvements, many VLBW infants do not tolerate exacerbation of AOP and require treatment.

TREATING ANEMIA OF PREMATURITY

Red Blood Cell Transfusion

The incidence of AOP has increased with the greater survival of VLBW infants, and treatment for symptomatic AOP has become common. For many years RBC transfusion was the only effective treatment for severe anemia. AOP is refractory to other therapies, including supplementation with iron, vitamin E, and folic acid. Early transfusion protocols called for infants to be transfused with "fresh" RBCs (less than 7 days old). The goal was to maximize the life of cells in vivo and to minimize the risk of hyperkalemia and acidosis. At approximately 15 mL/kg body weight, tiny babies require relatively small volumes of blood per transfusion. To conserve a valuable resource, a procedure termed the "cow technique" was used: multiple infants were cross-matched against a single RBC unit which was used to provide transfusions to multiple infants until depleted.[10] Because VLBW infants often received several transfusions to maintain adequate blood volume and hematocrit, exposure to multiple donors was common.

In the early 1990s blood banks serving neonatal units began to dedicate a single unit of blood to each infant. The unit is accessed and resealed under sterile conditions and can be used for multiple transfusions until the unit's original expiration date, 35 to 42 days after collection. This method limits each neonate's donor exposure.[11–15] Even with donor-sparing blood-banking techniques, blood transfusion has risks. Blood-borne infection is a primary concern. The risk of hepatitis B, hepatitis C, HIV, cytomegalovirus, and Epstein-Barr virus transmission is as low as it has ever been, because of donor screening and postcollection testing and processing techniques. Still, emerging infections exist and are a risk.[16] Treatments for AOP that further limit or eliminate the need for blood transfusion are desirable.

Until the 1990s the only treatment for symptomatic AOP was RBC transfusion. Most infants born prematurely before 30 weeks' gestation needed a RBC transfusion during their initial hospitalization. Early transfusions (in the first 1 to 2 weeks of life) typically were given for acute blood loss caused by blood sampling during critical illness. Late transfusions were given after 2 weeks of life for symptomatic AOP. Criteria for transfusion for AOP were largely unstandardized, however, and transfusion practices varied widely.[17–20] A common indication for transfusion was "blood out," or blood losses caused by phlebotomy (most likely to be seen in the smallest, sickest infants). It was assumed that replacing losses routinely would be beneficial. Likewise, many clinicians transfused RBCs based on an absolute hemoglobin or hematocrit level. Evidence accumulated that there was no benefit to either practice.[20–22]

Erythropoietin to Limit Red Blood Cell Transfusion

In 1987 the first clinical trial of r-EPO, in adults who had end-stage renal disease, demonstrated that r-EPO treatment was associated with an increased hematocrit and reduction in RBC transfusions.[23] There was reason to believe that the synthetic hormone could help VLBW infants. Although the pathophysiology of AOP was not understood completely, premature infants were known to have a low EPO level in the setting of a low hematocrit.[8] In addition, in vitro studies demonstrated that both circulating erythroid progenitor cells and those found in the bone marrow were highly sensitive to r-EPO.[24–26]

In 1990 the first pilot study of the effect of EPO on AOP was published.[27] Many subsequent randomized, controlled trials attempted to elucidate the effect of r-EPO on AOP and to develop optimal patient selection, dosing, nutritional supplementation, and timing of therapy with the goal of limiting RBC transfusion in premature neonates.[28–42] Ohls[43] summarized many of these studies in her excellent review in this journal in 2000.

The initial r-EPO trials in VLBW infants showed that administration of the drug resulted in reticulocytosis with subsequent increase in hematocrit.[30,33] Furthermore, most r-EPO–exposed infants received fewer and lower-volume RBC transfusion during the study period.[29,30,32–34,36] This finding was strongest in stable, growing preterm infants, most of whom had received multiple blood transfusions before study entry.[30,33] The first study of r-EPO administration to extremely low birth weight (ELBW, <1000 g) infants indicated that the hormone also helped avoid transfusion in these smallest, sickest infants.[34] Later randomized, controlled studies, however, did not find a significant reduction in RBC transfusion in ELBW patients.[40,42]

Two different timing strategies were employed in the r-EPO trials. "Early" treatment (before 8 days of age) with r-EPO was used to prevent AOP.[30,40] "Late" treatment (at or after 8 days of age) protocols were designed to treat AOP and to decrease RBC transfusions during convalescence.[28,33] Both regimens were shown to reduce RBC transfusion.[29,30,32–34,36] Despite hopes that early r-EPO administration would be superior to late administration in preventing RBC transfusion, subsequent studies comparing the two practices found no significant difference in this outcome.[39,41,44]

If r-EPO reduces RBC transfusion in VLBW infants, why, then, is its administration not routine? One answer lies in the magnitude of the drug's effect. Although r-EPO administration did reduce RBC transfusion in many trials, questions persist about whether the absolute reduction in transfusion volume achieved (milliliters per kilogram per patient) is of clinical significance in this era of single-donor, dedicated RBC unit transfusion protocols.[41,45–47] A more pertinent question today is whether r-EPO prevents exposure to multiple blood donors. To date, no multicenter randomized, controlled studies have answered this question.[42]

The initial r-EPO studies also shed light on optimal dosing and nutritional supplementation. The very first r-EPO studies used doses roughly equivalent to adult dosing protocols. These doses were found to be insufficient for premature infants, who require larger doses of the hormone per kilogram of bodyweight than adults because of a higher volume of distribution and faster elimination.[48,49] Although infants require relatively high doses of r-EPO, a therapeutic threshold does seem to exist above which no further EPO response is obtained. Head-to-head comparison showed that "high-dose" (1500 units/kg/wk) administration of r-EPO did not reduce RBC transfusion in ELBW infants more than "low dose" (750 units/kg/wk) administration.[38] Finally, it is well documented that infants receiving r-EPO have increased nutritional needs. Adequate protein and vitamin E administration, either enterally or parenterally, is essential to achieve full benefit of r-EPO. Infants receiving r-EPO have lower ferritin levels and hypochromic RBCs, necessitating supplementation with iron.[31] Both intravenous and oral iron supplementation have been shown to maintain serum ferritin levels and to support erythropoiesis.[33,35,37,50]

Restrictive Transfusion Criteria

Perhaps the most important finding of the first randomized, controlled trials of r-EPO was that implementing standard criteria for RBC transfusion alone safely reduced the number of transfusions administered, even for patients in the control group.[20,29,32,33] Before the r-EPO trials, investigators studied whether so-called "liberal" transfusion criteria would alleviate symptoms of AOP and reported mixed results. One study did not find a routine positive effect of RBC transfusion on tachypnea, tachycardia, or the incidence of apnea and bradycardia.[19] Another found a significant decrease in apnea and periodic breathing after RBC transfusion.[51]

In their multicenter study of r-EPO in growing preterm neonates, Shannon and colleagues[33] chose restrictive transfusion guidelines when standardizing their transfusion protocol across participating institutions. These conservative, staged transfusion criteria were based on oxygen and ventilatory requirements as well as on reticulocyte production and clinical symptoms (tachycardia, apnea and bradycardia, and somatic growth). Subsequently, comparative trials tipped the balance from liberal transfusion protocols toward restrictive criteria.[20–22,52,53] Bifano and colleagues[53] found no benefit in maintaining a hematocrit higher than 32 as compared with a lower hematocrit (<30) with regard to weight gain, days on a ventilator, total hospital days, 1-year weight gain and head growth, and neurodevelopmental outcome. Kirpalani and colleagues[52] found no difference in negative outcomes (death, ROP, bronchopulmonary dysplasia, brain ultrasound) with restrictive transfusion criteria. Although one study did find more apnea, intraventricular hemorrhage and periventricular leukomalacia in a restrictive transfusion group,[54] these risks have not been confirmed by others.[52,53,55] Compared with earlier liberal transfusion practices, these more restrictive criteria limit the number of transfusions (and, therefore, donor exposures) without apparent harm to the infant (**Box 1**).

Since their introduction, restrictive transfusion criteria have become the norm in many major newborn ICUs. Still, even with restrictive transfusion guidelines, there may be overtransfusion.[57] A recent review of transfusion practices and guidelines for neonates recommends further studies of "need-based transfusions" through the creation of a "transfusion marker" such as measurement of the adequacy of oxygen delivery, improvement in signs or symptoms of anemia, and resolution of cardiovascular impairment, possibly through echocardiographic measurement.[55] Ideally, such a marker would, simultaneously, limit RBC transfusions and the risks of anemia.

REFINING THE USE OF RECOMBINANT ERYTHROPOIETIN

In the new millennium attempts to refine the patient population and timing of r-EPO use for optimal benefit have been tempered by increasing evidence of potential harm caused by the drug. There still are no absolute indications for the use of r-EPO in the preterm population, and there are no data to suggest that r-EPO dramatically decreases or eliminates the need for RBC transfusions in preterm infants.[58] Some investigators have hypothesized that r-EPO will be of greatest benefit in the preterm population at highest risk for transfusion. Still, even in this select population, data suggest that r-EPO does not prevent a significant number or volume of transfusions.[4,42] In a subgroup analysis from Ohls'[40] 2001 report, r-EPO did prevent RBC transfusion in ELBW babies 1 month of age, leading to the hypothesis that the drug might prevent second-donor exposure in that population.[41]

Several meta-analyses have lent strength to this theory that r-EPO prevents late transfusion in preterm neonates, although the effect size is small.[45,47,59] One meta-analysis evaluated reduction in RBC transfusion in VLBW infants using late r-EPO. For this outcome 19 studies enrolling 912 infants were included. The composite number-needed-to-treat for benefit was 5. The weighted mean reduction in number of transfusions was 0.78 transfusions, and the total weighted mean RBC volume reduction was 7 mL. Post hoc analysis of the highest-quality studies showed a smaller effect size than seen in the primary analysis.[45] The clinical relevance of sparing this relatively small number and volume of late transfusions remains debatable, because most VLBW infants receive transfusions early in life.

Box 1
Transfusion criteria: then and now

Typical RBC transfusion criteria for VLBW infants before 1990[10]

Indications for transfusion:

When 5% to 10% of the infant's blood volume has been removed in a period of less than 48 hours, it should be replaced with packed RBCs.

In infants weighing less than 1500 g, hemoglobin values should be maintained in excess of 13 g/dL during the first week of life.

In convalescent infants (3–8 weeks of age), clinical symptoms or signs (persistent tachycardia or tachypnea, lethargy, easy fatigue with feedings, poor weight gain, central venous oxygen tension lower than 25 mm Hg) are indications for transfusion.

Current conservative RBC transfusion criteria for VLBW infants[56]

1. For infants requiring moderate or significant ventilation (defined as mean airway pressure > 8 cm H_2O and fraction of inspired oxygen [FIO_2] > 0.40): transfuse if hematocrit $\leq$ 35% (hemoglobin $\leq$ 11 g/dL).
2. For infants requiring minimal mechanical ventilation, defined as all other infants requiring (a) positive-pressure ventilation or (b) continuous positive airway pressure (endotracheal or nasal continuous positive airway pressure) of 6 cm H_2O or higher and FIO_2 higher than 0.40: transfuse if hematocrit is 30% or higher (hemoglobin $\leq$ 10 g/dL).
3. For infants receiving supplemental oxygen who do not require mechanical ventilation: transfuse if hematocrit 25% or higher (hemoglobin $\leq$ 8 g/dL) and one or more of the following is present:
   - Tachycardia (heart rate > 180 beats/min) or tachypnea (respiratory rate > 80 breaths/min) lasting more than 24 hours
   - An increased oxygen requirement from the previous 48 hours, defined as:
     (a) A fourfold or greater increase in nasal cannula flow (ie, from 0.25 L/min to 1 L/min) OR
     (b) An increase in nasal continuous positive airway pressure of 20% or more from previous 48 hours (ie, from 5 to 6 cm H_2O) OR
     (c) An absolute and sustained increase in FIO_2 of 0.10 or higher (via oxyhood, nasal continuous positive airway pressure, or cannula)
   - Weight gain of less than 10 g/kg/d over the previous 4 days while receiving 100 or more kcal/kg/d
   - Multiple episodes of apnea and bradycardia ($\geq$ 10 episodes in a 24-hour period or two or more episodes in a 24-hour period requiring bag-mask ventilation) while receiving therapeutic doses of methylxanthines
   - Undergoing surgery
4. For infants without any symptoms: transfuse if hematocrit is 20% or lower (hemoglobin < 7 g/dL) and the absolute reticulocyte count is lower than 100,000 cells/uL (<2%)

RISKS OF RECOMBINANT ERYTHROPOIETIN ADMINISTRATION

In the initial r-EPO trials a primary concern was whether administration of the hormone to premature infants would redirect hematopoiesis preferentially toward the erythrocyte line, resulting in neutropenia and increasing the rate of infection in exposed infants. Those studies found a decrease in circulating and myeloid neutrophils and precursors, but no increased rate of infection was reported.[27,28] These early results were confirmed by the randomized, controlled studies that found wide variation in the neutrophil counts of treated patients and did not show increased rates of infections in those receiving r-EPO.[33,36]

More recent studies in the adult literature have raised new concerns about r-EPO. In 2006 two studies published in the *New England Journal of Medicine* found that administration of increased amounts of r-EPO to patients who had chronic kidney disease did not improve survival and might be harmful. The first trial, Cardiovascular Risk Reduction by Early Anemia Treatment with Epoetin Beta, enrolled 603 patients who had stage III or IV chronic kidney disease in 94 different centers in 22 countries. Seventy-five percent of intervention subjects and 83% of control subjects were followed for 2 years after enrollment. The investigators found that administering r-EPO to achieve a target hemoglobin level of 13 to 15 g/dL compared with 10.5 to 11.5 g/dL did not reduce the incidence of first cardiovascular events, although those in the treatment group did report improved general health and physical function.[60]

The second trial, Correction of Hemogloblin and Outcomes in Renal Insufficiency, enrolled 1432 patients who had chronic kidney disease at 130 United States centers. The investigators found an increased risk of the composite primary outcome (time to death, myocardial infarction, hospitalization for congestive heart failure, or stroke) and no improvement in quality of life in the group that received r-EPO to achieve a higher hemoglobin level.[61] An editorial in the same issue of the *New England Journal of Medicine* recommended caution with regard to normalization of RBC levels via r-EPO in patients who had chronic kidney failure.[62] Extrapolating these results to VLBW infants, maintenance of a high-normal hematocrit through r-EPO administration may not be warranted, because an evaluation of liberal transfusion criteria to maintain a high-normal hematocrit did not show any benefit.[52,54]

Perhaps of more concern for neonates, r-EPO has been linked to neovascularization and tumor progression. Elucidation of the physiology of EPO indicates that its cellular pathways and targets result in angiogenesis.[63,64] EPO has been associated with pathologic blood vessel growth, (eg, in proliferative diabetic retinopathy).[65] Furthermore, in at least three published adult trials, r-EPO has been linked to decreased survival for some patients who had cancer because of tumor progression related to neovascularization.[66–69] Several clinical trials of darbepoetin (a modified r-EPO protein with a longer half life) were stopped when increased mortality was found in the treatment group.[69]

No studies have reported r-EPO–associated neoplasm in neonates, and, although a few studies have suggested that ROP, a disorder of vascular proliferation, may be exacerbated by r-EPO, there are no definitive data demonstrating this outcome.[44,70,71] A meta-analysis of early r-EPO administration and one comparing early versus late r-EPO reported unpublished data regarding ROP.[39,41,44,46] Only one study included in the meta-analyses found a statistically significant increase in any ROP with early compared with late administration of r-EPO.[39] No study included in the meta-analysis found the rate of ROP stage III or higher to be significantly different in infants treated early with r-EPO.[44] If there is a link between r-EPO and ROP, perhaps infants are at most risk if the drug is continued past 34 weeks' postmenstrual age, when both the vascular phase of ROP and endogenous reticulocytosis begin.

COST–BENEFIT ANALYSIS OF ERYTHROPOIETIN USE

Many studies in the 1990s attempted to capture the costs of EPO versus RBC transfusion.[30,32,72–75] The results varied, and the relative benefit of r-EPO for AOP is related to the study design (early versus late treatment; liberal versus restrictive transfusion criteria), patient population, and value assigned to complex outcomes. Not all studies took into account the risk of infection transmission, exclusion of which would lower the cost of transfusion.[32] Studies evaluating the cost of treating stable, growing premature infants with r-EPO are more likely to favor RBC transfusion over r-EPO than are studies focused on sicker premature infants at greater risk for RBC transfusion.[72,74] An up-to-date, comprehensive analysis could be helpful to clinicians and should include at least all the items listed in **Box 2**.

Perhaps the most difficult item to evaluate is the psychosocial burden imposed on the family, patient, and caregivers by transfusion or the potential risk of transfusion-related infection, however rare that transmission may be. Although most such infections now can be be cured (bacterial infection) or managed as chronic diseases (HIV, hepatitis C), significant social stigma and psychologic burden may be associated with acquisition. The value assigned to avoiding such infection is highly subjective and therefore is difficult to model accurately.

FUTURE DIRECTIONS

Current use of r-EPO in the VLBW population varies widely in the United States, and the future use of the medication is not easy to predict. New technologies, improvements in transfusion practice, and further understanding of the side effects of r-EPO may change the equation. Longer-acting darbepoetin has become the drug of choice for adult patients requiring EPO replacement. As yet there are no large multicenter, randomized, controlled trials to determine its safety and efficacy in the neonatal population. One study indicates that darbepoetin may increase reticulocytosis in convalescent VLBW infants. The cost savings achieved for adults treated with darbepoetin versus r-EPO may not hold true in the neonatal population, because newborns may require larger per-kilogram body weight doses at more frequent intervals than children or adults.[76,77] Still, the possibility of reduced dosing, necessitating fewer needle sticks, is attractive in this population that is susceptible to infection.

Strategies to increase autologous blood volume would tip the balance away from r-EPO. Autologous transfusion with banked cord blood is a logical adjunct, although most institutions are not equipped to offer this therapy.[55] A related practice is delayed umbilical cord clamping. Delaying clamping (eg, by 30 seconds) has been shown to

Box 2
Variables influencing cost–benefit studies of r-EPO treatment

r-EPO units/kg/wk

Weeks of r-EPO therapy

r-EPO price and administration costs (including waste of r-EPO)

Adverse effects of r-EPO (immediate and long term)

Number and volume of transfusion with/without r-EPO (using restrictive transfusion criteria)

Transfusion administration costs (typing and cross-matching, blood products, blood screening and processing, set-up charges, nursing costs)

Transfusion-related complications (infection, graft versus host disease, necrotizing enterocolitis)

Cost of technology to minimize transfusions

increase birth hematocrit and decrease the need for RBC transfusion in VLBW infants. In a few recent studies delayed clamping also has been associated with lower rates of intraventricular hemorrhage and improved neurodevelopmental outcome.[78–80]

Reducing blood sampling through microanalytical techniques and more judicious use of blood tests reduced the need for RBC transfusions in the 1990s. Further minimizing phlebotomy by using point-of-care technologies that use 0.1 mL of blood compared with the 0.3 to 0.5 mL needed for most laboratory microassays, in-line monitors, or noninvasive testing would reduce blood loss and transfusion requirements further. Developments that would tip the balance toward use of r-EPO are the emergence of new blood-borne infections or a compromise of the blood supply, other increases in costs of RBC administration, or the discovery of other beneficial effects of r-EPO.

SUMMARY

The jury is still out with regard to the role of r-EPO therapy in the VLBW population, and therefore the use of r-EPO varies widely throughout the United States. At the Newborn Special Care Unit, Yale New Haven Children's Hospital, VLBW infants are not routinely treated with r-EPO.

REFERENCES

1. Finne P, Halvorsen S. Regulation of erythropoiesis in the fetus and newborn. Arch Dis Child 1972;47(255):683–7.
2. Finne P. Erythropoietin levels in cord blood as an indicator of intrauterine hypoxia. Acta Paediatr Scand 1966;55(5):478–89.
3. Halvorsen S. Plasma erythropoietin levels in cord blood and in blood during the first weeks of life. Acta Paediatr 1963;52:425–35.
4. Ohls R. Erythropoietin to prevent and treat the anemia of prematurity. Curr Opin Pediatr 1999;11(2):108–14.
5. Stockman JA. Anemia of prematurity. Current concepts in the issue of when to transfuse. Pediatr Clin North Am 1986;33(1):111–28.
6. Brown M, Phibbs R, Garcia J, et al. Postnatal changes in erythropoietin levels in untransfused premature infants. J Pediatr 1983;103(4):612–7.
7. Stockman J, Garcia J, Oski F. The anemia of prematurity. Factors governing the erythropoietin response. N Engl J Med 1977;296(12):647–50.
8. Stockman JA, Graeber J, Clark D, et al. Anemia of prematurity: determinants of the erythropoietin response. J Pediatr 1984;105(5):786–92.
9. Brown M, Garcia J, Phibbs R, et al. Decreased response of plasma immunoreactive erythropoietin to "available oxygen" in anemia of prematurity. J Pediatr 1984;105(5):793–8.
10. Oski FA, Naiman JL. Hematologic problems in the newborn, vol. IV. 3rd edition. Philadelphia: W.B. Saunders Company; 1982.
11. Liu E, Mannino F, Lane T. Prospective, randomized trial of the safety and efficacy of a limited donor exposure transfusion program for premature neonates. J Pediatr 1994;125(1):92–6.
12. Wood A, Wilson N, Skacel P, et al. Reducing donor exposure in preterm infants requiring multiple blood transfusions. Arch Dis Child Fetal Neonatal Ed 1995;72(1):F29–33.
13. Cook S, Gunter J, Wissel M. Effective use of a strategy using assigned red cell units to limit donor exposure for neonatal patients. Transfusion 1993;33(5):379–83.

14. Jain R, Jarosz C, Myers T. Decreasing blood donor exposure in the neonates by using dedicated donor transfusions. Transfus Sci 1997;18(2):199–203.
15. Wang-Rodriguez J, Mannino F, Liu E, et al. A novel strategy to limit blood donor exposure and blood waste in multiply transfused premature infants. Transfusion 1996;36(1):64–70.
16. Bifano EM. Traditional and nontraditional approaches to the prevention and treatment of neonatal anemia. NeoReviews 2000;1(4):69–73.
17. Bifano E, Smith F, Borer J. Relationship between determinants of oxygen delivery and respiratory abnormalities in preterm infants with anemia. J Pediatr 1992; 120(2 Pt 1):292–6.
18. Ross M, Christensen R, Rothstein G, et al. A randomized trial to develop criteria for administering erythrocyte transfusions to anemic preterm infants 1 to 3 months of age. J Perinatol 1989;9(3):246–53.
19. Keyes W, Donohue P, Spivak J, et al. Assessing the need for transfusion of premature infants and role of hematocrit, clinical signs, and erythropoietin level. Pediatrics 1989;84(3):412–7.
20. Bifano E, Curran T. Minimizing donor blood exposure in the neonatal intensive care unit. Current trends and future prospects. Clin Perinatol 1995;22(3):657–69.
21. Lachance C, Chessex P, Fouron J, et al. Myocardial, erythropoietic, and metabolic adaptations to anemia of prematurity. J Pediatr 1994;125(2):278–82.
22. Bifano E. Defining symptomatology in anemia of prematurity. Pediatr Res 1993; 33:281a.
23. Eschbach J, Egrie J, Downing M, et al. Correction of the anemia of end-stage renal disease with recombinant human erythropoietin. Results of a combined phase I and II clinical trial. N Engl J Med 1987;316(2):73–8.
24. Shannon K, Naylor G, Torkildson J, et al. Circulating erythroid progenitors in the anemia of prematurity. N Engl J Med 1987;317(12):728–33.
25. Rhondeau S, Christensen R, Ross M, et al. Responsiveness to recombinant human erythropoietin of marrow erythroid progenitors from infants with the "anemia of prematurity". J Pediatr 1988;112(6):935–40.
26. Gallagher P, Ehrenkranz R. Erythropoietin therapy for anemia of prematurity. Clin Perinatol 1993;20(1):169–91.
27. Halpérin D, Wacker P, Lacourt G, et al. Effects of recombinant human erythropoietin in infants with the anemia of prematurity: a pilot study. J Pediatr 1990;116(5): 779–86.
28. Ohls R, Christensen R. Recombinant erythropoietin compared with erythrocyte transfusion in the treatment of anemia of prematurity. J Pediatr 1991;119(5): 781–8.
29. Carnielli V, Montini G, Da Riol R, et al. Effect of high doses of human recombinant erythropoietin on the need for blood transfusions in preterm infants. J Pediatr 1992;121(1):98–102.
30. Maier R, Obladen M, Scigalla P, et al. The effect of epoetin beta (recombinant human erythropoietin) on the need for transfusion in very-low-birth-weight infants. European Multicentre Erythropoietin Study Group. N Engl J Med 1994;330(17): 1173–8.
31. Meyer M, Meyer J, Commerford A, et al. Recombinant human erythropoietin in the treatment of the anemia of prematurity: results of a double-blind, placebo-controlled study. Pediatrics 1994;93(6 Pt 1):918–23.
32. Ohls R, Osborne K, Christensen R. Efficacy and cost analysis of treating very low birth weight infants with erythropoietin during their first two weeks of life: a randomized, placebo-controlled trial. J Pediatr 1995;126(3):421–6.

33. Shannon K, Keith JF III, Mentzer W, et al. Recombinant human erythropoietin stimulates erythropoiesis and reduces erythrocyte transfusions in very low birth weight preterm infants. Pediatrics 1995;95(1):1–8.
34. Al-Kharfy T, Smyth J, Wadsworth L, et al. Erythropoietin therapy in neonates at risk of having bronchopulmonary dysplasia and requiring multiple transfusions. J Pediatr 1996;129(1):89–96.
35. Bechensteen A, Hågå P, Halvorsen S, et al. Effect of low and moderate doses of recombinant human erythropoietin on the haematological response in premature infants on a high protein and iron intake. Eur J Pediatr 1997;156(1):56–61.
36. Ohls R, Harcum J, Schibler K, et al. The effect of erythropoietin on the transfusion requirements of preterm infants weighing 750 grams or less: a randomized, double-blind, placebo-controlled study. J Pediatr 1997;131(5):661–5.
37. Kumar P, Shankaran S, Krishnan R. Recombinant human erythropoietin therapy for treatment of anemia of prematurity in very low birth weight infants: a randomized, double-blind, placebo-controlled trial. J Perinatol 1998;18(3):173–7.
38. Maier R, Obladen M, Kattner E, et al. High-versus low-dose erythropoietin in extremely low birth weight infants. The European Multicenter rhEPO Study Group. J Pediatr 1998;132(5):866–70.
39. Donato H, Vain N, Rendo P, et al. Effect of early versus late administration of human recombinant erythropoietin on transfusion requirements in premature infants: results of a randomized, placebo-controlled, multicenter trial. Pediatrics 2000; 105(5):1066–72.
40. Ohls R, Ehrenkranz R, Wright L, et al. Effects of early erythropoietin therapy on the transfusion requirements of preterm infants below 1250 grams birth weight: a multicenter, randomized, controlled trial. Pediatrics 2001;108(4):934–42.
41. Maier R, Obladen M, Müller-Hansen I, et al. Early treatment with erythropoietin beta ameliorates anemia and reduces transfusion requirements in infants with birth weights below 1000 g. J Pediatr 2002;141(1):8–15.
42. Meyer M, Sharma E, Carsons M. Recombinant erythropoietin and blood transfusion in selected preterm infants. Arch Dis Child Fetal Neonatal Ed 2003;88(1): F41–5.
43. Ohls R. The use of erythropoietin in neonates. Clin Perinatol 2000;27(3):681–96.
44. Aher S, Ohlsson A. Early versus late erythropoietin for preventing red blood cell transfusion in preterm and/or low birth weight infants. Cochrane Database Syst Rev 2006;(3):CD004865.
45. Aher S, Ohlsson A. Late erythropoietin for preventing red blood cell transfusion in preterm and/or low birth weight infants. Cochrane Database Syst Rev 2006;(3):CD004868.
46. Ohlsson A, Aher S. Early erythropoietin for preventing red blood cell transfusion in preterm and/or low birth weight infants. Cochrane Database Syst Rev 2006;(3):CD004863.
47. Kotto-Kome A, Garcia M, Calhoun D, et al. Effect of beginning recombinant erythropoietin treatment within the first week of life, among very-low-birth-weight neonates, on "early" and "late" erythrocyte transfusions: a meta-analysis. J Perinatol 2004;24(1):24–9.
48. George J, Bracco C, Shannon K, et al. Age-related differences in erythropoietic response to recombinant human erythropoietin: comparison in adult and infant rhesus monkeys. Pediatr Res 1990;28(6):567–71.
49. Widness J, Veng-Pedersen P, Modi N, et al. Developmental changes in erythropoietin (EPO) pharmacokinetics in fetal and neonatal sheep. Pediatr Res 1990; 28(3):284A.

50. Meyer M, Haworth C, Meyer J, et al. A comparison of oral and intravenous iron supplementation in preterm infants receiving recombinant erythropoietin. J Pediatr 1996;129(2):258–63.
51. DeMaio J, Harris M, Deuber C, et al. Effect of blood transfusion on apnea frequency in growing premature infants. J Pediatr 1989;114(6):1039–41.
52. Kirpalani H, Whyte R, Andersen C, et al. The premature infants in need of transfusion (PINT) study: a randomized, controlled trial of a restrictive (low) versus liberal (high) transfusion threshold for extremely low birth weight infants. J Pediatr 2006;149(3):301–7.
53. Bifano E, Bode M, D'Eugenio D. Prospective randomized trial of high vs. low hematocrit in extremely low birth weight (ELBW) infants: one year growth and neurodevelopmental outcome. Pediatr Res 2002;51:325a.
54. Bell E, Strauss R, Widness J, et al. Randomized trial of liberal versus restrictive guidelines for red blood cell transfusion in preterm infants. Pediatrics 2005; 115(6):1685–91.
55. Ohls R. Transfusions in the preterm infant. NeoReviews 2007;8(9):e377–86.
56. Yale-New Haven Children's Hospital Newborn Special Care Unit Guidelines. Red blood cell transfusion criteria. New Haven (CT); 2006.
57. Widness J, Madan A, Grindeanu L, et al. Reduction in red blood cell transfusions among preterm infants: results of a randomized trial with an in-line blood gas and chemistry monitor. Pediatrics 2005;115(5):1299–306.
58. Strauss R. Controversies in the management of the anemia of prematurity using single-donor red blood cell transfusions and/or recombinant human erythropoietin. Transfus Med Rev 2006;20(1):34–44.
59. Garcia M, Hutson A, Christensen R. Effect of recombinant erythropoietin on "late" transfusions in the neonatal intensive care unit: a meta-analysis. J Perinatol 2002; 22(2):108–11.
60. Drüeke T, Locatelli F, Clyne N, et al. Normalization of hemoglobin level in patients with chronic kidney disease and anemia. N Engl J Med 2006;355(20):2071–84.
61. Singh A, Szczech L, Tang K, et al. Correction of anemia with epoetin alfa in chronic kidney disease. N Engl J Med 2006;355(20):2085–98.
62. Remuzzi G, Ingelfinger J. Correction of anemia—payoffs and problems. N Engl J Med 2006;355(20):2144–6.
63. Arcasoy M. The non-haematopoietic biological effects of erythropoietin. Br J Haematol 2008;141(1):14–31.
64. Morita M, Ohneda O, Yamashita T, et al. HLF/HIF-2α is a key factor in retinopathy of prematurity in association with erythropoietin. EMBO J 2003;22(5):1134–46.
65. Watanabe D, Suzuma K, Matsui S, et al. Erythropoietin as a retinal angiogenic factor in proliferative diabetic retinopathy. N Engl J Med 2005;353(8):782–92.
66. Henke M, Laszig R, Rübe C, et al. Erythropoietin to treat head and neck cancer patients with anaemia undergoing radiotherapy: randomised, double-blind, placebo-controlled trial. Lancet 2003;362(9392):1255–60.
67. Leyland-Jones B, Semiglazov V, Pawlicki M, et al. Maintaining normal hemoglobin levels with epoetin alfa in mainly nonanemic patients with metastatic breast cancer receiving first-line chemotherapy: a survival study. J Clin Oncol 2005;23(25): 5960–72.
68. Wright J, Ung Y, Julian J, et al. Randomized, double-blind, placebo-controlled trial of erythropoietin in non-small-cell lung cancer with disease-related anemia. J Clin Oncol 2007;25(9):1027–32.
69. Blau C. Erythropoietin in cancer: presumption of innocence? Stem Cells 2007; 25(8):2094–7.

70. Romagnoli C, Zecca E, Gallini F, et al. Do recombinant human erythropoietin and iron supplementation increase the risk of retinopathy of prematurity? Eur J Pediatr 2000;159(8):627–8.
71. Brown M, Barón A, France E, et al. Association between higher cumulative doses of recombinant erythropoietin and risk for retinopathy of prematurity. J AAPOS 2005;10(2):143–9.
72. Meyer M, Haworth C, McNeill L. Is the use of recombinant human erythropoietin in anaemia of prematurity cost-effective? S Afr Med J 1996;86(3):251–3.
73. Fain J, Hilsenrath P, Widness J, et al. A cost analysis comparing erythropoietin and red cell transfusions in the treatment of anemia of prematurity. Transfusion 1995;35(11):936–43.
74. Meyer M. Anaemia of prematurity. Epidemiology, management and costs. Pharmacoeconomics 1997;12(4):438–45.
75. Shireman T, Hilsenrath P, Strauss R, et al. Recombinant human erythropoietin vs transfusions in the treatment of anemia of prematurity. A cost-benefit analysis. Arch Pediatr Adolesc Med 1994;148(6):582–8.
76. Warwood T, Ohls R, Wiedmeier S, et al. Single-dose darbepoetin administration to anemic preterm neonates. J Perinatol 2005;25(11):725–30.
77. Warwood T, Ohls R, Lambert D, et al. Intravenous administration of darbepoetin to NICU patients. J Perinatol 2006;26(5):296–300.
78. Aladangady N, McHugh S, Aitchison T, et al. Infants' blood volume in a controlled trial of placental transfusion at preterm delivery. Pediatrics 2006;117(1):93–8.
79. Mercer J, Vohr B, McGrath M, et al. Delayed cord clamping in very preterm infants reduces the incidence of intraventricular hemorrhage and late-onset sepsis: a randomized, controlled trial. Pediatrics 2006;117(4):1235–42.
80. Philip A. Delayed cord clamping in preterm infants. Pediatrics 2006;117(4): 1434–5.

70. Romagnoli C, Zecca E, Gallini F, et al. Do recombinant human erythropoietin and iron supplementation increase the risk of retinopathy of prematurity? Eur J Pediatr 2000;159(8):627–8.
71. Brown MS, Baron AE, France EK, et al. Association between higher cumulative doses of recombinant erythropoietin and risk for retinopathy of prematurity. J AAPOS 2006;10(2):143–9.
72. Meyer MP, Haworth C, McNeill L. Is the use of recombinant human erythropoietin in anaemia of prematurity cost-effective? S Afr Med J 1996;86(3):251–3.
73. Fain J, Hilsenrath P, Widness JA, et al. A cost analysis comparing erythropoietin and red cell transfusions in the treatment of anemia of prematurity. Transfusion 1995;35(11):936–43.
74. Meyer M. Anaemia of prematurity. Epidemiology, management and costs. Pharmacoeconomics 1997;12(4):438–45.
75. Shireman TI, Hilsenrath PE, Strauss RG, et al. Recombinant human erythropoietin vs transfusions in the treatment of anemia of prematurity. A cost-benefit analysis. Arch Pediatr Adolesc Med 1994;148(6):582–8.
76. Warwood TL, Ohls RK, Wiedmeier SE, et al. Single-dose darbepoetin administration to anemic preterm neonates. J Perinatol 2005;25(11):725–30.
77. Warwood TL, Ohls RK, Lambert DK, et al. Intravenous administration of darbepoetin to NICU patients. J Perinatol 2006;26(5):296–300.
78. Aladangady N, McHugh S, Aitchison TC, et al. Infants' blood volume in a controlled trial of placental transfusion at preterm delivery. Pediatrics 2006;117(1):93–8.
79. Mercer JS, Vohr BR, McGrath MM, et al. Delayed cord clamping in very preterm infants reduces the incidence of intraventricular hemorrhage and late-onset sepsis: a randomized, controlled trial. Pediatrics 2006;117(4):1235–42.
80. Philip AG. Delayed cord clamping in preterm infants. Pediatrics 2006;117(4):1434–5.

Evaluation and Management of Stroke in the Neonate

Alan R. Barnette, MD[a], Terrie E. Inder, MBChB, MD, FRACP[a,b,c,*]

KEYWORDS

- Ischemic perinatal stroke • Seizures
- Thrombophilia • Venous thromboembolism
- Arterial ischemic stroke • Brain injury

Ischemic perinatal stroke (IPS) was defined in 2006 by an international group of experts as "a group of heterogeneous conditions in which there is focal disruption of cerebral blood flow secondary to arterial or cerebral venous thrombosis or embolization, between 20 weeks of fetal life through the 28th postnatal day, confirmed by neuroimaging or neuropathologic studies."[1]

This under-recognized condition occurs in 1 of 2300 to 5000 live births and is a major cause of long-term neurodisability. Approximately 15% of IPS occurs before term gestation.[2] Despite relatively low mortality (3%–10%, Canadian Stroke Study)[3] and low recurrence rates (3%–5%),[4,5] significant modifiable morbidity frequently follows IPS. Hemiplegic cerebral palsy develops in 37% of infants diagnosed in the newborn period and in 82% of infants with delayed diagnosis.[2] Although sensorimotor deficits are the most common, impairments in vision, cognition, behavior, and language also challenge the lives of 20% to 60% of this population.[1] Eighty-three percent of the arterial stokes involve the middle cerebral artery distribution, with two thirds involving the left middle cerebral artery and 10% having bilateral distribution.[6]

The pathophysiology of IPS is complex and multifactorial. It involves not only environmental but also maternal, fetal, placental, and neonatal factors. To prevent hemorrhagic complications of delivery, mothers and babies are especially prothrombotic in the 48 hours before and 24 hours after delivery.

The diagnosis of perinatal stroke often is delayed until late in the first year of life, when motor asymmetries prompt neuroimaging. Infants diagnosed as newborns most commonly present with seizures. Early diagnosis is associated more commonly with childhood epilepsy and mild motor abnormalities, whereas delayed diagnosis is

[a] Division of Newborn Medicine, Washington University School of Medicine, 660 South Euclid, Campus Box 8116, St. Louis, MO 63110, USA
[b] Division of Neurology, Washington University School of Medicine, St. Louis, MO 63110, USA
[c] Division of Radiology, Washington University School of Medicine, St. Louis, MO 63110, USA
* Corresponding author. Division of Newborn Medicine, Washington University School of Medicine, 660 South Euclid, Campus Box 8116, St. Louis, MO 63110.
E-mail address: inder_t@kids.wustl.edu (T.E. Inder).

Clin Perinatol 36 (2009) 125–136
doi:10.1016/j.clp.2008.09.008
perinatology.theclinics.com
0095-5108/08/$ – see front matter

associated with moderate to severe motor impairment.[7] Differences in presentation, diagnosis, and neurologic outcome may be caused by differences in severity, location, or timing of insult or may be completely different pathologically.[7] Care also must be taken to prevent prematurely and incorrectly labeling infants who have neonatal depression as having "birth asphyxia." This depression may be caused by an IPS that occurred weeks to months before delivery.

EVALUATION

History and Examination

Seizures are the most common clinical presentation leading to a diagnosis of perinatal stroke, but not all neonates who have strokes have seizures. Follow-up imaging studies of hemiplegic children who were born following a term gestation suggest that less than half the newborns who have perinatal stroke have neonatal seizures.[7] More subtle early findings associated with stroke on physical examination include poor feeding, hypotonia, lethargy, and asymmetric extremity tone and movements.[8] The daily assessment of general movements can assist in the early detection of evolving hemiplegia and subsequently can direct therapies to limit impairments.[9,10]

The etiology of perinatal stroke is multifactorial, and no obvious cause is identified in up to one half of the cases.[11,12] Antenatal, perinatal, and postnatal risk factors for stroke should be noted by caretakers. During pregnancy, a history of infertility, infection, thrombophilia, lupus, maternal heart disease, migraines, smoking, oligohydramnios, intrauterine growth restriction, placental abnormalities, cocaine use, primiparous gestation, and pregnancy with monozygotic twins have all been linked to a significantly increased risk of perinatal stroke.[13,14] During the perinatal interval, placental vasculopathy, difficult deliveries (cervical arterial dissections), premature rupture of membranes, chorioamnionitis, umbilical cord abnormalities, cesarean section, initial neonatal depression, and low Apgar scores are associated with an increased risk of perinatal stroke. After birth, polycythemia, dehydration, heart defects, extracorporeal membrane oxygenation, and infections are risk factors.[13,15]

Family histories of thrombophilias, strokes, and neurodevelopmental impairments should be ascertained. In addition to a thrombophilia evaluation, newborns that potentially have an IPS should be evaluated for heart defects, and vessels in which catheters have been employed should be investigated for thrombi with Doppler ultrasonography.

Neuroimaging

Although a thorough neurologic examination is important in diagnosing a perinatal stroke, its sensitivity is limited. Conventional and diffusion-weighted (DWI) MRI is imperative to improve the detection of IPS. The feasibility of MRI without sedation has been well demonstrated in infants.[16] Cranial ultrasound has poor sensitivity for the detection of strokelike lesions.[17] Drawbacks for CT include the exposure to ionizing radiation and limited anatomic definition, especially in the posterior fossa.[18]

The changes that occur in DWI and conventional T1- and T2-weighted MRIs can assist in determining the location and timing of the infarction. Evidence of perinatal stroke is detectable with DWI less than 24 hours after the insult. Although the DWI changes pseudonormalize over the following 7 days, alterations in the conventional T1 and T2 images develop (**Fig. 1**).[19–22] Metabolite ratios calculated from MR spectroscopy are sensitive in detecting brain injury in the first few days after an insult.[18,20,21] Serial imaging, with scans at less than 48 hours after birth and at 7 to 10 days of life are optimal for characterizing perinatal ischemic stroke and guiding subsequent therapies. MR

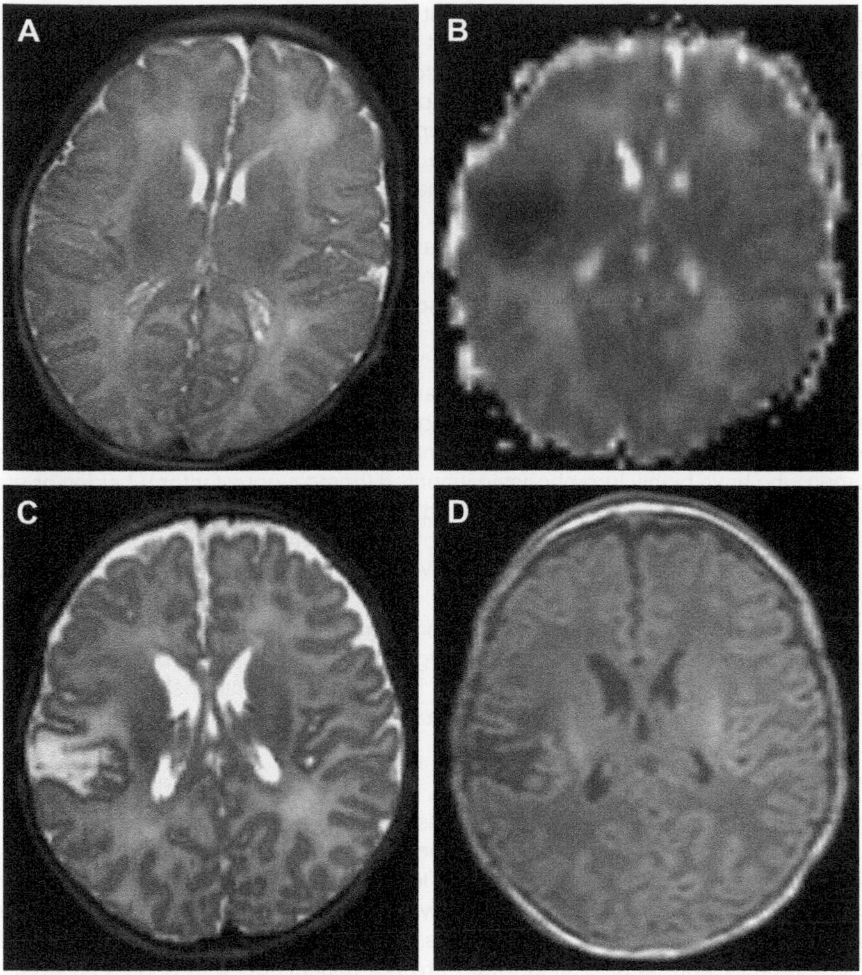

Fig. 1. At 4 days of life, (*A*) the T2-weighted image and (*B*) the apparent diffusion coefficient map display restricted diffusion in the right middle cerebral artery distribution. At 19 days of life, established injury is seen in both (*C*) T1- and (*D*) T2-weighted images.

angiography and venography assist further in determining the location, extent, and etiology of the infarction.

Early MRI changes have predictive value for long-term neurodevelopmental outcomes.[23,24] In addition, the presence of secondary Wallerian degeneration, with delayed white matter fiber tract abnormalities on diffusion, is highly predictive for motor deficits.[25] MRI changes in the thalamus and basal ganglia are predictive of motor deficits. Newborns who have significant subcortical white matter injury in addition to basal ganglia injury are predisposed to cognitive impairments. When large volumes of brain tissue are affected, the risks of neurodevelopmental impairment and epilepsy also increase.[18,24]

Evaluation of Thrombophilia

Numerous case reports exist of thrombophilia in patients who have IPS. In a multicenter, prospective, case-controlled study of symptomatic term neonates with stroke,

Gunther and colleagues[26] investigated eight neonatal prothrombotic factors at 6 to 16 weeks of age (**Table 1**). Sixty-eight percent of the 91 stroke patients and 24% of the 182 control patients had at least one of these risk factors; the greatest differences between stroke and control subjects were lipoprotein A and the factor V Leiden mutation. In a separate Canadian cohort, anticardiolipin antibodies were found to be elevated transiently after perinatal stroke (see **Table 1**).[27]

Although the role of testing remains unclear, measurements of thrombotic factors in the neonate should be delayed until at least 3 months of age to obtain reliable results. Normal pregnancy is a hypercoagulable state, especially in the days surrounding delivery, making interpretation of newborn and maternal prothrombotic mediators challenging.[13] With low recurrence rates and a lack of significant evidence to support the use of anticoagulation therapy acutely in arterial thrombosis, this delay will not change treatment.

Maternal prothrombotic states can increase the risk of fetal loss significantly. There are no randomized, controlled trials showing the effects of anticoagulation on prevention of maternal and fetal adverse outcomes. Obstetric literature supports treating women who have highly thrombogenic inherited (homozygous factor V Leiden or prothrombin G20210A mutations) or acquired (antiphospholipid syndrome) conditions with heparin and aspirin during pregnancy.[28] Maternal antiphospholipid antibody levels should be obtained soon after delivery, because levels change in the days following delivery.

In counseling parents, it is reassuring to note that the risk of recurrence of IPS in the both the newborn and in subsequent pregnancies is small.[14,29] To minimize risks further, mothers should be encouraged to avoid environmental risk factors such as smoking, dehydration, prolonged immobilization, oral contraceptives, and obesity.[14]

Detecting Seizure

Clinical neonatal seizures are the commonest presentation of IPS. The seizure often is multifocal clonic in nature and may be asymmetric, consistent with the hemispheric involvement (eg, right hand and face for a left middle cerebral artery infarction). The accurate recognition of seizures in the newborn is challenging. Activities diagnosed clinically as seizures in children and adults, such as repetitive rhythmic movements of an extremity and lip smacking, often are not associated with confirmed cortical electroencephalographic (EEG) seizures. Alternatively, EEG seizure activity occurs commonly in the absence of clinical manifestations, with 90% of EEG seizures in the neonatal ICU not being recognized clinically.[30] Current research is focusing on

Table 1
Summary of hypercoagulability risk factors in newborns with stroke

Author, Reference	N	Abnormal (%)	fVL	Protein C Deficiency	MTHFR	PT Variant	ACA	Lp (a)
Gunther et al (2000)[26]	91	32 (68)	17	6	15	4	—	20
Govaert et al (2000)[12]	40	3 (8)	3	0	—	—	—	—
Mercuri et al (2001)[77]	24	10 (42)	5	0	—	—	—	—
Golomb et al (2001)[27]	22	14 (64)	1	0	1	—	12[a]	—

Abbreviations: ACA, elevated anticardiolipin antibodies; fVL, factor V Leiden mutation; Lp (a), elevated lipoprotein (a); MTHFR, mutation of methyltetrahydrofolate reductase gene; PT variant, prothrombin G20210A variant.

[a] Ten of 12 normalized on repeat testing.

ways to improve the diagnosis and to understand the implications of subclinical seizures on outcomes in ischemic brain injury in the newborn.

TREATMENT

Therapeutic interventions address brain injury at multiple phases (**Fig. 2**).

Current Pharmacologic Therapies

Anticoagulation

Limited evidence and no randomized clinical trials exist to guide thrombolysis, antiplatelet, and anticoagulation therapy in neonates following a nonhemorrhagic ischemic perinatal stroke. Recommendations for therapy from an expert panel were published in a 2004 edition of *Chest*.[31] Because arterial ischemic strokes are pathophysiologically different from venous thromboembolism (VTE), respective treatments also differ. Thromboembolism develops more gradually and involves less turbulent flow.[5]

For arterial ischemic strokes, no anticoagulation or aspirin is recommended unless clear evidence of a thromboembolic event exists. If an embolus is identified, 3 months of unfractionated heparin (UFH) or low molecular weight heparin (LMWH) should be given. UFH, LMWH, and warfarin all seem to be safe for use in neonates. Doses of LMWH should be adjusted to maintain levels of anti-factor Xa antibodies at 0.5 to 1.0 units/mL.[5]

For a thromboembolism, treatment options include either 3 months of UFH or LMWH or radiographic monitoring and anticoagulation therapy if the thrombus extends. The use of LMWH should resume or a change to warfarin should occur if the thrombus extends after discontinuation of anticoagulation.

In the absence of critical compromise to major organs, thrombolytics such as tissue plasminogen activator are not recommended for use following IPS of any type. After the identification of an embolus, central catheters should be removed as soon as possible.

Anticonvulsants

Clinical seizures occur in 25% to 40% of cases of IPS, making this the most common presentation for infants diagnosed during the newborn period.[7,32] There is a lack of consensus on whether newborns at risk of seizures, including those who have strokes, should have continuous EEG monitoring and/or treatment of subclinical seizures. Seizures in neonates usually recur in the absence of treatment and often persist after

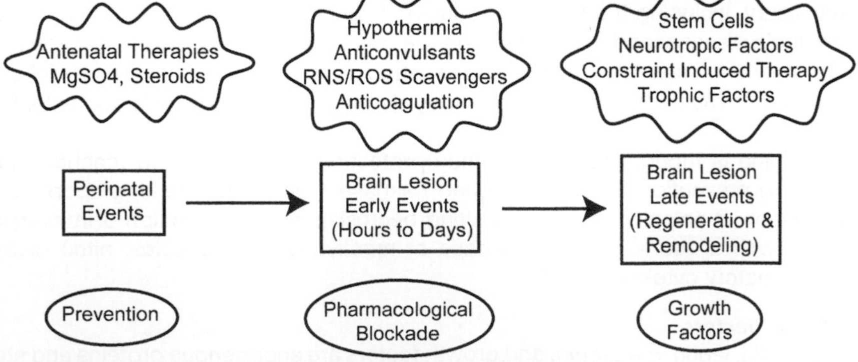

Fig. 2. Pathophysiology and therapeutic interventions for IPS.

initial treatment.[33] Seizures following infarction may amplify brain injury via multiple mechanisms, including increased metabolic demand, hyperthermia, increased release of reactive oxygen species, and disruption of endogenous repair mechanisms.[33,34]

Special considerations must be taken when using anticonvulsants in neonates. Phenobarbital and benzodiazepines may be ineffective in controlling neonatal seizures.[35] Glutamate receptor modifiers such as topiramate (an α-amino-3-hydroxy-5-methylisoxansole-proprionic acid antagonist) and MK801 (an N-methyl-D-aspartic acid antagonist) have been shown to control seizure in rodents, but caution must be used with pharmacotherapies that prevent hyperexcitability, because they may modify normal neurodevelopment. Animal data support the safety of topiramate[36] and levetiracetam,[37] but no randomized, controlled trials in neonates have been published.

Future Promising Pharmacologic Therapies

The agents discussed in this section have all shown efficacy in immature animal models, mature animal models, and/or adult stroke. There are, however, no clinical data on their neuroprotective efficacy in newborn stroke.

Statins

Statins (3-hydroxy-3-methylglutaril coenzyme A reductase inhibitors) can be neuroprotective when administered before an ischemic brain insult in immature rodents and before or after insult in more mature rodents.[38] In rodent models using simvastatin, decreases in the volume of brain injury and the prevention of long-term behavioral alterations have been observed. Multiple mechanisms have been proposed to explain the neuroprotective effects of statins, including (1) decreased inflammation via reduced expression of intercellular adhesion molecule-1, interkeukin1β, and tumor necrosis factor α; (2) prevention of apoptosis through inhibition of caspase-3 activation; and (3) enhancement of endothelial nitric oxide synthase expression.[39–41]

Anti-inflammatory agents

N-Acetylcysteine N-Acetylcysteine is a free radical scavenger that crosses the placenta and blood–brain barrier and is considered safe during pregnancy. In a neurologically immature rat model of inflammatory and ischemic brain injury, N-acetylcysteine provided protection from injury to both gray and white brain matter when given either before or immediately after the insult.[42] Its mechanisms of action include a multifactorial reduction in oxidative stress,[42] inflammation,[43] and apoptosis.[44]

Minocycline Minocycline has been used for neuroprotection in multiple rodent models of brain injury, including traumatic brain injury, multiple sclerosis, Parkinson disease, Huntington's disease, and lipopolysaccharide-induced injury. This drug has provided neuroprotection in neonatal rodent models when given before or immediately following an insult.[45] The degree of protection may depend on the magnitude and extent of the injury.

Minocycline is thought to provide neuroprotection though multiple mechanisms, including (1) prevention of caspase-3 and caspase-1 activation (limiting apoptosis); (2) prevention of calpain activation (limiting necrosis); and (3) inhibition of microglial activation with a decrease in the release of reactive oxygen species, nitric oxide, and inflammatory cytokines.[45,46]

Neurotropic factors

Erythropoietin, leptin, melatonin, and growth factors are endogenous proteins and steroids used primarily for non-neurologic purposes that may provide neuroprotection.

Erythropoietin Erythropoietin (EPO) is produced by the kidneys and fetal liver and regulates erythropoiesis. EPO receptors are present in the immature brains of rodents and mammals, including humans.[47] Multiple animal models have demonstrated a neuroprotective role for EPO following ischemic brain injury.[47–50] Possible mechanisms of protection include stabilizing cerebrovascular autoregulation, preventing apoptosis, and limiting inflammation, excitotoxic injury, and oxidative stress.[51,52] Additionally, EPO may promote endogenous neurogenesis and angiogenesis while suppressing gliogenesis following injury.[53] EPO is commercially available in a recombinant form; potential side effects include increasing iron deficiency, oxidative stress, and risk of retinopathy of prematurity.

Leptin Leptin is generated by adipose tissue and is involved in obesity and energy balance. Intracerebral and intraperitoneal injections of leptin are neuroprotective following excitotoxic brain injury in neonatal mice.[54] The potential mechanism of neuroprotection is hypothesized to be neuron receptor–mediated blunting of excitotoxic injury.

Melatonin Melatonin is a pineal hormone that provides circadian cues but also is a powerful antioxidant that scavenges reactive oxygen species, stabilizes mitochondrial membranes, and has demonstrated neuroprotective value in neonatal animal brain injury models[55,56] and in depressed human neonates.[57] Melatonin crosses the placenta and the blood–brain barrier, facilitating rapid and uninhibited delivery to the immature brain. It does not appear to inhibit fetal growth or cause malformations in fetal animal models[55] and seems to be safe for use in human neonates.[57,58]

Neuroprotective Devices

Hypothermia

Multicenter international randomized, controlled trials of hypothermia in newborn infants have demonstrated that cooling can be safe, significantly reduce infarct size, and improve of 18-month survival rates without neurologic disability.[59] Many centers now include cooling as part of the routine management of term newborns with moderate to severe encephalopathy. The mechanisms of action of therapeutic hypothermia involve a drop in cerebral metabolic demand as well as decreases in (1) excitatory neurotransmitter release, (2) free radical production, (3) edema, (4) coagulation activation, (5) neutrophil infiltration, and (6) cytokine release.

Hypothermia may prolong the therapeutic window for additional, currently undiscovered, neuroprotective interventions. The utility of hypothermia in perinatal stroke has not been studied and is unlikely to be studied because the rarity of early diagnosis of the condition limits randomized, controlled trials. Many of the pathways in perinatal stroke, however, are identical to the pathway of the more global hypoxic ischemic encephalopathy, and thus it is likely that therapeutic hypothermia also may benefit this population with minimal risk of adverse effects.

Functional Neurorehabilitation

Constraint-induced therapy

Constraint-induced movement therapy (CIMT) enhances the use of affected limbs by preventing the use of the dominant extremity while encouraging therapeutic use of the affected limb.[60] Children who have unilateral limb impairment often disregard the affected limb early in life, even when the impairment is mild.[61] This disregard, termed "learned non-use" for adults[62] or "developmental disregard" for infants and children,[63] can exacerbate motor impairment.[64]

Traditional treatment of hemiplegic cerebral palsy focuses on decreasing tone and spasticity while improving range of movement and function. The methods for accomplishing these goals include casting, splinting, stretching, surgery, and medications baclofen and botulinum toxin A.

The efficacy of CIMT was demonstrated in multiple primate experiments by Taub and colleagues[65] over the last 2 decades. These primates underwent surgical elimination of somatic sensation in a single forelimb, followed by immediate or delayed CIMT. More recently, prospective human trials demonstrated clinically beneficial short- and intermediate-term motor effects following CIMT in both adults and children who had asymmetric motor deficits after strokes. Other prospective, randomized pediatric trials evaluating the efficacy of CIMT[63,66] or forced use[67] have demonstrated trends favoring this therapy over conventional treatment for children at risk of developing upper limb hemiplegic cerebral palsy. Trials have varied considerably in method of constraint (from a restraining mitt to a long arm cast), time of restraint (for an hour a day to all day), and duration of therapy (from 10 days to 2 months),[60] but almost all demonstrate some degree of benefit following CIMT.[65] In adults, the therapy was associated with less reduction in cortical representation of the affected limb.[68] Although different tests are used to evaluate the effects in children and adults, improvements seem to be greater after perinatal stroke than after adult stroke.

Regenerative Interventions

Stem cells are relatively undifferentiated, multipotent, and have proliferative capacity. Over a decade ago, Bain and colleagues[69] differentiated neural stem cells into neural phenotypes capable of generating potential action. Histologic and MRI evidence of endogenous neurogenesis and subventricular zone (SVZ) growth exists for mammals and young rodents following brain injury, but this neurogenesis has not produced functional recovery.[70] Improvement in motor function,[71] spatial learning, and memory[72] have occurred after the injection of fetal cortical grafts into immature rat brains with focal infractions.

Multiple trophic factors (EPO, insulin growth factor 1, granulocyte colony-stimulating factor, transforming growth factor-α, and others) have been identified as playing a role in regulating SVZ neuron production, differentiation, and migration.[73,74] Additionally, rodent models have demonstrated that an enriched environment (with swings, blocks, and other sources of stimulation) enhances the survival of SVZ progenitors.[73] MR spectroscopy in the SVZ of humans and rodents has been used as a biomarker for in vivo serial monitoring of neurogenesis and migration after injury.[75]

Tremendous progress has been made in the understanding of stem cells and their application to neonatal brain injury. Unfortunately, clinical application of this emerging technology will not occur in the near future. Greater understanding of stem cell pathophysiology is needed before exogenous stem cells can be used to prevent immune rejection and promote the proliferation of neurons and their supporting cells in an efficient, regionally specific, and nontumorgenic manner.[73,76] Ethical considerations also must be addressed to allow continued investigation and application and prevent the propagation of incorrect information.

OUTCOMES

Although newborns who experience strokes recover better than older children or adults who have similar brain injuries, many still face long-term neurodevelopmental impairments. Almost half the IPS survivors have mild to moderate impairments, and one forth have severe long-term impairments.[18] Hemiplegic cerebral palsy develops in 37% of infants diagnosed in the newborn period and in 82% of infants who have a delayed diagnosis.[2] Although sensorimotor deficits are the most common, impairments in vision, cognition, behavior, and language also occur in 20% to 60%,[1] and epilepsy occurs in 25% to 50% of IPS survivors.[18]

SUMMARY

IPS is a common and underdiagnosed cause of encephalopathy. It is associated with major morbidity, including seizures and cognitive and motor impairments. These long-term impairments may be reduced with timely application of current and developing therapies.

When brain injury is suspected, conventional MRI and DWI should be used to assess the origin, timing, and location of brain injury. Along with clinical examinations and histories, neuroimaging and electroencephalographic monitoring provide information to guide treatment and give parents prognostic information. Additionally, with emerging pharmacotherapy and interventions such as therapeutic hypothermia and CIMT, rapid diagnosis and characterization of brain injury is vital to minimize injury and optimize neurodevelopmental outcomes. Further research is needed to understand better the mechanisms of perinatal stroke and to limit the associated morbidity.

REFERENCES

1. Raju TN, Nelson KB, Ferriero D, et al. Ischemic perinatal stroke: summary of a workshop sponsored by the National Institute of Child Health and Human Development and the National Institute of Neurological Disorders and Stroke. Pediatrics 2007;120(3):609–16.
2. Lee J, Croen LA, Lindan C, et al. Predictors of outcome in perinatal arterial stroke: a population-based study. Ann Neurol 2005;58(2):303–8.
3. Lynch JK, Nelson KB. Epidemiology of perinatal stroke. Curr Opin Pediatr 2001; 13(6):499–505.
4. deVeber GA, MacGregor D, Curtis R, et al. Neurologic outcome in survivors of childhood arterial ischemic stroke and sinovenous thrombosis. J Child Neurol 2000;15(5):316–24.
5. Kirton A, deVeber G. Therapeutic approaches and advances in pediatric stroke. NeuroRx 2006;3(2):133–42.
6. Miller V. Neonatal cerebral infarction. Semin Pediatr Neurol 2000;7(4):278–88.
7. Wu YW, March WM, Croen LA, et al. Perinatal stroke in children with motor impairment: a population-based study. Pediatrics 2004;114(3):612–9.
8. Chalmers EA. Perinatal stroke—risk factors and management. Br J Haematol 2005;130(3):333–43.
9. Guzzetta A, Mercuri E, Rapisardi G, et al. General movements detect early signs of hemiplegia in term infants with neonatal cerebral infarction. Neuropediatrics 2003;34(2):61–6.
10. Spittle AJ, Orton J, Doyle LW, et al. Early developmental intervention programs post hospital discharge to prevent motor and cognitive impairments in preterm infants. Cochrane Database Syst Rev 2007;(2):CD005495.
11. deVeber G, Monagle P, Chan A, et al. Prothrombotic disorders in infants and children with cerebral thromboembolism. Arch Neurol 1998;55(12):1539–43.
12. Govaert P, Matthys E, Zecic A, et al. Perinatal cortical infarction within middle cerebral artery trunks. Arch Dis Child Fetal Neonatal Ed 2000;82(1):F59–63.
13. Wu YW, Lynch JK, Nelson KB. Perinatal arterial stroke: understanding mechanisms and outcomes. Semin Neurol 2005;25(4):424–34.

14. Nelson KB. Thrombophilias, perinatal stroke, and cerebral palsy. Clin Obstet Gynecol 2006;49(4):875–84.
15. Fitzgerald KC, Williams LS, Garg BP, et al. Cerebral sinovenous thrombosis in the neonate. Arch Neurol 2006;63(3):405–9.
16. Mathur AM, Neil JJ, McKinstry RC, et al. Transport, monitoring, and successful brain MR imaging in unsedated neonates. Pediatr Radiol 2008;38(3):260–4.
17. Nelson KB. Perinatal ischemic stroke. Stroke 2007;38(2 Suppl):742–5.
18. Barkovich AJ. Pediatric neuroimaging. 4th edition. Philadelphia: Lippincott Williams & Wilkins; 2005.
19. Mader I, Schoning M, Klose U, et al. Neonatal cerebral infarction diagnosed by diffusion-weighted MRI: pseudonormalization occurs early. Stroke 2002;33(4):1142–5.
20. Barkovich AJ, Miller SP, Bartha A, et al. MR imaging, MR spectroscopy, and diffusion tensor imaging of sequential studies in neonates with encephalopathy. AJNR Am J Neuroradiol 2006;27(3):533–47.
21. Soul JS, Robertson RL, Tzika AA, et al. Time course of changes in diffusion-weighted magnetic resonance imaging in a case of neonatal encephalopathy with defined onset and duration of hypoxic-ischemic insult. Pediatrics 2001;108(5):1211–4.
22. McKinstry RC, Miller JH, Snyder AZ, et al. A prospective, longitudinal diffusion tensor imaging study of brain injury in newborns. Neurology 2002;59(6):824–33.
23. Hunt RW, Neil JJ, Coleman LT, et al. Apparent diffusion coefficient in the posterior limb of the internal capsule predicts outcome after perinatal asphyxia. Pediatrics 2004;114(4):999–1003.
24. Rutherford M, Srinivasan L, Dyet L, et al. Magnetic resonance imaging in perinatal brain injury: clinical presentation, lesions and outcome. Pediatr Radiol 2006;36(7): 582–92.
25. De Vries LS, Van der Grond J, Van Haastert IC, et al. Prediction of outcome in new-born infants with arterial ischaemic stroke using diffusion-weighted magnetic resonance imaging. Neuropediatrics 2005;36(1):12–20.
26. Gunther G, Junker R, Strater R, et al. Symptomatic ischemic stroke in full-term neonates: role of acquired and genetic prothrombotic risk factors. Stroke 2000; 31(10):2437–41.
27. Golomb MR, MacGregor DL, Domi T, et al. Presumed pre- or perinatal arterial ischemic stroke: risk factors and outcomes. Ann Neurol 2001;50(2):163–8.
28. Creasy RK, Resnik R, Iams JD. Maternal-fetal medicine. 5th edition. Philadelphia: WB Saunders; 2004.
29. Ferriero DM. Neonatal brain injury. N Engl J Med 2004;351(19):1985–95.
30. Murray DM, Boylan GB, Ali I, et al. Defining the gap between electrographic seizure burden, clinical expression, and staff recognition of neonatal seizures. published online. Arch Dis Child Fetal Neonatal Ed 11 Jul 2007;10.1136/ adc.2005.086314.
31. Monagle P, Chan A, Massicotte P, et al. Antithrombotic therapy in children: the Seventh ACCP Conference on Antithrombotic and Thrombolytic Therapy. Chest 2004;126(3 Suppl):645S–87S.
32. Nelson KB, Lynch JK. Stroke in newborn infants. Lancet Neurol 2004;3(3):150–8.
33. Silverstein FS, Jensen FE. Neonatal seizures. Ann Neurol 2007;62(2):112–20.
34. Wirrell EC, Armstrong EA, Osman LD, et al. Prolonged seizures exacerbate perinatal hypoxic-ischemic brain damage. Pediatr Res 2001;50(4):445–54.
35. Painter MJ, Scher MS, Stein AD, et al. Phenobarbital compared with phenytoin for the treatment of neonatal seizures. N Engl J Med 1999;341(7):485–9.
36. Glier C, Dzietko M, Bittigau P, et al. Therapeutic doses of topiramate are not toxic to the developing rat brain. Exp Neurol 2004;187(2):403–9.

37. Manthey D, Asimiadou S, Stefovska V, et al. Sulthiame but not levetiracetam exerts neurotoxic effect in the developing rat brain. Exp Neurol 2005;193(2):497–503.
38. Balduini W, Carloni S, Mazzoni E, et al. New therapeutic strategies in perinatal stroke. Curr Drug Targets CNS Neurol Disord 2004;3(4):315–23.
39. Balduini W, Mazzoni E, Carloni S, et al. Prophylactic but not delayed administration of simvastatin protects against long-lasting cognitive and morphological consequences of neonatal hypoxic-ischemic brain injury, reduces interleukin-1beta and tumor necrosis factor-alpha mRNA induction, and does not affect endothelial nitric oxide synthase expression. Stroke 2003;34(8):2007–12.
40. Endres M, Laufs U, Huang Z, et al. Stroke protection by 3-hydroxy-3-methylglutaryl (HMG)-CoA reductase inhibitors mediated by endothelial nitric oxide synthase. Proc Natl Acad Sci U S A 1998;95(15):8880–5.
41. Sironi L, Cimino M, Guerrini U, et al. Treatment with statins after induction of focal ischemia in rats reduces the extent of brain damage. Arterioscler Thromb Vasc Biol 2003;23(2):322–7.
42. Wang X, Svedin P, Nie C, et al. N-acetylcysteine reduces lipopolysaccharide-sensitized hypoxic-ischemic brain injury. Ann Neurol 2007;61(3):263–71.
43. Louwerse ES, Weverling GJ, Bossuyt PM, et al. Randomized, double-blind, controlled trial of acetylcysteine in amyotrophic lateral sclerosis. Arch Neurol 1995; 52(6):559–64.
44. Ferrari G, Yan CY, Greene LA. N-acetylcysteine (D- and L-stereoisomers) prevents apoptotic death of neuronal cells. J Neurosci 1995;15(4):2857–66.
45. Arvin KL, Han BH, Du Y, et al. Minocycline markedly protects the neonatal brain against hypoxic-ischemic injury. Ann Neurol 2002;52(1):54–61.
46. Cai Z, Lin S, Fan LW, et al. Minocycline alleviates hypoxic-ischemic injury to developing oligodendrocytes in the neonatal rat brain. Neuroscience 2006; 137(2):425–35.
47. Aydin A, Genc K, Akhisaroglu M, et al. Erythropoietin exerts neuroprotective effect in neonatal rat model of hypoxic-ischemic brain injury. Brain Dev 2003; 25(7):494–8.
48. Matsushita H, Johnston MV, Lange MS, et al. Protective effect of erythropoietin in neonatal hypoxic ischemia in mice. Neuroreport 2003;14(13):1757–61.
49. Sakanaka M, Wen TC, Matsuda S, et al. In vivo evidence that erythropoietin protects neurons from ischemic damage. Proc Natl Acad Sci U S A 1998;95(8): 4635–40.
50. Sadamoto Y, Igase K, Sakanaka M, et al. Erythropoietin prevents place navigation disability and cortical infarction in rats with permanent occlusion of the middle cerebral artery. Biochem Biophys Res Commun 1998;253(1):26–32.
51. Juul S, Felderhoff-Mueser U. Epo and other hematopoietic factors. Semin Fetal Neonatal Med 2007;12(4):250–8.
52. Jelkmann W. Biology of erythropoietin. Clin Investig 1994;72(6 Suppl):S3–S10.
53. Gonzalez FF, McQuillen P, Mu D, et al. Erythropoietin enhances long-term neuroprotection and neurogenesis in neonatal stroke. Dev Neurosci 2007;29(4–5):321–30.
54. Dicou E, Attoub S, Gressens P. Neuroprotective effects of leptin in vivo and in vitro. Neuroreport 2001;12(18):3947–51.
55. Miller SL, Yan EB, Castillo-Melendez M, et al. Melatonin provides neuroprotection in the late-gestation fetal sheep brain in response to umbilical cord occlusion. Dev Neurosci 2005;27(2–4):200–10.
56. Yon JH, Carter LB, Reiter RJ, et al. Melatonin reduces the severity of anesthesia-induced apoptotic neurodegeneration in the developing rat brain. Neurobiol Dis 2006;21(3):522–30.

57. Fulia F, Gitto E, Cuzzocrea S, et al. Increased levels of malondialdehyde and nitrite/nitrate in the blood of asphyxiated newborns: reduction by melatonin. J Pineal Res 2001;31(4):343–9.
58. Gitto E, Romeo C, Reiter RJ, et al. Melatonin reduces oxidative stress in surgical neonates. J Pediatr Surg 2004;39(2):184–9 [discussion: 184–9].
59. Jacobs S, Hunt R, Tarnow-Mordi W, et al. Cooling for newborns with hypoxic ischaemic encephalopathy. Cochrane Database Syst Rev 2007;(4):CD003311.
60. Hoare BJ, Wasiak J, Imms C, et al. Constraint-induced movement therapy in the treatment of the upper limb in children with hemiplegic cerebral palsy. Cochrane Database Syst Rev 2007;(2):CD004149.
61. Sundholm LK, Eliasson AC, Forssberg H. Obstetric brachial plexus injuries: assessment protocol and functional outcome at age 5 years. Dev Med Child Neurol 1998;40(1):4–11.
62. Taub E, Harger M, Grier HC, et al. Some anatomical observations following chronic dorsal rhizotomy in monkeys. Neuroscience 1980;5(2):389–401.
63. DeLuca S. Intensive movement therapy with casting for children with hemiparetic cerebral palsy: a randomized controlled trial [dissertation], The University of Alabama at Birmingham; 2002.
64. Damiano D, Mayston M, Scrutton D. Management of the motor disorders of children with cerebral palsy. 2nd edition. London: Cambridge University Press; 2004.
65. Taub E, Griffin A, Nick J, et al. Pediatric CI therapy for stroke-induced hemiparesis in young children. Dev Neurorehabil 2007;10(1):3–18.
66. Eliasson AC, Krumlinde-Sundholm L, Shaw K, et al. Effects of constraint-induced movement therapy in young children with hemiplegic cerebral palsy: an adapted model. Dev Med Child Neurol 2005;47(4):266–75.
67. Sung IY, Ryu JS, Pyun SB, et al. Efficacy of forced-use therapy in hemiplegic cerebral palsy. Arch Phys Med Rehabil 2005;86(11):2195–8.
68. Liepert J, Bauder H, Wolfgang HR, et al. Treatment-induced cortical reorganization after stroke in humans. Stroke 2000;31(6):1210–6.
69. Bain G, Kitchens D, Yao M, et al. Embryonic stem cells express neuronal properties in vitro. Dev Biol 1995;168(2):342–57.
70. Vawda R, Woodbury J, Covey M, et al. Stem cell therapies for perinatal brain injuries. Semin Fetal Neonatal Med 2007;12(4):259–72.
71. Sorensen JC, Grabowski M, Zimmer J, et al. Fetal neocortical tissue blocks implanted in brain infarcts of adult rats interconnect with the host brain. Exp Neurol 1996;138(2):227–35.
72. Hodges H, Sowinski P, Fleming P, et al. Contrasting effects of fetal CA1 and CA3 hippocampal grafts on deficits in spatial learning and working memory induced by global cerebral ischaemia in rats. Neuroscience 1996;72(4):959–88.
73. Curtis MA, Faull RL, Eriksson PS. The effect of neurodegenerative diseases on the subventricular zone. Nat Rev Neurosci 2007;8(9):712–23.
74. Barrett RD, Bennet L, Davidson J, et al. Destruction and reconstruction: hypoxia and the developing brain. Birth Defects Res C Embryo Today 2007;81(3):163–76.
75. Manganas LN, Zhang X, Li Y, et al. Magnetic resonance spectroscopy identifies neural progenitor cells in the live human brain. Science 2007;318(5852):980–5.
76. Kennea NL, Mehmet H. Perinatal applications of neural stem cells. Best Pract Res Clin Obstet Gynaecol 2004;18(6):977–94.
77. Mercuri E, Cowan F, Gupte G, et al. Prothrombotic disorders and abnormal neurodevelopmental outcome in infants with neonatal cerebral infarction. Pediatrics 2001;107(6):1400–4.

Screening for Maternal Depression in the Neonatal ICU

Kyle O. Mounts, MD, MPH[a,b,c,*]

KEYWORDS

• Depression • Screening • Neonatal • Intensive care

Postpartum depression is a common complication of pregnancy affecting between 10% and 15% of women during the postpartum period.[1] Postpartum depression rates of 28% to 48% have been reported in adolescent mothers[2] and rates up to 38% have been reported for women living in poverty.[3] In women with infants in the neonatal ICU (NICU), the rate of postpartum depression ranges from 28% to 70%.[4–6] The frequent occurrence of maternal depression and the potential long-term implications for their infants are the major arguments for identifying and referring women with depression who have infants in the NICU.

Depression is a significant health problem for women and can affect how a woman is able to care for herself[7] and her infant. Many women are not screened for depression during pregnancy, so screening women for depression while their infants are in the NICU may identify some women who have pre-existing, but undiagnosed, depression. Whether depression precedes delivery or occurs for the first time in the postpartum period does not decrease the importance of screening; either situation results in risk for the infant. Because many infants who have been discharged from the NICU are already at risk for growth and developmental problems, it is important to consider further the potential implications of unrecognized and untreated maternal depression.

BACKGROUND

Corticotropin-Releasing Hormone and the Neuroendocrinology of Depression

Corticotropin-releasing hormone (CRH) has been implicated in the pathophysiology of depression. Stress activates the hypothalamic–pituitary–adrenal (HPA) axis by

[a] Department of Pediatrics, Medical College of Wisconsin, 8701 Watertown Plank Road Milwaukee, WI 53226, USA
[b] Department of Pediatrics, University of Wisconsin-Madison, H4/442 Clinical Science Center, 600 Highland Avenue, Madison, WI 53792, USA
[c] Division of Neonatology, Wheaton Franciscan Healthcare St. Joseph, 5000 West Chambers Street, Milwaukee, WI 53210, USA
* Division of Neonatology, Wheaton Franciscan Healthcare St. Joseph, 5000 West Chambers Street, Milwaukee, WI 53210, USA.
E-mail address: kmounts@pol.net

Clin Perinatol 36 (2009) 137–152
doi:10.1016/j.clp.2008.09.014 perinatology.theclinics.com

increasing CRH.[8] The short-term effect of CRH activation is an increase in cardiovascular and metabolic activity, which, in turn, serves self-preservation and physiologic adaptive functions. Normally, increased production of cortisol terminates the stress response by negative feedback mechanisms mediated by corticosteroid receptors,[9,10] but in the presence of chronic stress there is evidence that these corticosteroid receptors are down-regulated.

Other neurotransmitters are also affected by CRH. Norepinephrine, which is important in the regulation of affect, is regulated by CRH. CRH stimulates tyrosine hydroxylase, an enzyme responsible for norepinephrine synthesis, increasing norepinephrine turnover. The relationship between the HPA axis and the serotonergic system is complex, but one potential effect is that as CRH and corticosteroids increase, specific changes in serotonin receptors occur[11] that affect mood and emotion. Norepinephrine reuptake inhibitors seem to block the effects of CRH directly; serotonin reuptake inhibitors seem to act indirectly to modulate CRH activity.[12]

Activation of the HPA axis results in an increase in cortisol production, which inhibits the inflammatory/immune response[13] by decreasing the production of cytokine and other inflammatory mediators as well as inhibiting their function in target tissues. At the same time, maternal infections can produce cytokines and inflammatory mediators that also are able to activate the HPA axis. CRH is known to interact with both prostaglandins and oxytocin, both of which mediate uterine contractility.[14] Thus, activation of the HPA axis, maternal depression, maternal infection, and preterm delivery share common pathways.

These changes take place in the mother, but experimental evidence suggests that similar biochemical changes take place in the fetus. Field and colleagues[15] assayed cortisol, norepinephrine, epinephrine, dopamine, and serotonin levels in depressed and non-depressed maternal neonatal dyads. Depressed mothers had significantly higher cortisol and norepinephrine and significantly lower dopamine levels at the prenatal and postnatal assessments. The newborns' hormonal concentrations, except for epinephrine, were higher than their mothers'. Elevated norepinephrine and cortisol concentrations were predictive of low birth weight and prematurity, respectively. In another study, Diego and colleagues[16] assessed the effects of the onset and chronicity of maternal depression on neonatal physiology in 80 pregnant women who were screened for depression during mid-pregnancy and shortly after delivery. At 1 week of age, infants of mothers who had prenatal and postnatal depressive symptoms had elevated cortisol and norepinephrine levels and lower dopamine levels. The effects of maternal depression on neonatal physiology depended more on prenatal than postnatal depression but also may have correlated with the duration of the depressive symptoms. These findings have implications for ongoing neonatal/child mental health development, because they demonstrate that fetuses are affected by exposure to maternal depression in utero. Essex and colleagues[17] longitudinally measured salivary cortisol levels in a group of children and found that preschoolers exposed to high levels of maternal stress had elevated cortisol concentrations. The strongest predictor of the children's' cortisol concentrations was the presence of maternal depression beginning in infancy. Thus, maternal depression may have long-term effects on future child development.

Relationship Between Depression and Prematurity and Low Birth Weight

Mancuso and colleagues[14] followed 282 pregnant women to investigate the effect of prenatal maternal anxiety and CRH on gestational length. They found that women who delivered prematurely had significantly higher levels of stress and CRH at both 18 to 20 weeks and 28 to 30 weeks gestation compared with women who delivered at term.

Dayan and colleagues[18] investigated the effects of antenatal depression and anxiety on spontaneous preterm birth resulting either from preterm labor or preterm premature rupture of membranes in a cohort of 681 singleton pregnancies. In their study the rate of spontaneous preterm birth was 9.7% in women who had high depression scores, compared with 4.0% in controls ($P = .02$). Field and colleagues[19] noted that women who had high cortisol levels had higher depression screening scores, and their fetuses had smaller head circumferences and weights. The infants also were born earlier and had lower birth weights. Suboptimal birth outcomes have been reported in other studies as well.[20–23]

On the other hand, Andersson and colleagues[24] reported the results of a study in Sweden that followed 1465 women and their infants. The women were assessed antenatally for depression and anxiety disorders. In their study there was no significant association between depressive and/or anxiety disorders and birth outcomes (growth restriction or prematurity). The investigators acknowledged, however, that their study may not be generalizable to other populations, in part because of the low incidence of premature delivery in Sweden (point prevalence 5.7%). Furthermore, they performed psychiatric assessments only one time during pregnancy, so they could not know the course of depressive and/or anxiety symptoms throughout pregnancy. Other studies also have demonstrated no significant association between maternal psychologic factors and birth outcome.[25–28]

EFFECTS OF POSTPARTUM DEPRESSION ON INFANT HEALTH

Mental Health

Maternal depression can affect infant attachment adversely. Attachment theory has become the dominant approach to understanding early socioemotional and personality development.[29] The central premise in attachment theory is that the need for human contact, reassurance, and comforting in the face of illness, injury, and threat is a normal response throughout the life span. This need is especially prominent early in development when physical and emotional survival depends on the care-giving relationship.[30] Field and colleagues[31] investigated interactions between depressed mothers and their infants at 3 and 5 months and found that, compared with control mothers, depressed mothers demonstrated less activity, less contented facial expressions, fewer imitative behaviors, fewer contingent responses, and less game playing during interactions. The infants of the depressed mothers, in turn, demonstrated more fussiness and fewer contented expressions. Beatson and Taryan[32] postulated that secure attachment may act as a buffer against HPA activation and that infants with insecure attachment, lacking this buffer, may be predisposed to depression and other psychiatric disorders in response to psychosocial stressors.

Behavioral, cognitive, and mental health development

Maternal reports of infant temperament have been found to differ significantly for depressed and non-depressed mothers, with depressed mothers reporting more difficult infants.[33,34] The severity and chronicity of maternal depressive symptoms are significantly related to more behavior problems at 5 years of age. The effect of maternal depression is uncertain, but there is some evidence that depression, or its effects on maternal interactions, can affect cognitive outcomes adversely. Murray and colleagues[35] found no evidence of an adverse effect for postnatal depression but did note that early experience of insensitive maternal interactions predicted poorer cognitive performance. Kurstjens and Wolke[36] found no significant effects of severity, timing of onset, duration, or chronicity of depression on cognitive development. They did note, however, that boys in families of low socioeconomic status and boys born at neonatal risk had lower intellectual development scores. Hay and colleagues[37] investigated the long-term sequelae in children of mothers who were depressed at 3 months postpartum and found that the children had significantly lower intelligence quotient scores than a control group with mothers who were not depressed. In addition, they also had attention problems, difficulties in mathematical reasoning, and a greater likelihood of special education needs. Boys were affected more severely than girls.

The children of mothers who are depressed also are at higher risk for psychopathology. Pawlby and colleagues[38] found a fourfold greater risk for psychiatric disorders in 11-year-old children whose mothers had postpartum depression. Of 129 children who were assessed for emotional and behavioral disorders, 11 had emotional disorders (separation anxiety, social anxiety, depressive episode), 11 had behavioral disorders (oppositional-defiant disorder, conduct disorder, attention-deficit and hyperactivity disorder), and 9 were comorbid for both types of disorders. Boys and girls were equally likely to be affected. In a related study, Hay and colleagues[39] reported that violence was associated with symptoms of attention-deficit/hyperactivity disorder and problems with anger management in children at age 11 years.

Physical Health

Maternal depression also can affect other areas of infant health. Successful feeding requires a cooperative relationship in which mother and infant must be able to interpret each other's cues. Maternal depression can affect that relationship adversely, preventing the interaction from developing and leading to poor infant feeding and growth.[40–42] In addition, mothers who are depressed are more likely to discontinue breastfeeding or to experience difficulties with breastfeeding.[43,44]

Maternal depression can affect health-seeking behaviors. Children of mothers who have depressive symptoms may have increased use of acute care, including emergency department visits, and decreased receipt of preventive services, including age-appropriate well-child visits and immunizations,[45,46] or they may use health care services more often without a clearly identifiable medical need.[47–49] Maternal depression also may affect compliance with health care recommendations. Bartlett and colleagues[50] reported that mothers who had high depressive symptoms had significantly more problems with their child using inhalers properly and forgetting doses.

RISK FACTORS FOR POSTPARTUM DEPRESSION

A number of risk factors for postpartum depression have been identified. The strongest predictors of postpartum depression are a history of depression[51] and a low level of partner support.[52,53] Other risk factors include anxiety during pregnancy,[54] stressful life events during pregnancy or in the early puerperium,[54] low self-esteem,[55] poor coping skills,[56] unwanted or unplanned pregnancy,[57] young age,[58] and nonwhite race.[59] Social risk factors include low socioeconomic status,[58–61] low levels of social support,[54–56,59] single marital status,[60] low educational level,[58,59] poor family functioning,[53] and recent immigration.[62] Mothers of multiples are also at higher risk for depression and anxiety disorders. Leonard[63] reported that 25% of mothers of multiples are affected by depression and anxiety during the prenatal and postpartum periods. Thorpe and colleagues[64] reported that 34% of mothers with two living twins and 53% of mothers with only one surviving twin were clinically depressed.

Neonatal ICU Risk Factors for Postpartum Depression

The infant, personal factors, situational variables and environmental stimuli have all been identified as potential sources of parental stressors.[65] Shields-Poë and Pinelli[66] measured parental stress and anxiety in 212 parents while the infant was in the NICU. The most powerful variable associated with stress scores was how parents perceived the severity of their infant's illness. Spear and colleagues[67] assessed family stress, coping strategies, and perceptions of infant health status on mood alterations in families with infants in the NICU who were born before 31 weeks' gestational age. High levels of depression symptoms were found in 53% of the study group. Higher levels of depression symptoms were associated with less effective coping strategies, greater parental stress, and a greater perception of disrupted parental role. Davis and colleagues[68] investigated the relationship between depression, stress, and perception of nursing support in 62 women who had infants less than 32 weeks' gestation. In the logistic regression model the relationship between maternal stress and depressive symptoms was statistically significant: for each one-point increase in stress score, the risk of depression increased by 14%. The relationship between a mother's perception of nursing support and depressive symptoms also was statistically significant: as the perception of nursing support decreased by one point, the risk of depression increased by 6%.

SIGNS AND SYMPTOMS

Signs and symptoms of postpartum depression are similar to those that would be expected with a major depressive illness. These symptoms can include either depressed mood or the loss of interest or pleasure in nearly all activities. In addition, changes in appetite or sleep patterns, decreased energy, feelings of worthlessness or guilt, difficulty thinking, concentrating, or making decisions, and recurrent thoughts of death or suicidal ideation may be present.[69] Depression can affect how a woman relates to those around her. In the context of the NICU, the manifestations of these symptoms may be reflected in the woman's interactions with staff and her infant, presenting as hostility,[70] aggressiveness,[71] anger,[72] and irritability.[73]

DEVELOPING A SCREENING PROGRAM FOR POSTPARTUM DEPRESSION

Women with infants in the NICU are at significant risk for depression, and failure to identify and treat women with depression is associated with a longer duration of depression.[74] Because maternal depression may not be identified before delivery,[75,76] and infants may remain in the NICU for a significant length of time, it is reasonable to consider the implementation of a universal screening program for depression in the NICU. Routine assessment will normalize the process, enhance awareness, and increase the health care providers' comfort level and competency.[77]

Preparation and Planning

Depression screening meets the criteria required for a screening program to be cost effective.[78] First, depression is a well-defined disorder, and diagnosis can be made using the diagnostic criteria described in the *Diagnostic and Statistical Manual-IV-TR*. Second, the incidence of depression in mothers with infants in the NICU is high, and the natural history of depression is reasonably well known. Third, women who have depression may not be identified readily by appearance alone and may not recover spontaneously. It has been reported that 46% of women who experience postpartum depressive symptoms continued to have depressive symptoms 1 year after the birth of their children.[79] Fourth, the infants of women who are depressed are at higher risk for attachment, behavioral, and cognitive disorders. Finally, depression is treatable, and a number of effective treatments exist.

The financial cost of screening itself is minimal. Screening requires little infrastructure, but the follow-up for women who require referral needs to be addressed. Some of the screens in use have been used extensively in the postpartum period and are well accepted by women.[80] Some of these instruments have been well validated for depression screening in a variety of clinical situations. The cost of treatment for depression must be considered within the larger context of the potential cost to society of lost productivity of women who are depressed and the potential lost productivity of their children. A growing body of literature suggests that identifying and treating depression appropriately could be cost effective by improving productivity in the work place.[81–87]

Barriers

A number of barriers to screening have been identified. Nutting and colleagues[88] provide a framework for addressing barriers by identifying three general types of barriers: (1) patient-centered; (2) physician-centered; and (3) systems-based. Gjerdingen and Yawn[89] also acknowledged that mothers may experience barriers that are unique to the postpartum period, including fear of judgment and referral to child protection, effects of medications on breastfeeding, and need for childcare during mental health visits. These barriers should be addressed in the planning stages for a depression screening program.

Patient-centered barriers

Dennis and Chung-Lee[90] reviewed the literature on the barriers to seeking help. A common barrier was a woman's inability to disclose her feelings, and this barrier was often reinforced by family members' and health professionals' reluctance to respond to the woman's needs. Another barrier was lack of knowledge or the acceptance of myths about postpartum depression. Other patient-centered barriers include social stigma,[91,92] access, and cost.[93,94] Providing accurate anticipatory information about depression for all mothers early in the hospitalization may help "normalize" the feelings that they may have, provide an opportunity for discussion about their feelings, and help decrease the stigma associated with mental health. The cost of and access to treatment will remain barriers for some women until mental health services are made available to all.

Physician-centered/staff-centered barriers

Pediatricians have cited lack of time to identify and treat maternal depression, unfamiliarity with screening instruments, concern about liability, and lack of community resources as significant barriers to screening.[95] Despite these concerns depression screening in the pediatric outpatient setting has been found to be feasible and successful.[96–100] The same concerns may also influence the decision to introduce screening in the NICU. Time constraints are less important because infants may be inpatients for extended periods of time, and other providers can perform the screening. Familiarity with postpartum depression and screening instruments can be overcome through education.

Liability remains a significant concern. At this time, depression screening is not considered standard of care in the NICU, but as more information is collected and guidelines are developed, this situation may change.[101] Liability issues also may include the follow-up after screening and the nature of the referral. A well-established but adaptable plan for referrals will help decrease the liability after screening occurs.

Some of the barriers for other staff members may be similar to the concerns of pediatricians, including lack of information and concern about liability. Informational needs can be met through education,[102] and liability can be minimized by attending to the process of screening and referral.

Systems-based barriers

Systems-based barriers may include the availability and accessibility of mental health resources. Many hospitals have a behavioral health department that may be interested in developing a relationship with the NICU to facilitate the screening–referral process. Insurers and managed care organizations may share a similar interest in the process, recognizing the implications of maternal mental health. Outside the professional sector, postpartum depression support groups may be available to some women. Chen and colleagues[103] have demonstrated that participation in support groups for women who have postpartum depression provides quantifiable psychosocial benefits. Another systems-based barrier at the hospital level may include the hospital's concern about liability. In some situations, involving the hospital's risk management and/or legal departments in the planning process could address their concerns and elicit their support.

It could be argued that maternal depression screening is beyond the scope of practice of the NICU; however, care of the neonate should include consideration of the environment to which the infant will be discharged. Other potentially sensitive information that is considered necessary to defining the infant's environment is collected routinely on nursing and social work assessments throughout the infant's hospitalization and is recorded in the infant's chart. Maternal mental health should be considered as important as any other environmental factor because of its potential effect on the infant's development and health.

Screening

A number of screening tools are available to screen for depression during the postnatal period.[104]

The Center for Epidemiologic Studies–Depression (CES-D)[105] is a screening tool that was developed for the general population but has been used in the postpartum period.[106–109] The CES-D is a 20-question instrument in which a score greater than or equal to 16 (out of 30) is considered indicative of depressive symptoms. Its sensitivity and specificity for detecting depression are 60% and 92%, respectively.[110] The CES-D has been translated into a number of languages, including Spanish, Italian, Greek, and Chinese.

The 10-item Edinburgh Postnatal Depression Survey (EPDS) was developed to address a perceived need for an acceptable, simple self-report scale specifically designed to be administered to women in the postpartum period.[111] In the original study, using a threshold of 12/13, the sensitivity of the EPDS was 86% and the specificity was 78%.[111] Reducing the threshold score to 9/10 decreased the false-negative rate to 10%. Eberhard-Gran and colleagues[112] recently reviewed 18 validation studies and concluded that most studies showed that the EPDS has a high sensitivity, but differences in study design and the large range of confidence intervals limited comparisons of the sensitivity and specificity among the different versions of the EPDS. The tool has been used extensively in the postpartum period and has been translated into many languages, including Spanish, French, German, Vietnamese, and Thai.

The Postpartum Depression Screening Scale (PDSS)[113] is a 35-item instrument that gives a total score as well as scores on seven dimensions (sleeping/eating disturbances, anxiety/insecurity, emotional lability, cognitive impairment, loss of self, guilt/shame, and contemplating harming oneself) of postpartum depression. The instrument is available in English and Spanish and is written at a seventh grade level. Sensitivity and specificity have been reported to be between 84% and 94% and 72% and 98%, respectively.[114–116]

Other self-report, general population screening tools have been used, including the Hamilton Depression Rating Scale,[117] the Beck Depression Inventory,[118] the General Health Questionnaire,[119] the Inventory of Depressive Symptomatology,[120] and the Zung Self-Rating Depression Scale.[121]

Identifying the most appropriate screening instrument to use in the NICU requires an assessment of the population needs, because no single test has been universally accepted. It may be necessary to consider cultural needs in screening some groups. Screening the postpartum adolescent population requires additional considerations. DeRosa and Logsdon[122] recently reviewed the screening tools available from the perspective of adolescent needs. They concluded that there was not an ideal instrument for the adolescent but recommended using both the CES-D and the EPDS because that combination could be used to evaluate the response to treatment and the progression of mental health of women into adulthood.

Deciding who will screen and when

Screening should be a multidisciplinary endeavor. An NICU culture that recognizes the importance of screening and accepts the role that screening plays in supporting women should underlie the screening program. In an environment that is openly supportive of women who have depression, it is reasonable to consider a range of providers who could administer the screening instrument. A woman interacts with many care providers during her infant's hospitalization, and during that time she may develop stronger relationships with some care providers than with others. It is important to acknowledge that it may be the woman's perception of her support that is most important in determining who should administer the screening instrument, because a trusting relationship may increase the acceptability of the offer for screening. Therefore, the most appropriate person to administer the screening instrument should reflect the woman's need rather than being defined specifically by the health care providers. At the same time, the health care team member who administers the instrument to the woman should be aware of the available resources to facilitate referral when needed. This aspect of the screening process may involve input from the NICU social worker or other contact person.

During the first 2 weeks postpartum women are at risk for postpartum blues, which are characterized by symptoms consistent with depression but are considered transitory.[123] Therefore, screening after 2 weeks should be considered.[104] It currently is unknown, however, how the impact of an admission to the NICU can affect the course of depression for women with infants in the NICU. Further research is needed to determine the optimal time(s) for screening in this population.

After screening has been completed, the results and the recommended follow-up should be documented.

Follow-Up

One of the prerequisites to developing a screening program is to ensure that appropriate follow-up is available to women who need it. Follow-up care can be provided by a number of care providers who have interest and competency in depression management. Some obstetric care providers and family practice care providers have the necessary skills and interest to assume care for the women who are referred. Other considerations could include behavioral health providers within the hospital, health care system, or community. Insurers and managed care organizations may have an interest in mental health care provision and may be willing to identify resources within their organizations for women who have postpartum depression. Finally, postpartum depression support groups could play a significant role in the follow-up of the women.

Singer and colleagues[124] measured maternal psychologic distress, parenting stress, family impact, and life stressors in mothers of very low birth weight (VLBW) infants in a longitudinal study over 3 years. They found that mothers of VLBW infants had more psychologic distress than mothers of term infants at 1 month. At 2 years, mothers of low-risk VLBW infants did not differ from term mothers, but mothers of high-risk VLBW infants continued to report psychologic distress. By 3 years, mothers of high-risk VLBW infants did not differ from mothers of term infants in distress symptoms, but parenting stress remained greater. They concluded that neonatal follow-up programs should incorporate psychologic screening and support services for mothers of VLBW infants in the immediate postnatal period, and should continue monitoring mothers of high-risk VLBW infants.

Data collection should be incorporated into the screening program for ongoing assessment of the process. The Quality Assurance/Quality Improvement department in the hospital may be able to provide valuable infrastructure for data collection. In addition, screening and referral results could be incorporated into NICU-specific data collection systems.

PATERNAL DEPRESSION

Postpartum depression can affect men whose infants are in the NICU. A number of studies have demonstrated that the greatest predictor of paternal postpartum depression is maternal postpartum depression.[125–127] Other risk factors for the fathers include a previous history of depression.[125] Field and colleagues[128] investigated prenatal depressive symptoms, anxiety, anger, and daily hassles in 156 depressed and non-depressed pregnant women and their depressed and non-depressed partners. They found that depressed partners had higher anxiety and daily hassle scores than non-depressed partners. Paternal depression seemed to have less effect than maternal depression on their partners' scores, a finding that might be attributable to the increase in maternal cortisol. Depression in fathers during the postnatal period has been found to be associated with adverse emotional and behavioral outcomes in children and an increased risk of conduct problems in boys after controlling for maternal depression and other factors.[129] The effects of paternal postpartum depression on infant health and development are not fully known and require further investigation. Therefore, it is important to consider the mental health of both parents of infants in the NICU.

SUMMARY

Depression is common among women who have infants in the NICU. Screening for depression in the NICU can be considered part of the care of the infant, because unrecognized and untreated depression has the potential to affect infant health and development adversely. Screening programs for maternal depression can be developed in the NICU but require adequate planning and preparation to ensure that screening is acceptable to women and that appropriate follow-up is available to them. More research is necessary to optimize the screening process and to establish its role in neonatal care.

ACKNOWLEDGMENTS

The author gratefully acknowledges the contributions of the Wisconsin Association for Perinatal Care, the Perinatal Foundation, Postpartum Support International, the neonatal ICU nurses and staffs of Wheaton Franciscan Healthcare St. Joseph, Columbia-St. Mary's Milwaukee, Aurora Sinai Medical Center, and the Aurora Women's Pavilion, and, especially, all the women who have shared their experiences.

REFERENCES

1. O'Hara MW, Swain AM. Rates and risk of postpartum depression—a meta-analysis. Int Rev Psychiatry 1996;8(1):37–56.
2. Deal LW, Holt VL. Young maternal age and depressive symptoms: results from the 1988 National Maternal and Infant Health Survey. Am J Public Health 1998;88(2):266–70.
3. Sequin L, Potvin L, St. Denis M, et al. Depressive symptoms in the late postpartum among low socioeconomic status women. Birth 1999;26(3):157–63.
4. Meyer EC, Garcia Coll CT, Seifer R, et al. Psychological distress in mothers of preterm infants. J Dev Behav Pediatr 1995;11(6):412–7.
5. Miles MS, Holditch-Davis D, Burchinal P, et al. Distress and growth outcomes in mothers of medically fragile infants. Nurs Res 1999;48(3):129–40.
6. Miles MS, Holditch-Davis D, Schwartz TA, et al. Depressive symptoms in mothers of prematurely born infants. J Dev Behav Pediatr 2007;28(1):36–44.
7. Murray L, Woolgar M, Murray J, et al. Self-exclusion from health care in women at high risk for postpartum depression. J Public Health Med 2003;25(2):131–7.
8. Feijo de Mello AA, Feijo de Mello M, Carpenter LL, et al. Update on stress and depression: the role of the hypothalamic–pituitary–adrenal (HPA) axis. Rev Bras Psiquiatr 2003;25(4):231–8.
9. Barden N. Implication of the hypothalamic–pituitary–adrenal axis in the physiopathology of depression. J Psychiatry Neurosci 2004;29(3):185–93.
10. Checkley S. The neuroendocrinology of depression and chronic stress. Br Med Bull 1996;52(3):597–617.
11. Lopez JF, Vazquez DM, Chalmers DT, et al. Regulation of 5-HT receptors and the hypothalamic–pituitary–adrenal axis. Implications for the neurobiology of suicide. Ann N Y Acad Sci 1997;836:106–34.
12. Leonard BE. Stress, norepinephrine and depression. J Psychiatry Neurosci 2001;26(Suppl):S11–6.
13. Tsigos C, Chrousos GP. Hypothalamic–pituitary axis, neuroendocrine factors and stress. J Psychosom Res 2002;53(4):865–71.
14. Mancuso RA, Schetter CD, Rini CM, et al. Maternal prenatal anxiety and corticotropin-releasing hormone associated with timing of delivery. Psychosom Med 2004;66(5):762–9.
15. Field T, Diego M, Hernandez-Reif M, et al. Prenatal maternal biochemistry predicts neonatal biochemistry. Int J Neurosci 2004;114(8):933–45.
16. Diego MA, Field T, Hernandez-Reif M, et al. Prepartum, postpartum, and chronic depression effects on newborns. Psychiatry 2004;67(1):63–80.
17. Essex MJ, Klein MH, Cho E, et al. Maternal stress beginning in infancy may sensitize children to later stress exposure: effects on cortisol and behavior. Biol Psychiatry 2002;52(8):776–84.
18. Dayan J, Creveuil C, Marks MN, et al. Prenatal depression, prenatal anxiety, and spontaneous preterm birth: a prospective cohort study among women with early and regular care. Psychosom Med 2006;68(6):938–46.

19. Field T, Hernandez-Reif M, Diego M, et al. Prenatal cortisol, prematurity and low birthweight. Infant Behav Dev 2006;29(3):268–75.
20. Keenan K, Sheffield R, Boeldt D. Are prenatal psychological or physical stressors associated with suboptimal outcomes in neonates born to adolescent mothers? Early Hum Dev 2007;83(9):623–7.
21. Bhagwanani SG, Seagraves K, Dierker LJ, et al. Relationship between prenatal anxiety and perinatal outcome in nulliparous women: a prospective study. J Natl Med Assoc 1997;89(2):93–8.
22. Field T, Diego M, Hernandez-Reif M, et al. Chronic prenatal depression and neonatal outcome. Int J Neurosci 2008;118(1):95–103.
23. Misri S, Oberlander TF, Fairbrother N, et al. Relation between prenatal maternal mood and anxiety and neonatal health. Can J Psychiatry 2004;49(10):684–9.
24. Andersson L, Sundstrom-Poromaa I, Wulff M, et al. Neonatal outcome following maternal antenatal depression and anxiety: a population-based study. Am J Epidemiol 2004;159(9):872–81.
25. Perkin MR, Bland JM, Peacock JL, et al. The effect of anxiety and depression during pregnancy on obstetric complications. Br J Obstet Gynaecol 1993; 100(7):629–34.
26. Hedegaard M, Henriksen TB, Sabroe S, et al. The relationship between psychological distress during pregnancy and birth weight for gestational age. Acta Obstet Gynecol Scand 1996;75(1):32–9.
27. Jacobsen G, Schei B, Hoffman HJ. Psychological factors and small-for-gestational-age infants among parous Scandinavian women. Acta Obstet Gynecol Scand Suppl 1997;165:14–8.
28. Kent A, Hughes P, Ormerod L, et al. Uterine artery resistance and anxiety in the second trimester of pregnancy. Ultrasound Obstet Gynecol 2002;19(2):177–9.
29. Thompson RA. The legacy of early attachments. Child Dev 2000;71(1):145–52.
30. Carlson EA, Sampson MC, Sroufe LA. Implications of attachment theory and research for developmental–behavioral pediatrics. J Dev Behav Pediatr 2003; 24(5):364–79.
31. Field TA, Sandberg D, Garcia R, et al. Pregnancy problems, postpartum depression, and early mother–infant interactions. Dev Psychol 1985;21:1152–6.
32. Beatson J, Taryan S. Predisposition to depression: the role of attachment. Aust N Z J Psychiatry 2003;37(4):219–25.
33. McMahon C, Barnett B, Kowalenko N, et al. Postnatal depression, anxiety and unsettled infant behavior. Aust N Z J Psychiatry 2001;35(5):581–8.
34. McGrath JM, Records K, Rice M. Maternal depression and infant temperament characteristics. Infant Behav Dev 2008;31(1):71–80.
35. Murray L, Hipwell A, Hooper R, et al. The cognitive development of 5-year-old children of postnatally depressed mothers. J Child Psychol Psychiatry 1996; 37(8):927–35.
36. Kurstjens S, Wolke D. Effects of maternal depression on cognitive development of children over the first 7 years of life. J Child Psychol Psychiatry 2001;42(5): 623–36.
37. Hay DF, Pawlby S, Sharp D, et al. Intellectual problems shown by 11-year-old children whose mothers had postnatal depression. J Child Psychol Psychiatry 2001;42(7):871–89.
38. Pawlby S, Sharp D, Hay D, et al. Postnatal depression and child outcome at 11 years: the importance of accurate diagnosis. J Affect Disord 2008;107(1–3):241–5.
39. Hay D, Pawlby S, Angold A, et al. Pathways to violence in the children of mothers who were depressed postpartum. Dev Psychol 2003;39(6):1083–94.

40. O'Brien LM, Heycock EG, Hanna M, et al. Postnatal depression and faltering growth: a community study. Pediatrics 2004;113(5):1242–7.
41. Patel V, DeSouza N, Rodrigues M. Postnatal depression and infant growth and development in low income countries: a cohort study from Goa, India. Arch Dis Child 2003;88(1):34–7.
42. Rahman A, Iqbal Z, Bunn J, et al. Impact of maternal depression on infant nutritional status and illness. Arch Gen Psychiatry 2004;61(9):946–52.
43. Dennis CL, McQueen K. Does maternal postpartum depressive symptomatology influence infant feeding outcomes? Acta Paediatr 2007;96(4):590–4.
44. McLearn KT, Minkovitz CS, Strobino DM, et al. Maternal depressive symptoms at 2 to 4 months post partum and early parenting practices. Arch Pediatr Adolesc Med 2006;160(3):279–84.
45. Minkovitz CS, Strobino D, Scharfstein D, et al. Maternal depressive symptoms and children's receipt of health care in the first 3 years of life. Pediatrics 2005; 115(2):306–14.
46. Flynn HA, Davis M, Marcus SM, et al. Rates of maternal depression in pediatric emergency department and relationship to child service utilization. Gen Hosp Psychiatry 2004;26(4):316–22.
47. Chee CY, Chong YS, NG TP, et al. The association between maternal depression and frequent non-routine visits to the infant's doctor—a cohort study. J Affect Disord 2008;107(1–3):247–53.
48. Dennis CL. Influence of depressive symptomatology on maternal health service utilization and general health. Arch Womens Ment Health 2004;7(3):183–92.
49. Mandl KD, Tronick EZ, Brennan TA, et al. Infant health care use and maternal depression. Arch Pediatr Adolesc Med 1999;153(8):808–13.
50. Bartlett SJ, Krishnan JA, Riekert KA, et al. Maternal depressive symptoms and adherence to therapy in inner-city children with asthma. Pediatrics 2004; 113(2):229–37.
51. Leigh B, Milgrom J. Risk factors for antenatal depression, postnatal depression and parenting stress. BMC Psychiatry 2008;8:24–35.
52. Milgrom J, Gemmill AW, Bilszta JL, et al. Antenatal risk factors for postnatal depression: a large prospective study. J Affect Disord 2008;108(1–2):147–57.
53. O'Brien M, Heron Asay J, McCluskey-Fawcett K. Family functioning and maternal depression following premature birth. J Reprod Infant Psychol 1999;17(2): 175–88.
54. Robertson E, Grace S, Wallington T, et al. Antenatal risk factors for postpartum depression: a synthesis of recent literature. Gen Hosp Psychiatry 2004;26(4): 289–95.
55. Logsdon MC, Davis DW, Birkimer JC, et al. Predictors of depression in mothers of preterm infants. J Soc Behav Pers 1997;12(1):73–88.
56. Veddovi M, Kenny DT, Gibson F, et al. The relationship between depressive symptoms following premature birth, mothers' coping style, and knowledge of infant development. J Reprod Infant Psychol 2001;19(4):313–23.
57. Rich-Edwards JW, Kleinman K, Abrams A, et al. Sociodemographic predictors of antenatal and postpartum depressive symptoms among women in a medical group practice. J Epidemiol Community Health 2006;60(3):221–7.
58. Field T, Hernandez-Reif M, Diego M. Risk factors and stress variables that differentiate depressed from nondepressed pregnant women. Infant Behav Dev 2006;29(2):169–74.
59. Howell EA, Mora P, Leventhal H. Correlates of early postpartum depressive symptoms. Matern Child Health J 2006;10(2):149–57.

60. Beeghly M, Olson KL, Weinberg MK, et al. Prevalence, stability, and sociodemographic correlates of depressive symptoms in black mothers during the first 18 months postpartum. Matern Child Health J 2003;7(3):157–68.
61. Secco ML, Profit S, Kennedy E, et al. Factors affecting postpartum depressive symptoms of adolescent mothers. J Obstet Gynecol Neonatal Nurs 2007; 36(1):47–54.
62. Dennis CL, Janssen PA, Singer J. Identifying women at-risk for postpartum depression in the immediate postpartum period. Acta Psychiatr Scand 2004; 110(5):338–46.
63. Leonard L. Depression and anxiety disorders during multiple pregnancy and parenthood. J Obstet Gynecol Neonatal Nurs 1998;27(3):329–37.
64. Thorpe K, Golding J, MacGillivray I, et al. Comparison of prevalence of depression in mothers of twins and mothers of singletons. BMJ 1991;302(6781):875–8.
65. Miles M, Carter M. Assessing parental stress in intensive care unit. MCN Am J Matern Child Nurs 1983;8:354–9.
66. Shields-Poë D, Pinelli J. Variables associated with parental stress in neonatal intensive care units. Neonatal Netw 1997;16(1):29–37.
67. Spear ML, Leef K, Epps S, et al. Family reactions during infants' hospitalization in the neonatal intensive care unit. Am J Perinatol 2002;19(4):205–13.
68. Davis L, Edwards H, Mohay H, et al. The impact of very premature birth on the psychological health of mothers. Early Hum Dev 2003;73(1–2):61–70.
69. American Psychiatric Association. Diagnostic and statistical manual of mental disorders. 4th edition, Text Revision. Washington, DC: American Psychiatric Association; 2000. p. 349.
70. Doering LV, Moser DK, Dracup K. Correlates of anxiety, hostility, depression, and psychosocial adjustment in parents of NICU infants. Neonatal Netw 2000;19(5):15–23.
71. Pasquini M, Picardi A, Biondi M, et al. Relevance of anger and irritability in outpatients with major depressive disorder. Psychopathology 2004;37(4):155–60.
72. Hand IL, Noble L, North A, et al. Psychiatric symptoms among postpartum women in an urban hospital setting. Am J Perinatol 2006;23(6):329–34.
73. Shanok AF, Miller L. Depression and treatment with inner city pregnant and parenting teens. Arch Womens Ment Health 2007;10(5):199–210.
74. England SJ, Ballard C, George S. Chronicity in postnatal depression. Eur J Psychiatr 1994;8:93–6.
75. Heneghan AM, Johnson Silver E, Bauman LJ, et al. Do pediatricians recognize mothers with depressive symptoms? Pediatrics 2000;106(6):1367–73.
76. Heneghan A, Morton S, DeLeone NL. Paediatricians' attitudes about discussing maternal depression during a paediatric primary care visit. Child Care Health Dev 2006;33(3):333–9.
77. Beck CT. Recognizing and screening for postpartum depression in mothers of NICU infants. Adv Neonatal Care 2003;3(1):37–46.
78. Cuckle HS, Wald NJ. Principles of screening. In: Wald NJ, editor. Antenatal and neonatal screening. Oxford (UK): Oxford University Press; 1984.
79. Horwitz SM, Briggs-Gowan MJ, Storfer-Isser A, et al. Prevalence, correlates, and persistence of maternal depression. J Womens Health 2007;16(5):678–91.
80. Gemmill AW, Leigh B, Ericksen J, et al. A survey of the clinical acceptability of screening for postnatal depression in depressed and non-depressed women. BMC Public Health 2006;6:211–9.
81. Kessler RC, Barber C, Birnbaum HG, et al. Depression in the workplace: effects on short-term disability. Health Aff (Millwood) 1999;18(5):163–71.

82. Greenberg PE, Stiglin LE, Finkelstein SN, et al. The economic burden of depression in 1990. J Clin Psychiatry 1993;54(11):405–18.
83. Williams RA, Strasser PB. Depression in the workplace. Impact on employees. AAOHN J 1999;47(11):526–37.
84. Conti DJ, Burton WN. The economic impact of depression in a workplace. J Occup Med 1994;36(9):983–8.
85. Dewa CS, Goering P, Lin E, et al. Depression-related short-term disability in an employed population. J Occup Environ Med 2002;44(7):628–33.
86. Simon GE, Barber C, Birnbaum HG, et al. Depression and work productivity: the comparative costs of treatment versus nontreatment. J Occup Environ Med 2001;43(1):2–9.
87. Stewart WF, Ricci JA, Chee E, et al. Cost of lost productive work time among US workers with depression. JAMA 2003;289(23):3135–44.
88. Nutting PA, Rost K, Dickinson M, et al. Barriers to initiating depression treatment in primary care practice. J Gen Intern Med 2002;17(2):103–11.
89. Gjerdingen DK, Yawn BP. Postpartum depression screening: importance, methods, barriers, and recommendations for practice. J Am Board Fam Med 2007;20(3):280–8.
90. Dennis CL, Chung-Lee L. Postpartum depression help-seeking barriers and maternal treatment preferences: a qualitative systematic review. Birth 2006;33(4):323–31.
91. Scholle SH, Haskett RF, Janusa BH, et al. Addressing depression in obstetrics/gynecology practice. Gen Hosp Psychiatry 2003;25(2):83–90.
92. Katon WJ, Ludman EJ. Improving services for women with depression in primary care settings. Psychol Women Q 2003;27:114–20.
93. LaRocco-Cockburn A, Melville J, Bell M, et al. Depression screening attitudes and practices among obstetrician–gynecologists. Obstet Gynecol 2003;101 (5 Pt 1):892–8.
94. Bambauer KZ, Safran DG, Ross-Degnan D, et al. Depression and cost-related medication non-adherence in Medicare beneficiaries. Arch Gen Psychiatry 2007;64(5):602–8.
95. Horwitz SM, Kelleher KJ, Stein REK, et al. Barriers to the identification and management of psychosocial issues in children and maternal depression. Pediatrics 2007;119(1):e208–18.
96. Olson AL, Dietrich AJ, Prazar G, et al. Brief maternal depression screening at well-child visits. Pediatrics 2006;118(1):207–16.
97. Currie ML, Rademacher R. The pediatrician's role in recognizing and intervening in postpartum depression. Pediatr Clin North Am 2004;51(3):785–801.
98. Chaudron LH, Szilagyi PG, Kitzman HJ, et al. Detection of postpartum depressive symptoms by screening at well-child visits. Pediatrics 2004;113(3):551–8.
99. Freeman MP, Wright R, Watchman M, et al. Postpartum depression assessments at well-baby visits: screening feasibility, prevalence, and risk factors. J Womens Health 2005;14(10):929–35.
100. Dubowitz H, Feigelman S, Lane W, et al. Screening for depression in an urban pediatric primary care clinic. Pediatrics 2007;119(3):435–42.
101. Chaudron LH, Szilagyi PG, Campbell AT, et al. Legal and ethical considerations: risks and benefits of postpartum depression screening at well-child visits. Pediatrics 2007;119(1):123–8.
102. Logsdon MC, Wisner K, Billings DM, et al. Raising the awareness of primary care providers about postpartum depression. Issues Ment Health Nurs 2006; 27(1):59–73.

103. Chen C-H, Tseng Y-F, Chou F-H, et al. Effects of support group intervention in postnatally distressed women: a controlled study in Taiwan. J Psychosom Res 2000;49(6):395–9.
104. Boyd RC, Le HN, Somberg R. Review of screening instruments for postpartum depression. Arch Womens Ment Health 2005;8(3):141–54.
105. Radloff LS. The CES-D Scale: a self-report depression scale for research in the general population. Appl Psychol Meas 1977;1:385–401.
106. Beeghly M, Weinberg MK, Olson KL, et al. Stability and change in level of maternal depressive symptomatology during the first postpartum year. J Affect Disord 2002;71(1–3):169–80.
107. Chaudron LH, Klein MH, Remington P, et al. Predictors, prodromes and incidence of postpartum depression. J Psychosom Obstet Gynaecol 2001;22(2): 103–12.
108. Logsdon MC, McBride AB, Birkimer JC. Social support and postpartum depression. Res Nurs Health 1994;17(6):449–57.
109. Bozoky I, Corwin EJ. Fatigue as a predictor of postpartum depression. J Obstet Gynecol Neonatal Nurs 2002;31(4):436–43.
110. Campbell SB, Cohn JF. Prevalence and correlates of postpartum depression in first-time mothers. J Abnorm Psychol 1991;100(4):594–9.
111. Cox JL, Holden JM, Sagovsky R. Detection of postnatal depression: development of the 10-item Edinburgh Postnatal Depression Scale. Br J Psychiatry 1987;150:782–6.
112. Eberhard-Gran M, Eskild A, Tambs K, et al. Review of validation studies of the Edinburgh Postnatal Depression Scale. Acta Psychiatr Scand 2001;104(4): 243–9.
113. Beck CT, Gable RK. Postpartum Depression Screening Scale: development and psychometric testing. Nurs Res 2000;49(5):272–82.
114. Beck CT, Gable RK. Comparative analysis of the performance of the Postpartum Depression Screening Scale with two other depression instruments. Nurs Res 2001;50(4):242–50.
115. Beck CT, Gable RK. Further validation of the Postpartum Depression Screening Scale. Nurs Res 2001;50(3):155–64.
116. Beck CT, Gable RK. Screening performance of the Postpartum Depression Screening Scale—Spanish version. J Transcult Nurs 2005;16(4):331–8.
117. Hamilton M. A rating scale for depression. J Neurol Neurosurg Psychiatry 1960; 23:56–62.
118. Beck AT, Ward CH, Mendelson M, et al. An inventory for measuring depression. Arch Gen Psychiatry 1961;4:561–71.
119. Goldberg DP. The detection of psychiatric illness by questionnaire; a technique for the identification and assessment of non-psychotic psychiatric illness. London: Oxford University Press; 1972.
120. Rush AJ, Giles DE, Schlesser MA, et al. The Inventory for Depressive Symptomatology (IDS): preliminary findings. Psychiatry Res 1986;18(1):65–87.
121. Zung WWK. A self-rating depression scale. Arch Gen Psychiatry 1965;12: 63–70.
122. DeRosa N, Logsdon MC. A comparison of screening instruments for depression in postpartum adolescents. J Child Adolesc Psychiatr Nurs 2006;19(1):13–20.
123. O'Hara MW. Post-partum blues, depression, and psychosis: a review. J Psychosom Obstet Gynaecol 1987;7:205–27.

124. Singer LT, Salvator A, Guo S, et al. Maternal psychological distress and parenting stress after the birth of a very low-birth-weight infant. JAMA 1999;281(9):799–805.
125. Areias MEG, Kumar R, Barros H, et al. Correlates of postnatal depression in mothers and fathers. Br J Psychiatry 1996;169(1):36–41.
126. Goodman JH. Paternal postpartum depression, its relationship to maternal depression, and implications for family health. J Adv Nurs 2004;45(1):26–35.
127. Pinheiro RT, Magalhaes PVS, Horta BL, et al. Is paternal postpartum depression associated with maternal postpartum depression? Population-based study in Brazil. Acta Psychiatr Scand 2006;113(3):230–2.
128. Field T, Diego M, Hernandez-Reif M, et al. Prenatal paternal depression. Infant Beh Dev 2006;29(4):579–83.
129. Ramchandani P, Stein A, Evans J, et al. Paternal depression in the postnatal period and child development: a prospective population study. Lancet 2005;365(9478):2201–5.

Controversies in the Treatment of Gastroesophageal Reflux Disease in Preterm Infants

Neelesh A. Tipnis, MD[a,b,*], Sajani M. Tipnis, MD[b,c]

KEYWORDS

- Gastroesophageal reflux disease • Preterm infant • Apnea
- Bronchopulmonary dysplasia • Proton pump inhibitor

Gastroesophageal reflux (GER) is the retrograde movement of gastrointestinal contents into the esophagus. It typically is a physiologic process and is common in term and premature infants. When this retrograde movement of gastrointestinal contents results in injury to the esophagus or supra-esophageal structures, however, GER is considered pathologic, and the infant is identified as having gastrointestinal reflux disease (GERD). The reported incidence of GER varies based on the criteria used for diagnosis and ranges from 22% to 85% of premature infants.[1–4] Recent studies have found that the use of acid-suppression therapy for GERD in infants younger than 1 year of age is increasing[5] and that nearly 25% of very low birth weight infants are treated with reflux medications at discharge.[6] Differentiating between physiologic and pathologic GER, understanding the mechanisms that result in the generation of and the protection against GER, and understanding the rationale for treatment are important for the effective management of GERD in premature infants.

MECHANISMS OF GASTROESOPHAGEAL REFLUX IN PRETERM INFANTS

The most common mechanism of GER in the preterm infant is transient relaxation of the lower esophageal sphincter.[7] During an episode of transient lower esophageal

[a] Division of Pediatric Gastroenterology and Nutrition, Department of Pediatrics, Children's Hospital of Wisconsin and the Medical College of Wisconsin, 8701 Watertown Plank Road, Suite B610, Milwaukee, WI 53226, USA
[b] Children's Hospital of Wisconsin, 9000 W. Wisconsin Avenue, Milwaukee, WI 53226, USA
[c] Division of Neonatology, Department of Pediatrics, Children's Hospital of Wisconsin and the Medical College of Wisconsin, 8701 Watertown Plank Road, Suite C410, Milwaukee, WI 53226, USA
* Corresponding author. Division of Pediatric Gastroenterology and Nutrition, Department of Pediatrics, 8701 Watertown Plank Road, Suite B610, Milwaukee, WI 53226.
E-mail address: ntipnis@mcw.edu (N.A. Tipnis).

Clin Perinatol 36 (2009) 153–164
doi:10.1016/j.clp.2008.09.011 perinatology.theclinics.com

sphincter relaxation, the pressure of the lower esophageal sphincter is reduced spontaneously to less than the intragastric pressure, forming a common cavity between the stomach and esophagus. Because the intragastric pressure typically exceeds the intra-esophageal pressure, gas or liquid contents resting in the fundus of the stomach can reflux into the esophagus. Increased intra-abdominal pressure and decreased baseline lower esophageal sphincter pressure also are associated with GER and may play a more significant role in infants who have respiratory or neurologic disease.

PROTECTION FROM GASTROESOPHAGEAL REFLUX IN THE PRETERM INFANT

Mechanisms to protect the esophagus from GER are present even in the preterm infant. Abnormalities in any of these protection mechanisms can predispose an infant to the consequences of GER. Regurgitation of gastric contents into the esophagus triggers several esophageal and laryngeal reflexes to counteract GER and to protect the airway from acid exposure.[8] Distension of the esophagus by refluxate results in the induction of a secondary peristaltic wave that propels the material back into the stomach and in reflexive closure of the upper esophageal sphincter to prevent migration of refluxed material into the posterior pharynx (the esophagopharyngeal closure reflex). If refluxate reaches the upper esophagus, however, the upper esophageal sphincter opens reflexively to allow expulsion of the material into the pharynx, but the glottis closes spontaneously to prevent airway aspiration, and the closure is accompanied by a period of apnea. Entry of refluxate into the pharynx also results in primary peristalsis.[9] The esophageal epithelium serves as the main barrier for limiting the effects of acid exposure to the esophagus. Intercellular phospholipids and bicarbonate secretion from mucous glands in the esophagus and salivary glands neutralize the gastric acid in refluxed materials.[10] Exposure of the esophageal mucosa to acid and bile causes the breakdown of tight junctions, leading to edema and dilatation of the intracellular spaces of Disse.[11]

CLINICAL FEATURES OF GASTROESOPHAGEAL REFLUX IN PRETERM INFANTS

Many clinical signs and symptoms in preterm infants have been attributed to GER, including apnea, chronic lung disease, poor weight gain, and behavioral symptoms. The literature supporting and refuting these clinical features is discussed in the following sections.

Apnea

Apnea often occurs during or following feeding periods, leading to the assumption that apnea occurs as a result of GER. It is postulated that refluxate during the GER episodes stimulates laryngeal chemoreflexes.[12] Laryngeal stimulation in preterm infants results in obstructive, central, and mixed apneas as well as other reflex activities including cough, increased swallowing, and arousal.[13] Several studies in the 1970s demonstrated an association between esophageal acidification and apnea in preterm infants.[14,15] Aggressive treatment of GER with medication (prokinetic agents, antacids) or surgery resolved the apneas.[16,17] Several studies using prolonged pH monitoring or impedance monitoring have failed to demonstrate a temporal relationship between GER and apnea, however. In a study of 14 infants, Walsh and colleagues[18] found no difference in the frequency of apnea during periods of GER and during non-GER periods. Barrington and colleagues[19] evaluated 45 preterm infants at the time of discharge and found no statistical correlation between apnea lasting longer than 10 seconds and the number of GER episodes or total duration of GER. Less than 1% of apneas recorded in 119 preterm infants evaluated by DiFiore and colleagues[20] were associated with GER. Using multiple intraluminal impedance monitoring, Peter and colleagues[21] evaluated 19 preterm infants and found no difference in the frequency of apnea associated with GER during reflux periods and of episodes of apnea occurring during reflux-free periods. These studies demonstrate that both GER and apnea do occur together in preterm infants but occur as separate rather than simultaneous events, suggesting that common risk factors for both apnea and GER are present in these individuals. Last, treatment with prokinetic agents has not been shown to improve apnea.[22] The effects of acid suppression using newer proton-pump inhibitor (PPI) agents have not been studied.

Bronchopulmonary Dysplasia

Bronchopulmonary dysplasia (BPD) or chronic lung disease affects 30% of preterm infants with a birth weight under 1 kg.[23] Analysis of tracheal aspirates for lipid-laden macrophages, gastric pepsin, and acid-denatured bile salts shows evidence of a relationship between chronic aspiration and chronic lung disease.[24] Furthermore, treatment of GER improves the pulmonary status of older children who have chronic lung disease and of adults who have pulmonary fibrosis.[25–28]

Current studies in neonates fail to show a clear causal relationship between GER and chronic lung disease. Researchers have used the amount of acid exposure in the esophagus during sleep as a method of assessing chronic lung disease risk. Jolley and colleagues[29] found high GER scores in 28 infants who had BPD, but in most of these infants exposure to esophageal acid during sleep was not prolonged. The infants who had prolonged exposure to esophageal acid during sleep improved more with reflux treatment than those who had normal exposure to esophageal acid during sleep. Akinola and colleagues[30] retrospectively reviewed 629 preterm infants of whom 137 had pH testing. Sixty-three percent of these infants had abnormal pH scores; however, there was no correlation of BPD status with GER status in this cohort. Omari and colleagues[31] found no difference in the mechanism of GER in infants who had BPD compared with healthy infants.

The method used to detect GER may play a role in helping to identify those at risk for BPD. Starosta and colleagues[24] reported higher pepsin levels in a heterogeneous group of children who had chronic lung diseases and proximal GER detected by pH-metry than in children who did not have proximal GER. A recent study by Farhath and colleagues[32] found that pepsin levels in tracheal aspirates were higher in ventilated very low birth weight infants that went on to develop BPD than in those who did not develop BPD. The studies involving pepsin also may indicate that nonacid reflux is an important mediator of lung disease in preterm infants. Treatment trials showing an improvement in pulmonary status are needed to establish better a relationship between GERD and BPD.

Growth

Failure to thrive is a sign often attributed to GER in infants. A retrospective case-control study evaluated the impact of GER on growth and hospital stay in a cohort of 23 preterm infants and an in equal number of control infants matched for gestational age, birth weight, gender, and severity of BPD. The diagnosis of GER was based on clinical symptoms. Investigators found no significant difference between patients and control infants in average weekly weight gain, caloric intake, grams gained per calorie given, or weekly increments gained in length and head circumference. Infants who had clinical GER took more than twice as many days to achieve full feeds than control infants, and the length of stay for infants who had GER was nearly a third longer than for the control infants.[33] Another study correlated clinical features in 150 preterm infants evaluated by pH-metry.[34] Infants were categorized into three groups based on the pH testing: normal, mild GER, and severe GER. The groups did not differ in clinical characteristics, including birth weight, gestational age, incidence of patent ductus arteriosus, intraventricular hemorrhage, necrotizing enterocolitis, chronic lung disease, or treatment with xanthines. Infants who had mild or severe GER based on pH testing had more clinical symptoms of GER (increased gastric residue or emesis). Infants who had severe GER had a longer length of hospital stay, a higher incidence of respiratory distress syndrome, and lower hematocrits than infants who had no or mild GER. It was not clear whether there is a causal relationship between GER and these symptoms or if the increased reflux scores were reflective of underlying disease. There are no studies evaluating the efficacy of GERD treatment using growth as a clinical research end point.

Behavior

Several behaviors such as irritability, facial grimacing, head arching, and frequent swallowing have been attributed to GER, particularly in older infants.[35] A double-blind, withdrawal study using famotidine demonstrated a reduction in crying time and regurgitation episodes; however, many infants experienced neurologic symptoms such as increased irritability.[36] Since then, case-controlled and placebo-controlled studies have found poor correlation of these behavioral symptoms with GER in preterm infants[37] and have found no difference in symptom scores after treatment with cisapride[38] or omeprazole.[39] Therefore, it is unlikely that these behavioral symptoms are the result of GER in preterm infants.

EVALUATION OF GASTROESOPHAGEAL REFLUX IN PRETERM INFANTS

Because GER is a normal physiologic event, the role of diagnostic testing is to determine if GER is causing disease and to exclude other pathologic conditions that mimic GER.[40] Therefore the value of specific diagnostic tests varies, depending on the clinical presentation.

History and physical examination alone may be adequate to diagnose GERD and initiate management in some cases. In general, physiologic GER in infants is easy to recognize, and no treatment is necessary. Common signs and symptoms attributed to GER include regurgitation (milk in the pharynx), vomiting, irritability, arching, grimacing, apnea, bradycardia, desaturation, and respiratory symptoms. Many of these clinical features, however, are common to other disorders such as milk protein allergy; as discussed previously, studies have failed to correlate these symptoms with GER, and treatment has not been shown to be efficacious. Signs and symptoms that suggest a diagnosis other than GER include bilious vomiting, gastrointestinal bleeding, consistently forceful vomiting, failure to thrive, diarrhea, constipation, fever, lethargy, hepatosplenomegaly, bulging fontanelle, macro/microcephaly, seizures, abdominal tenderness or distension, documented or suspected genetic/metabolic syndromes, and associated chronic disease.[40]

Radiographic upper gastrointestinal series are useful to detect anatomic abnormalities, such as aspiration with swallowing, esophageal rings or webs, hiatal hernia, or malrotation, that may cause respiratory complications, dysphagia, or vomiting. The upper gastrointestinal series is not useful for the diagnosis of GERD, because the observation of gastric reflux may represent physiologic GER, and observed mucosal abnormalities may be caused by conditions that mimic GERD.[40]

Esophageal pH monitoring determines when the esophageal lumen becomes acidified. Interpretation of these studies generally involves calculations of the amount of time that the esophageal pH is below 4 and/or the number and length of episodes. The percentage of time in a 24-hour study that the esophageal pH is less than 4, also called the "reflux index" (RI), is considered the most valid measure of reflux because it reflects the cumulative exposure of the esophagus to acid. Commonly, an RI greater than 11% is considered to indicate pathologic GERD in infants.[41] A recent British study, however, reported variability in the location of pH catheter and threshold values for significant RI scores at tertiary referral centers.[1] Esophageal pH monitoring also may be performed to determine whether an episodic symptom such as apnea or pain is caused by GER. In such cases the occurrence of the symptom and esophageal pH are monitored simultaneously so that a symptom index (the percentage of GER episodes associated with the symptom) can be evaluated.[42] Studies using prolonged esophageal pH monitoring show poor correlation between the severity of symptoms and response to therapy. In infants in whom GERD is suspected, an abnormal pH study (RI >10%) was associated only with pneumonia, apnea with fussing, and constipation.[43]

Esophageal electrical impedance monitoring, also known as the "multichannel intra-esophageal impedance test" (MII), is relatively new. Electrical impedance changes when a bolus of fluid or air passes between electrical sensors along a catheter. When combined with esophageal pH monitoring, the MII test allows detection of both acid and nonacid episodes of GER.[44] Unfortunately, despite the improved detection of GER episodes, this new technology has not yet influenced clinical management in pediatric patients, especially those who have airway symptoms in whom a cause–effect relationship is difficult to establish.[21,45] More recently, normative values have been established for acidic and weakly acidic reflux in preterm infants;[46] however, the usefulness of pH/MII testing has not been evaluated in preterm infants.

Upper endoscopy with biopsy evaluates whether GER has caused damage to the esophagus by allowing visualization of mucosal surface. A number of endoscopic and histologic findings have been reported in the esophagus of preterm infants, including erythema, erosions, and mucosal inflammation;[47] however, 39% of infants who had a pathologic RI score by pH testing had normal esophageal biopsies, and 50% of infants who had histologic esophagitis had normal esophageal pH scores.[48] Therefore, histology alone was not predictive of GERD in this study.

Nuclear scintigraphy is performed by the oral ingestion or instillation of technetium-labeled formula or food into the stomach; then the number of episodes of postprandial GER and any episodes of aspiration into the lung are observed. Scintigraphy also provides information about gastric emptying, which may be delayed in some children who have GERD. A lack of standardized techniques, the absence of age-specific normative data, and a lack of sensitivity limit the value of this test.[40] Furthermore, although nuclear scintigraphy identified GER in preterm infants, there was no correlation with the proximal extent of the episodes with clinical symptoms.[49]

Empiric therapy without diagnostic evaluation has been validated in adults as a cost-effective approach for diagnosis of the likely relationship between acid reflux and symptoms of cough,[50] heartburn, noncardiac chest pain,[51] and dyspepsia.[52] In preterm infants, however, there are no data evaluating the effects of empiric GERD therapy before diagnostic testing for traditional GERD-related symptoms. Caution should be used, because the pharmacokinetics and dosing of PPI drugs are not well understood in this population. If a trial of empiric therapy is initiated, it should be time limited to determine whether there is a symptomatic response and to evaluate whether symptoms relapse off drug.

TREATMENT OF GASTROESOPHAGEAL REFLUX DISEASE IN PRETERM INFANTS

Compared with adults, few studies have evaluated the treatment of GERD in preterm infants. Most infants who have frequent regurgitation have physiologic reflux, and no interventions are required.[40] It is important to balance the potential risks of GERD with those of therapy when deciding on appropriate treatment in the individual patient.

Nonpharmacologic Treatments

Nonpharmacologic options for GER therapy in infants include positioning changes, thickening of feeds, trial use of hypoallergenic or high-calorie formulas, and alterations in the mode of feeding.

Positioning

In a randomized, crossover study of infants younger than 5 months of age, semisupine positioning (sitting) in an infant seat was found to exacerbate GER, whereas the prone position was superior.[53] More recently, van Wijk and colleagues[54] found faster gastric emptying and less liquid reflux with a strategy of feeding infants in the right decubitus position followed by position change to the left decubitus position 1 hour later. Caution should be used when placing infants in nonsupine positions because of the risk of sudden infant death syndrome.[40]

Manipulation of feeds

Thickening of feeds with guar gum or cereals or the use of newer milk-based formulas that thicken upon acidification in the stomach reduces the number and height of non-acid reflux episodes and regurgitation but does not decrease acid reflux events.[55] The addition of thickeners may result in changes in formula osmolarity and caloric density, resulting in excessive caloric intake. A 2-week trial of a hypoallergenic formula (protein hydrolysate– or amino acid–based) can be considered to exclude intolerance to cow's milk protein as a cause of reflux symptoms.[40] Continuous drip feeding reduces vomiting and reflux symptoms, but chronic use of indwelling tubes that cross the gastroesophageal junction is associated with increased regurgitation and esophagitis.[56] This problem may be avoided by intermittent orogastric tube placement.

Pharmacologic Treatments

Pharmacotherapy focuses on reducing the exposure to esophageal acid, either by buffering or reducing secreted gastric acid. None of the available currently available agents prevents regurgitation.

Acid neutralizers and surface agents

Oral antacids and surface agents such as alginates have been poorly studied in preterm infants. The availability of alginate preparations is limited. Because of the risk of heavy-metal toxicity, chronic antacid use in preterm infants is not recommended.[40]

Prokinetic therapies

Prokinetic agents have limited role in the treatment of GERD in preterm infants because of their lack of efficacy demonstrated in large meta-analyses (metoclopramide) and potential cardiac (domperidome and cisapride) or neurologic (metoclopramide and domperidome) side effects. Bethanachol has been used for treatment, but its efficacy is questionable, and the side effects generally outweigh any potential benefit.[40] Erythromycin increases antral contractility via the motilin receptor but has had mixed results in improving reflux scores and feeding tolerance in preterm infants.[57] During early infancy, however, the use of erythromycin is associated with the development of hypertrophic pyloric stenosis and cardiac arrhythmias.[58] Baclofen, a gamma butyric acid receptor agonist, reduced the frequency of transient lower esophageal sphincter relaxation, decreased acid reflux, and accelerated gastric emptying in a placebo- controlled study in infants.[59] The development of baclofen analogues has been hampered by neurologic side effects in early adult studies.[60]

Acid-Suppression Therapies

H2-receptor antagonists

H2-receptor antagonists (H2Ras) decrease acid secretion by inhibiting the histamine-2 receptor on the gastric parietal cell. The pharmacokinetics of ranitidine has been studied in preterm infants; and ranitidine has been shown to protect against steroid-induced ulcers in patients who have chronic lung disease.[61,62] Famotidine used at a dose of 0.5 mg/kg reduced the frequency of regurgitation and at a dose of 1 mg/kg reduced crying time in preterm infants;[36] however, the pharmacokinetics and efficacy of famotidine have not been studied in preterm infants. Neither the pharmacokinetic properties of other H2RAs, nor their efficacies in the treatment of signs or symptoms of GERD have been evaluated in preterm infants.

Proton-pump inhibitors

PPIs covalently bind and deactivate the H+, K+ -ATPase pumps in the stomach, providing more effective gastric suppression than H2RAs.[63] Genetic and developmental variability in the expression of cytochrome P450 metabolic pathways may result in differences in the pharmacokinetic properties of PPIs in preterm infants.[64] The pharmacokinetic and pharmacodynamic properties of lansoprazole and omeprazole have been studied only recently in a small number of neonates.[65,66] In a double-blind, placebo-controlled, cross-over study in preterm neonates, omeprazole dosed at 0.7 mg/kg once daily normalized the reflux index in six of seven infants who had abnormal pH scores and reduced the percentage of the time where the intragastric pH was less than 4. This study, however, found no difference in the frequency of reflux symptoms in the placebo and omeprazole arms at the end of the treatment.[66]

Risks of acid suppression

Although acid-suppression therapy is beneficial for individuals who have proven GERD, data now indicate that there are potential adverse consequences of chronic suppression of gastric acid. Although there were limits in the study design, antecedent H2RA exposure was associated with an increased risk of necrotizing enterocolitis.[67] Infants who had late-onset sepsis were seven times more likely to have been exposed to ranitidine.[68] In children, acid suppression with either H2RAs or PPIs was associated with an increased incidence of acute gastroenteritis and community-acquired pneumonia.[69] Studies in adults have found an increased risk of *Clostridium difficile*, *Salmonella*, and *Campylobacter* infections[70] in persons taking acid suppressants and an association between PPI use and decreased absorption and calcium and vitamin B_{12} and hip fracture.[71,72] The effects of chronic acid suppression on vitamin or mineral absorption have not been evaluated in younger populations, particularly in preterm infants.

Antireflux Surgery

Current medical therapy almost always provides adequate treatment for esophageal complications of GER, but surgical options for the treatment of GERD, such as fundoplication, enteral feeding tube placement, and esophagogastric disassociation, can be considered when medical therapy fails.[40] The decision to subject a child to the risks of antireflux surgery requires that outcome will be substantially better than with medical therapy. Although recent studies suggest that potential risks are associated with long-term medical therapy, these risks are small compared with the potential complications of fundoplication surgery. The operative complication rate in a European study evaluating outcomes in infants undergoing fundoplication for GER related to esophageal atresia, for GER related to congenital diaphragmatic hernia, and for GER without other underlying disease was between 1.6% and 4.6%, and the postoperative complication rate was between 8.2% and 10.6%.[73] GERD-related symptoms can persist in up to two thirds of children who undergo antireflux surgery. Many of these children continue to receive GERD medical therapy 2 months following the procedure.[74]

SUMMARY

GER is common in preterm infants and usually is a physiologic phenomenon with little clinical consequence. Correlation of clinical signs and symptoms with GER has been poor in most studies. The efficacy of GERD therapy has not been studied systematically in preterm infants. Furthermore, GERD therapy, particularly with prokinetic agents, acid-suppression therapy, and surgery, is fraught with recognized complications and potentially with other complications that currently are unknown. Therefore, clinicians must weigh carefully the risks, benefits, and alternatives of GERD therapy before initiating treatment. Potential alternative diagnoses, pretreatment diagnostic testing, and desired treatment outcomes should be considered before initiating GERD therapy. Cessation of GERD therapy should be considered, particularly if treatment does not result in the desired clinical outcome.

REFERENCES

1. Dhillon AS, Ewer AK. Diagnosis and management of gastro-oesophageal reflux in preterm infants in neonatal intensive care units. Acta Paediatr 2004;93(1):88–93.
2. Kohelet D, Boaz M, Serour F, et al. Esophageal pH study and symptomatology of gastroesophageal reflux in newborn infants. Am J Perinatol 2004;21(2):85–91.
3. Marino AJ, Assing E, Carbone MT, et al. The incidence of gastroesophageal reflux in preterm infants. J Perinatol 1995;15(5):369–71.
4. Newell SJ, Booth IW, Morgan ME, et al. Gastro-oesophageal reflux in preterm infants. Arch Dis Child 1989;64(6):780–6.
5. Barron JJ, Tan H, Spalding J, et al. Proton pump inhibitor utilization patterns in infants. J Pediatr Gastroenterol Nutr 2007;45(4):421–7.
6. Malcolm WF, Gantz M, Martin RJ, et al. Use of medications for gastroesophageal reflux at discharge among extremely low birth weight infants. Pediatrics 2008; 121(1):22–7.
7. Omari TI, Barnett C, Snel A, et al. Mechanisms of gastroesophageal reflux in healthy premature infants. J Pediatr 1998;133(5):650–4.
8. Jadcherla SR, Duong HQ, Hoffmann RG, et al. Esophageal body and upper esophageal sphincter motor responses to esophageal provocation during maturation in preterm newborns. J Pediatr 2003;143(1):31–8.
9. Jadcherla SR, Gupta A, Stoner E, et al. Correlation of glottal closure using concurrent ultrasonography and nasolaryngoscopy in children: a novel approach to evaluate glottal status. Dysphagia 2006;21(1):75–81.
10. Orlando RC. Review article: oesophageal mucosal resistance. Aliment Pharmacol Ther 1998;12(3):191–7.
11. Tobey NA, Carson JL, Alkiek RA, et al. Dilated intercellular spaces: a morphological feature of acid reflux–damaged human esophageal epithelium. Gastroenterology 1996;111(5):1200–5.

12. Thach BT. Maturation and transformation of reflexes that protect the laryngeal airway from liquid aspiration from fetal to adult life. Am J Med 2001;111(Suppl. 8A): 69S–77S.
13. Davies AM, Koenig JS, Thach BT. Upper airway chemoreflex responses to saline and water in preterm infants. J Appl Phys 1988;64(4):1412–20.
14. Leape LL, Holder TM, Franklin JD, et al. Respiratory arrest in infants secondary to gastroesophageal reflux. Pediatrics 1977;60(6):924–8.
15. Herbst JJ, Book LS, Bray PF. Gastroesophageal reflux in the "near miss" sudden infant death syndrome. J Pediatr 1978;92(1):73–5.
16. Herbst JJ, Minton SD, Book LS. Gastroesophageal reflux causing respiratory distress and apnea in newborn infants. J Pediatr 1979;95(5 Pt 1):763–8.
17. Spitzer AR, Boyle JT, Tuchman DN, et al. Awake apnea associated with gastroesophageal reflux: a specific clinical syndrome. J Pediatr 1984;104(2):200–5.
18. Walsh JK, Farrell MK, Keenan WJ, et al. Gastroesophageal reflux in infants: relation to apnea. J Pediatr 1981;99(2):197–201.
19. Barrington KJ, Tan K, Rich W. Apnea at discharge and gastro-esophageal reflux in the preterm infant. J Perinatol 2002;22(1):8–11.
20. Di Fiore JM, Arko M, Whitehouse M, et al. Apnea is not prolonged by acid gastroesophageal reflux in preterm infants. Pediatrics 2005;116(5):1059–63.
21. Peter CS, Sprodowski N, Bohnhorst B, et al. Gastroesophageal reflux and apnea of prematurity: no temporal relationship. Pediatrics 2002;109(1):8–11.
22. Kimball AL, Carlton DP. Gastroesophageal reflux medications in the treatment of apnea in premature infants. J Pediatr 2001;138(3):355–60.
23. Allen J, Zwerdling R, Ehrenkranz R, et al. Statement on the care of the child with chronic lung disease of infancy and childhood. Am J Respir Crit Care Med 2003; 168(3):356–96.
24. Starosta V, Kitz R, Hartl D, et al. Bronchoalveolar pepsin, bile acids, oxidation, and inflammation in children with gastroesophageal reflux disease. Chest 2007; 132(5):1557–64.
25. Chen PH, Chang MH, Hsu SC. Gastroesophageal reflux in children with chronic recurrent bronchopulmonary infection. J Pediatr Gastroenterol Nutr 1991;13(1): 16–22.
26. Davis RD Jr, Lau CL, Eubanks S, et al. Improved lung allograft function after fundoplication in patients with gastroesophageal reflux disease undergoing lung transplantation. J Thorac Cardiovasc Surg 2003;125(3):533–42.
27. Foglia RP, Fonkalsrud EW, Ament ME, et al. Gastroesophageal fundoplication for the management of chronic pulmonary disease in children. Am J Surg 1980; 140(1):72–9.
28. Raghu G, Yang ST, Spada C, et al. Sole treatment of acid gastroesophageal reflux in idiopathic pulmonary fibrosis: a case series. Chest 2006;129(3):794–800.
29. Jolley SG, Herbst JJ, Johnson DG, et al. Esophageal pH monitoring during sleep identifies children with respiratory symptoms from gastroesophageal reflux. Gastroenterology 1981;80(6):1501–6.
30. Akinola E, Rosenkrantz TS, Pappagallo M, et al. Gastroesophageal reflux in infants < 32 weeks gestational age at birth: lack of relationship to chronic lung disease. Am J Perinatol 2004;21(2):57–62.
31. Omari TI, Barnett CP, Benninga MA, et al. Mechanisms of gastro-oesophageal reflux in preterm and term infants with reflux disease. Gut 2002;51(4):475–9.
32. Farhath S, He Z, Nakhla T, et al. Pepsin, a marker of gastric contents, is increased in tracheal aspirates from preterm infants who develop bronchopulmonary dysplasia. Pediatrics 2008;121(2):e253–9.

33. Frakaloss G, Burke G, Sanders MR. Impact of gastroesophageal reflux on growth and hospital stay in premature infants. J Pediatr Gastroenterol Nutr 1998;26(2):146–50.
34. Khalaf MN, Porat R, Brodsky NL, et al. Clinical correlations in infants in the neonatal intensive care unit with varying severity of gastroesophageal reflux. J Pediatr Gastroenterol Nutr 2001;32(1):45–9.
35. Orenstein SR. Gastroesophageal reflux. Curr Probl Pediatr 1991;21(5):193–241.
36. Orenstein SR, Shalaby TM, Devandry SN, et al. Famotidine for infant gastro-oesophageal reflux: a multi-centre, randomized, placebo-controlled, withdrawal trial. Aliment Pharmacol Ther 2003;17(9):1097–107.
37. Snel A, Barnett CP, Cresp TL, et al. Behavior and gastroesophageal reflux in the premature neonate. J Pediatr Gastroenterol Nutr 2000;30(1):18–21.
38. Barnett CP, Omari T, Davidson GP, et al. Effect of cisapride on gastric emptying in premature infants with feed intolerance. J Paediatr Child Health 2001;37(6):559–63.
39. Moore DJ, Tao BS, Lines DR, et al. Double-blind placebo-controlled trial of omeprazole in irritable infants with gastroesophageal reflux. J Pediatr 2003;143(2):219–23.
40. Rudolph CD, Mazur LJ, Liptak GS, et al. Guidelines for evaluation and treatment of gastroesophageal reflux in infants and children: recommendations of the North American Society for Pediatric Gastroenterology and Nutrition. J Pediatr Gastroenterol Nutr 2001;32(Suppl. 2):S1–31.
41. Vandenplas Y, Goyvaerts H, Helven R, et al. Gastroesophageal reflux, as measured by 24-hour pH monitoring, in 509 healthy infants screened for risk of sudden infant death syndrome. Pediatrics 1991;88(4):834–40.
42. Vandenplas Y, Hassall E. Mechanisms of gastroesophageal reflux and gastroesophageal reflux disease. J Pediatr Gastroenterol Nutr 2002;35(2):119–36.
43. Salvatore S, Hauser B, Vandemaele K, et al. Gastroesophageal reflux disease in infants: how much is predictable with questionnaires, pH-metry, endoscopy and histology? J Pediatr Gastroenterol Nutr 2005;40(2):210–5.
44. Rosen R, Lord C, Nurko S. The sensitivity of multichannel intraluminal impedance and the pH probe in the evaluation of gastroesophageal reflux in children. Clin Gastroenterol Hepatol 2006;4(2):167–72.
45. Condino AA, Sondheimer J, Pan Z, et al. Evaluation of gastroesophageal reflux in pediatric patients with asthma using impedance-pH monitoring. J Pediatr 2006;149(2):216–9.
46. Lopez-Alonso M, Moya MJ, Cabo JA, et al. Twenty-four-hour esophageal impedance-pH monitoring in healthy preterm neonates: rate and characteristics of acid, weakly acidic, and weakly alkaline gastroesophageal reflux. Pediatrics 2006;118(2):e299–308.
47. Maki M, Ruuska T, Kuusela AL, et al. High prevalence of asymptomatic esophageal and gastric lesions in preterm infants in intensive care. Crit Care Med 1993;21(12):1863–7.
48. Heine RG, Cameron DJ, Chow CW, et al. Esophagitis in distressed infants: poor diagnostic agreement between esophageal pH monitoring and histopathologic findings. J Pediatr 2002;140(1):14–9.
49. Morigeri C, Bhattacharya A, Mukhopadhyay K, et al. Radionuclide scintigraphy in the evaluation of gastroesophageal reflux in symptomatic and asymptomatic preterm infants. Eur J Nucl Med Mol Imaging 2008.
50. Ours TM, Kavuru MS, Schilz RJ, et al. A prospective evaluation of esophageal testing and a double-blind, randomized study of omeprazole in a diagnostic

and therapeutic algorithm for chronic cough. Am J Gastroenterol 1999;94(11): 3131–8.
51. Fass R, Fennerty MB, Ofman JJ, et al. The clinical and economic value of a short course of omeprazole in patients with noncardiac chest pain. Gastroenterology 1998;115(1):42–9.
52. Johnsson F, Weywadt L, Solhaug JH, et al. One-week omeprazole treatment in the diagnosis of gastro-oesophageal reflux disease. Scand J Gastroenterol 1998;33(1):15–20.
53. Orenstein SR, Whitington PF, Orenstein DM. The infant seat as treatment for gastroesophageal reflux. N Engl J Med 1983;309(13):760–3.
54. van Wijk MP, Benninga MA, Dent J, et al. Effect of body position changes on postprandial gastroesophageal reflux and gastric emptying in the healthy premature neonate. J Pediatr 2007;151(6):585–90.
55. Wenzl TG, Schneider S, Scheele F, et al. Effects of thickened feeding on gastroesophageal reflux in infants: a placebo-controlled crossover study using intraluminal impedance. Pediatrics 2003;111(4 Pt 1):e355–9.
56. Peter CS, Wiechers C, Bohnhorst B, et al. Influence of nasogastric tubes on gastroesophageal reflux in preterm infants: a multiple intraluminal impedance study. J Pediatr 2002;141(2):277–9.
57. Aly H, Abdel-Hady H, Khashaba M, et al. Erythromycin and feeding intolerance in premature infants: a randomized trial. J Perinatol 2007;27(1):39–43.
58. Chicella MF, Batres LA, Heesters MS, et al. Prokinetic drug therapy in children: a review of current options. Ann Pharmacother 2005;39(4):706–11.
59. Omari TI, Benninga MA, Sansom L, et al. Effect of baclofen on esophagogastric motility and gastroesophageal reflux in children with gastroesophageal reflux disease: a randomized controlled trial. J Pediatr 2006;149(4):468–74.
60. Boeckxstaens GE, Beaumont H, Rydholm H, et al. Effect of the $GABA_B$ receptor agonist AZD9343 on transient lower esophageal sphincter relaxations and acid reflux in healthy volunteers: a phase 1 trial. Gastroenterology 2008;134(4(S1)): A126.
61. Kelly EJ, Chatfield SL, Brownlee KG, et al. The effect of intravenous ranitidine on the intragastric pH of preterm infants receiving dexamethasone. Arch Dis Child 1993;69(1 Spec No):37–9.
62. Kuusela AL, Ruuska T, Karikoski R, et al. A randomized, controlled study of prophylactic ranitidine in preventing stress-induced gastric mucosal lesions in neonatal intensive care unit patients. Crit Care Med 1997;25(2):346–51.
63. Sachs G, Shin JM, Howden CW. Review article: the clinical pharmacology of proton pump inhibitors. Aliment Pharmacol Ther 2006;23(Suppl. 2):2–8.
64. Springer M, Atkinson S, North J, et al. Safety and pharmacodynamics of lansoprazole in patients with gastroesophageal reflux disease aged <1 year. Paediatr Drugs 2008;10(4):255–63.
65. Zhang W, Kukulka M, Witt G, et al. Age-dependent pharmacokinetics of lansoprazole in neonates and infants. Paediatr Drugs 2008;10(4):265–74.
66. Omari TI, Haslam RR, Lundborg P, et al. Effect of omeprazole on acid gastroesophageal reflux and gastric acidity in preterm infants with pathological acid reflux. J Pediatr Gastroenterol Nutr 2007;44(1):41–4.
67. Guillet R, Stoll BJ, Cotten CM, et al. Association of H2-blocker therapy and higher incidence of necrotizing enterocolitis in very low birth weight infants. Pediatrics 2006;117(2):e137–42.
68. Bianconi S, Gudavalli M, Sutija VG, et al. Ranitidine and late-onset sepsis in the neonatal intensive care unit. J Perinat Med 2007;35(2):147–50.

69. Canani RB, Cirillo P, Roggero P, et al. Therapy with gastric acidity inhibitors increases the risk of acute gastroenteritis and community-acquired pneumonia in children. Pediatrics 2006;117(5):e817–20.
70. Leonard J, Marshall JK, Moayyedi P. Systematic review of the risk of enteric infection in patients taking acid suppression. Am J Gastroenterol 2007;102(9):2047–56, quiz 2057.
71. Yang YX, Lewis JD, Epstein S, et al. Long-term proton pump inhibitor therapy and risk of hip fracture. J Am Med Assoc 2006;296(24):2947–53.
72. O'Connell MB, Madden DM, Murray AM, et al. Effects of proton pump inhibitors on calcium carbonate absorption in women: a randomized crossover trial. Am J Med 2005;118(7):778–81.
73. Holschneider P, Dubbers M, Engelskirchen R, et al. Results of the operative treatment of gastroesophageal reflux in childhood with particular focus on patients with esophageal atresia. Eur J Pediatr Surg 2007;17(3):163–75.
74. Gilger MA, Yeh C, Chiang J, et al. Outcomes of surgical fundoplication in children. Clin Gastroenterol Hepatol 2004;2(11):978–84.

Optimizing Growth in the Preterm Infant

Michael R. Uhing, MD*, Utpala (Shonu) G. Das, MD

KEYWORDS

- Enteral nutrition • Parenteral nutrition • Protein
- Amino acid • Expressed breast milk

In the neonatal ICU (NICU), the nutritional support provided to each preterm infant is addressed daily. Despite this attention, postnatal growth failure continues to be a ubiquitous problem in these infants. In a 1995–1996 cohort of very low birth weight (VLBW) infants in the National Institute of Health and Child Development Research Network, 22% of the cohort was small for gestational age (SGA) at birth; however, by 36 weeks' postmenstrual age (PMA), 97% of the cohort was below the 10th percentile in weight.[1] Although growth velocity can be improved by the implementation of standardized nutritional regimens, the most appropriate approach to the nutritional management of premature infants is not known.[2] This article examines several of the controversies regarding the nutritional management of preterm infants, including what growth velocity achieves the best outcome, the role of early, aggressive parenteral nutrition, the most appropriate time and method to initiate enteral nutrition, and methods to improve growth once full enteral nutrition has been achieved.

WHAT IS THE OPTIMAL GROWTH RATE FOR THE PRETERM INFANT?

The trend in recent years has been to provide earlier and more aggressive nutritional support to decrease the incidence of growth failure and avoid the catabolic state that occurs when the provision of sufficient nutritional intake is delayed. This more aggressive approach often has resulted in less postnatal weight loss and decreased time to the regaining of birth weight.[3] Research now, however, suggests that a dilemma exists with far-reaching ramifications: one can provide inadequate nutritional support and increase the risk of neurodevelopmental impairment and bone disease[4–6] or provide better nutritional support and increase the risk of cardiovascular disease in later childhood and adulthood.[7,8] Where the balance lies is not known. Is there a point at which neurologic outcome can be optimized without sacrificing cardiovascular health? Furthermore, weight gain is the growth parameter most often followed; is there another parameter that may determine better where this balance lies?

Medical College of Wisconsin, Children's Corporate Center, Suite C410, 999 North 92nd Street, Milwaukee, WI 53226, USA
* Corresponding author.
E-mail address: muhing@mcw.edu (M.R. Uhing).

Clin Perinatol 36 (2009) 165–176
doi:10.1016/j.clp.2008.09.010 perinatology.theclinics.com

The standard most commonly used to help determine optimal postnatal growth is intrauterine growth velocity. The intrauterine growth velocity decreases from approximately 21 g/kg/d (15 g/d) between 23 and 27 weeks' gestation to 12 g/kg/d (33 g/d) between 35 and 37 weeks' gestation.[9] The average growth velocity for the entire period from 23 to 37 weeks' gestation is approximately 16 g/kg/d (25 g/d). Mimicking intrauterine growth patterns may seem attractive, but whether this velocity is appropriate during extrauterine life is not known. In addition, because infants lose weight after birth and often do not regain birth weight for 1 to 2 weeks, recreating the intrauterine growth velocity after this period of weight loss automatically leads to relative growth retardation at term PMA when compared with infants not born prematurely.[10]

Maximizing growth is of paramount importance to minimize the risk of poor neurologic outcomes. In extremely low birth weight (ELBW) infants, Ehrenkranz and colleagues[4] found that the risk of neurologic impairment at 18 months of age increased from 29% in infants gaining an average of 21 g/kg/d to 55% in those gaining an average of only 12 g/kg/d. In this study, the rate of weight gain was calculated from the time that the infants regained their birth weight until hospital discharge. Although many potential confounding variables, such as intraventricular hemorrhage, sepsis, and necrotizing enterocolitis (NEC), were included in the analysis, the retrospective nature of the study does not preclude the possibility that the infants who demonstrated better weight gain may have been less "sick" than those who had poorer weight gain. In a randomized trial of preterm infants receiving either an enriched or a standard formula, Lucas and colleagues[8] found that infants with birth weights less than 1850 g who were fed the standard formula had a greater incidence of cerebral palsy and lower intelligence quotients. In VLBW SGA infants, Latal-Hajnal and colleagues[6] found that neurologic outcomes at 2 years of age correlated better with postnatal growth than with appropriateness of weight for gestational age at birth.

In contrast, greater weight gain may compromise cardiovascular health. Low birth weight infants who demonstrate greater postnatal catch-up growth have been found to have higher systolic blood pressures at 3 years of age.[11] In a follow-up of the randomized trial by Lucas,[8] Singhal and colleagues[7] found that, although the preterm infants fed the enriched formula had better neurologic outcomes, the incidence of insulin resistance at 13 to 16 years of age was greater in the group fed enriched formulas as infants than in group fed the standard formula. In term infants, the rate of weight gain in the first 4 months of life correlates with obesity at 7 years of age.[12] Low birth weight infants who had the greatest weight gain during childhood had the highest blood pressure as adults,[13] but weight gain in the first year of life did not affect blood pressure as an adult. Eriksson and colleagues[14] found that death from coronary artery disease was associated with low birth weight and was most pronounced in the individuals who achieved catch-up growth to the 50th percentile or higher by 7 years of age. Therefore, better nutrition as an infant may lead to insulin resistance, increased blood pressure, and increased mortality from coronary artery disease later in life. It is difficult, however, to differentiate the relative influences of intrauterine programming, early neonatal nutrition, and later childhood nutrition on the subsequent development of cardiovascular disease in adulthood.

Weight gain alone provides only a single view of growth and does not indicate the type of growth (ie, fat versus lean body mass). Compared with term infants, preterm infants have an altered distribution of adipose tissue which persists into school age.[15,16] Because the alterations found in this study correlate best with the severity of disease, the impact of variation in nutritional support on the distribution of adipose tissue is not known.[15] Monitoring linear and head circumference growth rates, which should average 0.9 to 1.0 cm/wk, can help ensure that growth is associated with increasing lean body mass.[10] The ability to determine body composition now is becoming available and may help establish nutritional regimens that optimize body composition as well as growth velocity.

What then is the optimal target weight gain for preterm infants? This criterion is not known, but at this time it seems prudent to favor improved neurologic outcome over other outcomes. Currently it is the authors' practice to strive for a weight gain of 15 to 20 g/kg/d for infants with a PMA of less than 35 weeks and 15 g/kg/d for infants with a PMA of more 35 weeks. Linear and head growth are measured weekly and compared with the infant's weight gain to help assess changes in lean body mass.

DOES EARLY NUTRITION MAKE A DIFFERENCE?

Compared with the recommended intakes, preterm infants younger than 30 weeks' gestation accumulate an energy deficit of 813 kcal/kg in the first 5 weeks of life.[17] More than half of this deficit occurs in the first week of life. Using stepwise regression analysis, this energy deficit accounts for 45% of the variation in hospital growth rates.[17] By minimizing postnatal weight loss and decreasing the time to the regaining of birth weight, the risk of subsequent growth retardation at term PMA when intrauterine growth velocity is achieved is lessened.[10]

Because there are many confounding variables when evaluating the outcome of preterm infants, especially ELBW infants, it is difficult to determine the independent effects of nutritional support in the first week of life. In infants with birth weights of 750 to 1500 g, an aggressive nutritional approach starting on the first day of life leads to less postnatal weight loss, improved overall weight gain, improved linear growth, and improved head growth at hospital discharge.[18] In a randomized study, Wilson and colleagues[19] found that growth during hospitalization as measured by weight, length, and head circumference improved when total parenteral nutrition (TPN) was started earlier and more aggressively. There was also less weight loss after birth, and no adverse effects were found. In a retrospective study of VLBW SGA infants, Brandt and colleagues[20] found that higher energy intake in the first 10 days of life was associated with greater increases in head circumference measured at 12 months of age. The average gestational age of these infants was approximately 33 weeks, and most calories were provided enterally.[20] Because head growth correlates with improved neurologic outcome, it is speculated that more aggressive early nutrition may improve long-term neurologic outcome. With a more aggressive nutritional approach, the postnatal growth grid shows less postnatal weight loss and overall greater weight gain.[3]

Again, the benefits of early aggressive nutrition must be balanced against the possible adverse effects. Preterm infants with greater weight gain in the first 2 weeks of life may develop greater insulin resistance later in life.[7] At this time, however, the benefits of improved neurologic outcome seem to outweigh the possible harm of poorer cardiovascular health.

EARLY NUTRITION: WHAT SHOULD IT BE?

In the fetus, amino acid (aa) uptake is relatively high, whereas fetal carbohydrate and fat uptake is relatively low. Studies in fetal sheep suggest that umbilical aa uptake ranges from 5.6 to 8.3 g/kg/d,[21,22] with aa oxidation contributing 40% of the energy needs of the fetus.[22] Although studies in humans do not exist, Hay and colleagus[23] estimated that umbilical aa uptake in humans is 3.6 to 4.8 g/kg/d by correcting for differences in body composition between sheep and humans. Consistent with high fetal uptake, aa metabolism in preterm infants does not seem to be immature when compared with term infants.[24] Therefore, the practice of delaying the initiation of aas or starting at low rates of administration is a marked deviation from the intrauterine environment. It is estimated that infants younger than 30 weeks' gestation develop a protein deficit of 23 g/kg in the first 5 weeks of life, with more than half occurring in the first week.[17]

Current evidence suggests that aggressive early aa administration and consequent prevention of endogenous aa loss are beneficial. Prevention of a negative nitrogen balance is achieved in preterm infants by providing aas at a rate of 1 to 1.5 g/kg/d.[25–28] In a randomized trial of 135 VLBW infants, initiating aa infusions at 2.4 g/kg/d within 1 hour after birth, compared with a stepwise progression to reach this same level on day of life 3, led to normalized plasma aa profiles on day of life 2.[29] Initiating aa infusions at 3 to 3.5 g/kg/d has been shown to be safe and leads to protein accretion and plasma aa concentrations close to those achieved during intrauterine life.[25,30] This result can be achieved with a nonprotein energy intake as little as 30 kcal/kg/d.[24] In VLBW infants, increasing aa administration to 4 g/kg/d within the first week also has been shown to be safe and to improve weight gain, longitudinal growth, and head growth.[18,31]

Several benefits of early aggressive aa administration have been shown. In a retrospective analysis, Poindexter and colleagues[32] found that preterm infants reaching an intake of at least 3 g/kg/d within the first 5 days of life had a decreased risk of having a head circumference measurement in less than the 10th percentile at discharge and in the fifth percentile at 18 months of age. In a retrospective review of six NICUs, Olsen and colleagues[33] found that growth velocity in the first 28 days of life in infants of less than 30 weeks' gestation was correlated significantly with protein intake. Each additional 1 g/kg/d of protein was associated with an additional weight gain of 4.1 g/kg/d and had a greater effect on growth than increasing caloric intake. Several studies show that a more aggressive infusion of aa in the first few days of life leads to improved growth.[34]

Although most studies show improved growth with early aa administration, this finding is not universal. In a recent randomized study of 122 VLBW infants comparing a more aggressive regimen of aa infusion (initial rate of 1.5 g/kg/d and advancing to 3.5 g/kg/d by day of life 3) and a less aggressive approach (initial rate of 1.0 g/kg/d advancing to a maximum of 2.5 g/kg/d by day of life 4), no differences were found in any growth parameters at 28 days of age.[35] The higher aa group did have higher serum urea nitrogen (BUN) concentrations and also had plasma levels of five aas that were above the 90th percentile of their reference values. The authors commented, however, that true reference values for preterm infants are not established.

One factor thought to be important in the pathogenesis of bronchopulmonary dysplasia is poor nutrition. Interestingly, Porcelli and colleagues[31] also found that providing aas at 4 g/kg/d decreased the incidence of bronchopulmonary dysplasia from 28% to 5% in ELBW infants. This finding has not been corroborated by other studies.[18]

An additional benefit of early aa administration is improved glucose tolerance caused at least in part by increased insulin secretion.[19,27] Thureen and colleagues[25] found that insulin concentrations were almost twofold greater in VLBW infants receiving aas at 3 g/kg/d than in infants receiving aas at 1 g/kg/d. Concentrations of C-peptide and insulin-like growth factor-1 also correlate with protein intake.[36,37]

Concerns raised about early aggressive aa administration relate to possible metabolic derangements, including metabolic acidosis, hyperammonemia, and elevated BUN. These problems were associated primarily with the previous use of protein hydrolysate aa solutions and not currently available crystalline aa solutions.[38,39] Recent studies show no evidence of increased risk of significant acidosis or hyperammonemia. Protein intakes of 5 g/kg/d or more can lead to poorer intellectual function and abnormal plasma aa profiles, however, and should be avoided.[40,41]

The effect of early and aggressive aa intake on BUN has been inconsistent. Most studies show no effect[25,32,34,42] or an effect that is statistically significant but not particularly clinically significant.[31,35] In a retrospective study of 121 VLBW infants receiving parenteral nutrition in the first 3 days of life with aa intakes ranging from 0 to 3.7 g/kg/d, there was no correlation between aa intake and BUN concentrations.[43] Higher BUN concentrations were more likely in infants who had a lower gestational age, indicating that factors such as immature renal function, alterations in hydration status, and a fetal aa oxidation pattern for energy use may have the most influence on BUN concentrations.

In the most aggressive nutritional approach studied thus far, Ibrahim and colleagues[30] initiated aas at 3.5 g/kg/d and intralipids at 3 g/kg/d within 1 hour of birth in 32 VLBW ventilator-dependent infants. Compared with the control group in which TPN was not initiated until 48 hours of age, there were no differences in plasma cholesterol, triglycerides, BUN, creatinine, or bicarbonate concentrations.

The available evidence suggests that aas should be provided as soon after birth as possible at a minimum of 1.5 g/kg/d but preferably with infusions of 3 g/kg/d.[44,45] The authors' practice is to begin TPN immediately after birth using a standard solution of 7.5% dextrose and 3% aa. This standard solution is premixed and available 24 hours per day. When infused between 60 and 100 mL/kg/d, 1.8 to 3 g/kg/d of aa is provided. Within 24 hours, an individualized TPN solution is ordered with an initial aa concentration of 3 g/kg/d. In ELBW infants, aa intake is advanced to 4 g/kg/d within the first few days of life. If concerns regarding significant renal ischemia or dysfunction exist, a less aggressive approach is used.

ENTERAL FEEDING FOR THE VERY LOW BIRTH WEIGHT INFANT: WHEN AND BY HOW MUCH?

When Should Enteral Feeds be Initiated?

The timing for initiation of enteral feedings remains controversial. Studies attempting to answer the question regarding the safety of "early" versus "delayed" initiation of enteral nutrition do not have consistent definitions of "early" and often are combined with other changes in the nutritional regimen. Early enteral feedings have a trophic effect on intestinal structure and integrity. Retrospective studies, however, have raised concerns that early enteral nutrition of preterm infants may lead to an increased risk of NEC.[46] Most prospective, randomized trials show that initiating enteral nutrition within the first 3 days of life compared with a more delayed introduction improves time to reaching full enteral nutrition and improves weight gain.[19,47–49] Other potential benefits include decreased incidence of osteopenia,[49,50] decreased need for central venous catheters,[51] decreased cholestasis,[49] and decreased incidence of sepsis.[47,51,52] None of these studies showed an increased risk of NEC.

Delays in the introduction of enteral nutrition often are intertwined with the controversy regarding the safety of enteral nutrition when an umbilical artery catheter (UAC) is in place. In theory, the presence of a catheter in the aorta may alter intestinal blood flow and increase risk of ischemia. Intestinal blood flow does not seem to be affected by the presence of a UAC, however.[53] Several studies show no association between the incidence of NEC and early feedings with a UAC in place.[19,35,48,51] A survey of neonatal medical directors showed that approximately 80% believed that it was safe to provide trophic feeding ($\leq$ 20 mL/kg/d) most or some of the time to infants with a UAC in place, and 51% believed that it was safe most or some of the time to provide greater than trophic feeding volumes with a UAC in place.[54]

Should Infants Receive Trophic Feedings with Delayed Feeding Advancement?

Most studies examining the effects of trophic feeding on patient outcome compare variable periods of trophic feeding with delayed feeding. These studies are very heterogeneous but overall show a reduction in days to full feeding, total days that feedings were held, and length of hospital stay in the trophic feeding group, without a significant effect on the incidence of NEC.[55]

One study, however, comparing trophic feeding for 10 days versus regular advancement of feedings in infants of less than 32 weeks' gestation showed that the incidence of NEC was greater in the group with regular advancement of feedings (10% versus 1.4%).[56] The study also found significant increases in the days that a central venous catheter was required (13 days versus 37 days), age at attainment of full enteral feeds (19 days versus 36 days), and length of stay (64 days versus 76 days) in the trophic feeding group. This study is difficult to interpret, because it was terminated early, and several infants with ileal perforation were excluded. In addition, enteral feedings were delayed in both groups, to an average age of 10 days, until after study entry. This prolonged period of delayed enteral feeding may have influenced the outcome of the study.

How Quickly Should Feedings be Advanced?

Early studies suggested that increasing enteral feedings at a rate more than 20 mL/kg/d increased the risk of NEC.[57] Several prospective, randomized trials have not found this association, however. In VLBW infants, advancing feedings at a rate of 35 mL/kg/d compared with 15 mL/kg/d led to earlier attainment of full enteral feedings and time to the regaining of birth weight without an increased incidence of NEC.[58] In a study of 155 infants with birth weights between 1 and 2 kg, infants in which feedings were advanced by 30 mL/kg/d attained birth weight earlier, reached full-volume enteral feedings earlier, and required fewer days of intravenous fluids than the infants in whom feedings were advanced only by 20 mL/kg/d.[59] Again, no difference in the incidence of NEC was found.

Are there Benefits to a Standardized Feeding Regimen?

From the point of view of optimizing growth, feeding preterm infants earlier and faster improves time to full feeds and growth velocity. The effect on the incidence of NEC is unclear, however. Interestingly, rather than concentrating on the actual feeding regimen itself, there is evidence that simply implementing a feeding regimen that standardizes nutritional support in an NICU may be the most important factor in optimizing growth while minimizing the risk of NEC.[60] An additional advantage of an aggressive approach to enteral feeding is that the need for central venous access is minimized, decreasing the risk of catheter-associated infections and complications.

PROMOTING GROWTH USING ENTERAL FEEDINGS

Human milk is the enteral feeding of choice for preterm infants.[61] The addition of human milk fortifiers to expressed breast milk (EBM) provides additional nutrient supplementation in the form of protein, calcium, phosphorus, carbohydrate, vitamins, and minerals. Supplementation with these fortifiers improves weight gain, linear growth, and head growth without adverse effects.[62,63]

For some infants growth remains suboptimal despite this supplementation. Assumptions regarding nutrient intake often are made using estimates of the average nutrient content of human milk. This estimate may not provide an accurate nutritional assessment for individual infants, because the fat and protein content of human milk is highly variable.[64]

The initial step in optimizing growth in preterm infants fed EBM is to increase the volume provided. Often enteral feedings are provided at a maximum value of 150 mL/kg/d. For most stable preterm infants, this volume is an arbitrary ceiling that leads to the potential for growth failure. To meet sufficient nutrient requirements, it is estimated that preterm infants may require 180 mL/kg/d of fortified human milk.[23] In a randomized study of infants of less than 30 weeks' gestation, enteral feedings at a volume of 200 mL/kg/d improved weight gain at 35 weeks' PMA compared with infants receiving only 150 mL/kg/d and did so without adverse effects.[65] In a prospective study of fortified human milk, intakes of 200 mL/kg/d were well tolerated and improved weight gain.[66]

When the volume of the feedings cannot be increased, several options are available to improve the nutrient content of EBM. The first option is to assess the caloric density of the EBM and manipulate its expression to increase caloric density. An easy way to estimate the caloric density of EBM is to determine its lipid content by measuring the creamatocrit.[67–69] A sample of fresh EBM is spun in a centrifuge, separating the lipid portion (cream). The caloric density is determined from the percentage of lipid volume to total milk volume. If an infant is not growing adequately, and the creamatocrit measurement indicates that the EBM has a low caloric density, hindmilk (milk expressed several minutes after flow is initiated) or milk expressed later in the day, both of which have a higher fat content, can be used to improve caloric density.[70–72] It is important to realize that the creamatocrit varies during the day, and therefore a single measurement is only an estimate at one particular time point.[70] In addition, the creamatocrit is an estimate only of fat content; it does not measure the concentrations of other nutrients that may affect growth.

The delivery of fat to an infant receiving EBM also needs to be optimized. Intermittent bolus feeding improves delivery of fat to the infants compared with continuous tube feeding.[73] If continuous tube feedings are required, the syringe should be maintained in a vertical position with the tip upright.[73]

If growth remains suboptimal despite adequate caloric intake, additional protein supplementation may be considered. The recommended protein intake for enterally fed preterm infants is between 3.4 g/kg/d and 4.3 g/kg/d.[74] Based on an average protein content of EBM of approximately 1.9 g/dL, fortified EBM provides approximately 3 g/100 kcal or 3.6 g/kg/d if enteral intake is 120 kcal/kg/d.[64] Because the protein content of EBM is highly variable and therefore often is lower than 1.9 g/dL, many infants do not receive this recommended intake of protein. Multiple studies show that higher protein intake increases nitrogen retention, weight gain, linear growth, and head growth.[75–77] Therefore, additional protein supplementation should be considered an option in achieving the recommended intake. In a prospective randomized study, Arslanoglu and colleagues[78] found that adjusting the fortification of human milk to optimize protein intake improved weight gain and head growth. The fortification was adjusted to maintain BUN concentrations between 9 and 14 mg/dL; fortification was increased if the BUN was lower than 9 mg/dL and was decreased if the BUN was higher than 14 mg/dL.

As more sophisticated techniques become increasingly available, the protein, fat, and energy content of EBM can be determined more accurately, allowing even better modulation of nutrient intake while preserving the benefits of human milk. In the authors' practice, EBM is fortified when enteral intake reaches 100 mL/kg/d. To ensure that adequate energy intake is being provided, the creamatocrit is measured weekly in all VLBW infants and more often in infants that do not demonstrate adequate weight gain. If weight gain is inadequate, the volume of enteral feedings is increased, if possible. If the creamatocrit indicates low caloric density, the expression of milk is altered to provide more calories using hindmilk. If the provision of hindmilk and greater energy intake fails to improve weight gain, additional protein is supplemented at 1 g/kg/d, and the BUN is followed. With this practice virtually all preterm infants can achieve adequate growth using human milk.

SUMMARY

Optimizing growth in the preterm infant continues to be a difficult task and is complicated by a lack of knowledge of the optimal growth pattern. Adequate growth is necessary to optimize neurologic outcome even in the face of potential cardiovascular complications later in life. Prevention of postnatal growth failure requires a comprehensive nutritional regimen that provides adequate nutritional support as soon after birth as possible and is maintained throughout an infant's hospital course.

REFERENCES

1. Lemons JA, Bauer CR, Oh W, et al. Very low birth weight outcomes of the National Institute of Child health and human development neonatal research network, January 1995 through December 1996. NICHD Neonatal Research Network. Pediatrics 2001;107(1):E1–8.
2. Bloom BT, Mulligan J, Arnold C, et al. Improving growth of very low birth weight infants in the first 28 days. Pediatrics 2003;112(1 Pt 1):8–14.
3. Christensen RD, Henry E, Kiehn TI, et al. Pattern of daily weights among low birth weight neonates in the neonatal intensive care unit: data from a multihospital health-care system. J Perinatol 2006;26(1):37–43.
4. Ehrenkranz RA, Dusick AM, Vohr BR, et al. Growth in the neonatal intensive care unit influences neurodevelopmental and growth outcomes of extremely low birth weight infants. Pediatrics 2006;117(4):1253–61.
5. Lapillonne A, Salle BL, Glorieux FH, et al. Bone mineralization and growth are enhanced in preterm infants fed an isocaloric, nutrient-enriched preterm formula through term. Am J Clin Nutr 2004;80(6):1595–603.
6. Latal-Hajnal B, von Siebenthal K, Kovari H, et al. Postnatal growth in VLBW infants: significant association with neurodevelopmental outcome. J Pediatr 2003;143(2):163–70.
7. Singhal A, Fewtrell M, Cole TJ, et al. Low nutrient intake and early growth for later insulin resistance in adolescents born preterm. Lancet 2003;361(9363):1089–97.
8. Lucas A, Morley R, Cole TJ. Randomised trial of early diet in preterm babies and later intelligence quotient. BMJ 1998;317(7171):1481–7.
9. Kramer MS, Platt RW, Wen SW, et al. A new and improved population-based Canadian reference for birth weight for gestational age. Pediatrics 2001;108(2):E35–42.
10. Ehrenkranz RA, Younes N, Lemons JA, et al. Longitudinal growth of hospitalized very low birth weight infants. Pediatrics 1999;104(2 Pt 1):280–9.
11. Min JW, Kong KA, Park BH, et al. Effect of postnatal catch-up growth on blood pressure in children at 3 years of age. J Hum Hypertens 2007;21(11):868–74.
12. Stettler N, Zemel BS, Kumanyika S, et al. Infant weight gain and childhood overweight status in a multicenter, cohort study. Pediatrics 2002;109(2):194–9.
13. Law CM, Shiell AW, Newsome CA, et al. Fetal, infant, and childhood growth and adult blood pressure: a longitudinal study from birth to 22 years of age. Circulation 2002;105(9):1088–92.

14. Eriksson JG, Forsen T, Tuomilehto J, et al. Catch-up growth in childhood and death from coronary heart disease: longitudinal study. BMJ 1999;318(7181):427–31.
15. Uthaya S, Thomas EL, Hamilton G, et al. Altered adiposity after extremely preterm birth. Pediatr Res 2005;57(2):211–5.
16. Gianni ML, Mora S, Roggero P, et al. Regional fat distribution in children born preterm evaluated at school age. J Pediatr Gastroenterol Nutr 2008;46(2):232–5.
17. Embleton NE, Pang N, Cooke RJ. Postnatal malnutrition and growth retardation: an inevitable consequence of current recommendations in preterm infants? Pediatrics 2001;107(2):270–3.
18. Dinerstein A, Nieto RM, Solana CL, et al. Early and aggressive nutritional strategy (parenteral and enteral) decreases postnatal growth failure in very low birth weight infants. J Perinatol 2006;26(7):436–42.
19. Wilson DC, Cairns P, Halliday HL, et al. Randomised controlled trial of an aggressive nutritional regimen in sick very low birthweight infants. Arch Dis Child Fetal Neonatal Ed 1997;77(1):F4–11.
20. Brandt I, Sticker EJ, Lentze MJ. Catch-up growth of head circumference of very low birth weight, small for gestational age preterm infants and mental development to adulthood. J Pediatr 2003;142(5):463–8.
21. Marconi AM, Battaglia FC, Meschia G, et al. A comparison of amino acid arteriovenous differences across the liver and placenta of the fetal lamb. Am J Physiol 1989;257(6 Pt 1):E909–15.
22. Lemons JA, Schreiner RL. Amino acid metabolism in the ovine fetus. Am J Physiol 1983;244(5):E459–66.
23. Hay WW Jr, Lucas A, Heird WC, et al. Workshop summary: nutrition of the extremely low birth weight infant. Pediatrics 1999;104(6):1360–8.
24. Denne SC, Karn CA, Ahlrichs JA, et al. Proteolysis and phenylalanine hydroxylation in response to parenteral nutrition in extremely premature and normal newborns. J Clin Invest 1996;97(3):746–54.
25. Thureen PJ, Melara D, Fennessey PV, et al. Effect of low versus high intravenous amino acid intake on very low birth weight infants in the early neonatal period. Pediatr Res 2003;53(1):24–32.
26. Thureen PJ, Anderson AH, Baron KA, et al. Protein balance in the first week of life in ventilated neonates receiving parenteral nutrition. Am J Clin Nutr 1998;68(5):1128–35.
27. Rivera A Jr, Bell EF, Bier DM. Effect of intravenous amino acids on protein metabolism of preterm infants during the first three days of life. Pediatr Res 1993;33(2):106–11.
28. Van Goudoever JB, Colen T, Wattimena JL, et al. Immediate commencement of amino acid supplementation in preterm infants: effect on serum amino acid concentrations and protein kinetics on the first day of life. J Pediatr 1995;127(3):458–65.
29. te Braake FW, van den Akker CH, Wattimena DJ, et al. Amino acid administration to premature infants directly after birth. J Pediatr 2005;147(4):457–61.
30. Ibrahim HM, Jeroudi MA, Baier RJ, et al. Aggressive early total parental nutrition in low-birth-weight infants. J Perinatol 2004;24(8):482–6.
31. Porcelli PJ Jr, Sisk PM. Increased parenteral amino acid administration to extremely low-birth-weight infants during early postnatal life. J Pediatr Gastroenterol Nutr 2002;34(2):174–9.
32. Poindexter BB, Langer JC, Dusick AM, et al. Early provision of parenteral amino acids in extremely low birth weight infants: relation to growth and neurodevelopmental outcome. J Pediatr 2006;148(3):300–5.

33. Olsen IE, Richardson DK, Schmid CH, et al. Intersite differences in weight growth velocity of extremely premature infants. Pediatrics 2002;110(6):1125–32.
34. Maggio L, Cota F, Gallini F, et al. Effects of high versus standard early protein intake on growth of extremely low birth weight infants. J Pediatr Gastroenterol Nutr 2007;44(1):124–9.
35. Clark RH, Chace DH, Spitzer AR. Effects of two different doses of amino acid supplementation on growth and blood amino acid levels in premature neonates admitted to the neonatal intensive care unit: a randomized, controlled trial. Pediatrics 2007;120(6):1286–96.
36. Smith WJ, Underwood LE, Keyes L, et al. Use of insulin-like growth factor I (IGF-I) and IGF-binding protein measurements to monitor feeding of premature infants. J Clin Endocrinol Metab 1997;82(12):3982–8.
37. Jackson JK, Biondo DJ, Jones JM, et al. Can an alternative umbilical arterial catheter solution and flush regimen decrease iatrogenic hemolysis while enhancing nutrition? A double-blind, randomized, clinical trial comparing an isotonic amino acid with a hypotonic salt infusion. Pediatrics 2004;114(2):377–83.
38. Johnson JD, Albritton WL, Sunshine P. Hyperammonemia accompanying parenteral nutrition in newborn infants. J Pediatr 1972;81(1):154–61.
39. Heird WC, Dell RB, Driscoll JM Jr, et al. Metabolic acidosis resulting from intravenous alimentation mixtures containing synthetic amino acids. N Engl J Med 1972; 287(19):943–8.
40. Goldman HI, Goldman J, Kaufman I, et al. Late effects of early dietary protein intake on low-birth-weight infants. J Pediatr 1974;85(6):764–9.
41. Menkes JH, Welcher DW, Levi HS, et al. Relationship of elevated blood tyrosine to the ultimate intellectual performance of premature infants. Pediatrics 1972;49(2): 218–24.
42. Kotsopoulos K, Benadiba-Torch A, Cuddy A, et al. Safety and efficacy of early amino acids in preterm <28 weeks gestation: prospective observational comparison. J Perinatol 2006;26(12):749–54.
43. Ridout E, Melara D, Rottinghaus S, et al. Blood urea nitrogen concentration as a marker of amino-acid intolerance in neonates with birthweight less than 1250 g. J Perinatol 2005;25(2):130–3.
44. Koletzko B, Goulet O, Hunt J, et al. Guidelines on paediatric parenteral nutrition of the european society of paediatric gastroenterology, hepatology and nutrition (ESPGHAN) and the european society for clinical nutrition and metabolism (ESPEN). J Pediatr Gastroenterol Nutr 2005;41(Suppl 2):S1–87.
45. Hay WW. Early postnatal nutritional requirements of the very preterm infant based on a presentation at the NICHD-AAP workshop on research in neonatology. J Perinatol 2006;26(Suppl 2):S13–8.
46. McKeown RE, Marsh TD, Amarnath U, et al. Role of delayed feeding and of feeding increments in necrotizing enterocolitis. J Pediatr 1992;121(5 Pt 1):764–70.
47. McClure RJ, Newell SJ. Randomised controlled study of clinical outcome following trophic feeding. Arch Dis Child Fetal Neonatal Ed 2000;82(1):F29–33.
48. Troche B, Harvey-Wilkes K, Engle WD, et al. Early minimal feedings promote growth in critically ill premature infants. Biol Neonate 1995;67(3):172–81.
49. Dunn L, Hulman S, Weiner J, et al. Beneficial effects of early hypocaloric enteral feeding on neonatal gastrointestinal function: preliminary report of a randomized trial. J Pediatr 1988;112(4):622–9.
50. Weiler HA, Fitzpatrick-Wong SC, Schellenberg JM, et al. Minimal enteral feeding within 3 d of birth in prematurely born infants with birth weight < or = 1200 g improves bone mass by term age. Am J Clin Nutr 2006;83(1):155–62.

51. Davey AM, Wagner CL, Cox C, et al. Feeding premature infants while low umbilical artery catheters are in place: a prospective, randomized trial. J Pediatr 1994;124(5 Pt 1):795–9.
52. Flidel-Rimon O, Friedman S, Lev E, et al. Early enteral feeding and nosocomial sepsis in very low birthweight infants. Arch Dis Child Fetal Neonatal Ed 2004;89(4):F289–92.
53. Havranek T, Johanboeke P, Madramootoo C, et al. Umbilical artery catheters do not affect intestinal blood flow responses to minimal enteral feedings. J Perinatol 2007;27(6):375–9.
54. Tiffany KF, Burke BL, Collins-Odoms C, et al. Current practice regarding the enteral feeding of high-risk newborns with umbilical catheters in situ. Pediatrics 2003;112(1 Pt 1):20–3.
55. Tyson JE, Kennedy KA. Trophic feedings for parenterally fed infants. Cochrane Database Syst Rev 2005;(3):CD000504.
56. Berseth CL, Bisquera JA, Paje VU. Prolonging small feeding volumes early in life decreases the incidence of necrotizing enterocolitis in very low birth weight infants. Pediatrics 2003;111(3):529–34.
57. Anderson DM, Kliegman RM. The relationship of neonatal alimentation practices to the occurrence of endemic necrotizing enterocolitis. Am J Perinatol 1991;8(1):62–7.
58. Rayyis SF, Ambalavanan N, Wright L, et al. Randomized trial of "slow" versus "fast" feed advancements on the incidence of necrotizing enterocolitis in very low birth weight infants. J Pediatr 1999;134(3):293–7.
59. Caple J, Armentrout D, Huseby V, et al. Randomized, controlled trial of slow versus rapid feeding volume advancement in preterm infants. Pediatrics 2004;114(6):1597–600.
60. Patole SK, de Klerk N. Impact of standardised feeding regimens on incidence of neonatal necrotising enterocolitis: a systematic review and meta-analysis of observational studies. Arch Dis Child Fetal Neonatal Ed 2005;90(2):F147–51.
61. Vohr BR, Poindexter BB, Dusick AM, et al. Persistent beneficial effects of breast milk ingested in the neonatal intensive care unit on outcomes of extremely low birth weight infants at 30 months of age. Pediatrics 2007;120(4):e953–9.
62. Moody GJ, Schanler RJ, Lau C, et al. Feeding tolerance in premature infants fed fortified human milk. J Pediatr Gastroenterol Nutr 2000;30(4):408–12.
63. Kuschel CA, Harding JE. Multicomponent fortified human milk for promoting growth in preterm infants. Cochrane Database Syst Rev 2004;(1):CD000343.
64. Weber A, Loui A, Jochum F, et al. Breast milk from mothers of very low birthweight infants: variability in fat and protein content. Acta Paediatr 2001;90(7):772–5.
65. Kuschel CA, Harding JE. Protein supplementation of human milk for promoting growth in preterm infants. Cochrane Database Syst Rev 2000;(2):CD000433.
66. Doege C, Bauer J. Effect of high volume intake of mother's milk with an individualized supplementation of minerals and protein on early growth of preterm infants <28 weeks of gestation. Clin Nutr 2007;26(5):581–8.
67. Meier PP, Engstrom JL, Murtaugh MA, et al. Mothers' milk feedings in the neonatal intensive care unit: accuracy of the creamatocrit technique. J Perinatol 2002;22(8):646–9.
68. Wang CD, Chu PS, Mellen BG, et al. Creamatocrit and the nutrient composition of human milk. J Perinatol 1999;19(5):343–6.
69. Ferris AM, Jensen RG. Lipids in human milk: a review. 1: sampling, determination, and content. J Pediatr Gastroenterol Nutr 1984;3(1):108–22.

70. Lubetzky R, Mimouni FB, Dollberg S, et al. Consistent circadian variations in creamatocrit over the first 7 weeks of lactation: a longitudinal study. Breastfeed Med 2007;2(1):15–8.
71. Valentine CJ, Hurst NM, Schanler RJ. Hindmilk improves weight gain in low-birth-weight infants fed human milk. J Pediatr Gastroenterol Nutr 1994;18(4):474–7.
72. Daly SE, Di Rosso A, Owens RA, et al. Degree of breast emptying explains changes in the fat content, but not fatty acid composition, of human milk. Exp Physiol 1993;78(6):741–55.
73. Greer FR, McCormick A, Loker J. Changes in fat concentration of human milk during delivery by intermittent bolus and continuous mechanical pump infusion. J Pediatr 1984;105(5):745–9.
74. Klein CJ. Nutrient requirements for preterm infant formulas. J Nutr 2002;132(6 Suppl 1):1395S–577S.
75. Zello GA, Menendez CE, Rafii M, et al. Minimum protein intake for the preterm neonate determined by protein and amino acid kinetics. Pediatr Res 2003;53(2):338–44.
76. Premji SS, Fenton TR, Sauve RS. Higher versus lower protein intake in formula-fed low birth weight infants. Cochrane Database Syst Rev 2006;(1):CD003959.
77. Cooke R, Embleton N, Rigo J, et al. High protein pre-term infant formula: effect on nutrient balance, metabolic status and growth. Pediatr Res 2006;59(2):265–70.
78. Arslanoglu S, Moro GE, Ziegler EE. Adjustable fortification of human milk fed to preterm infants: does it make a difference? J Perinatol 2006;26(10):614–21.

Postnatal Corticosteroids for Bronchopulmonary Dysplasia

Alan H. Jobe, MD, PhD

KEYWORDS

• Lung injury • Alveoli • Premature • Neurodevelopment
• Mechanical ventilation

All who drink of this treatment recover in a short time, except those whom it does not help, who all die. Therefore, it is obvious that it fails only in incurable cases.

—Galen, 200 AD

A PERSPECTIVE

Are corticosteroids being used today in the uninformed way that Galen used his potion to treat patients almost 2000 years ago, and are treatment failures the result of the disease or the drug? Galen seemed to discount drug toxicity for those unfortunate incurable cases. There really are only two core questions that need to be asked about the use of postnatal corticosteroids for bronchopulmonary dysfunction (BPD): do they work, and do they have clinically concerning adverse effects? The challenge is to define what "work" means, what adverse effects are of concern, and what "they" are, because multiple corticosteroids are used in different doses at different postnatal ages for different treatment durations. The use of postnatal corticosteroids for BPD has been widely evaluated by randomized, controlled trials, but these trials have multiple treatment schedules and have produced limited and inconsistent information about outcomes. Ultimately, the clinician must weigh the statistical and population-based evidence and decide if corticosteroids might help a particular infant and if the risks are acceptable.

The Food and Drug Administration has not approved the use of corticosteroid drugs for the treatment of bronchopulmonary dysplasia.

Division of Pulmonary Biology, Cincinnati Children's Hospital, University of Cincinnati, 3333 Burnet Avenue, Cincinnati, OH 45229-3039, USA
E-mail address: alan.jobe@cchmc.org

Clin Perinatol 36 (2009) 177–188
doi:10.1016/j.clp.2008.09.016 perinatology.theclinics.com

HOW FREQUENTLY ARE CORTICOSTEROIDS USED?

The use of postnatal corticosteroids has been a bit like women's hemlines, rising and falling based on fashion or perceived benefits and risks. In 1990, about 17% of very low birth weight (VLBW) infants cared for in the Vermont Oxford Network received postnatal corticosteroids, and the rate of use was 7% for VLBW infants in the National Institute for Child Health and Human Development Neonatal Research Network.[1] The peak rate of use was 28% for Vermont Oxford Network and 23% for the Neonatal Research Network in 1997. As follow-up information about adverse effects of corticosteroids on neurodevelopment began to appear, the American Academy of Pediatrics and the Canadian Pediatric Association strongly recommended against the use of corticosteroids to prevent or treat BPD in 2002.[2] Since then, use has decreased. In 2006 8% of VLBW infants overall in the Vermont Oxford Network registry and 23% of the infants in the group at highest risk (those with birth weights between 501 and 750 g) received postnatal corticosteroids (R. Soll, personal communication, 2008). Therefore, postnatal corticosteroids continue to be used selectively in infants. Infants also receive corticosteroids for indications other than BPD. In 62 neonatal ICUs in California in 2003, 19% of VLBW infants received postnatal steroids, but only 3.6% received steroids for BPD alone; the other uses were for treatment of hypotension, airway management after extubation, or a combination of indications.[3] Some ICUs also use aerosolized corticosteroids. Thus the risks and benefits of corticosteroid use remain a concern. Corticosteroids are used preferentially in the smaller and earlier gestational age infants because those infants are at highest risk for developing severe BPD.

DO CORTICOSTEROIDS WORK FOR BRONCHOPULMONARY DYSPLASIA?

One way of interpreting the question whether corticosteroids work for BPD is whether the use of corticosteroids improves lung function in ventilator-dependent infants at risk for BPD sufficiently to permit extubation. Corticosteroids now are used less frequently soon after birth to "prevent" BPD because of concerns about the risk and interactions with other drugs such as indomethacin.[4,5] The summary conclusions of the meta-analyses by Halliday and colleagues[6–8] indicate that postnatal corticosteroids do not decrease death, although there is a trend for a death benefit for treatments started at 7 to 14 days of age (**Table 1**). Corticosteroids decrease BPD and decrease extubation failures independently of the age at which treatments are started. The trials included in these meta-analyses dated mostly from the era before surfactant treatment was available, and some of the trials were done before the use of antenatal corticosteroids was common. The infants in these studies were larger than many of the infants who receive postnatal corticosteroids today. Also, there have been changes in the techniques used for mechanical ventilation and in ventilatory goals. Higher P_{CO_2} values may be accepted for infants requiring mechanical ventilation for severe respiratory failure. A therapy that was effective in a different era and in a different patient population may not work now. If postnatal corticosteroids do not work in current practice, a further discussion of their use is not relevant.

The American Academy of Pediatrics and Canadian Pediatric Association joint condemnation of postnatal corticosteroid use for BPD curtailed enthusiasm for further studies.[2] Nevertheless, two studies were attempted, and both were closed before full enrollment. Watterberg and colleagues[5] randomly assigned ventilated infants with birth weights between 500 and 999 g to a 15-day tapered course of hydrocortisone or placebo within 2 days of birth. The hypothesis was that hydrocortisone would treat the adrenal insufficiency that commonly occurs soon after birth, would improve survival, and would decrease BPD. The trial was stopped because of increased

Table 1
Postnatal corticosteroids: association with death/chronic lung disease

Time of Treatment	# Studies	# Patients	Relative Risk	Significance
Death				
<96 h	21	3068	1.01 (0.89–1.15)	—
7–14 d	6	288	0.66 (0.40–1.09)	—
>3 wk	8	54	0.99 (0.71–1.39)	—
Chronic lung disease				
<96 h	15	2415	0.69 (0.60–.80)	*
7–14 d	5	247	0.62 (0.47–.82)	*
> 3 wk (home O_2)	5	481	0.66 (0.47–.92)	*
Failure to extubate at 7 d				
<96 h	6	936	0.76 (0.66–.88)	*
7–14 d	2	84	0.62 (0.46–.84)	*
>3 wk	5	288	0.69 (0.58–.82)	*

Data from Refs.[6–8]

intestinal perforations in hydrocortisone-treated infants who also received indomethacin as prophylaxis for patent ductus arteriosus. Although there was no overall death or BPD benefit, a prospectively planned analysis of infants exposed to histologic chorioamnionitis did demonstrate decreased BPD and death in infants randomly assigned to hydrocortisone. This trial demonstrated benefit in a subpopulation of infants managed by current practices.

The Dexamethasone: A Randomized Trial (DART) study randomly assigned 70 ventilator-dependent infants with average birth weights less than 700 g to a 10-day tapered dose of dexamethasone or placebo at a mean postnatal age of 23 days.[9] The initial dexamethasone dose of 0.15 mg/kg was lower than that used in previous trials. Enrollment was stopped because infants could not be recruited, in part because of concerns about risks. This study was underpowered and did not demonstrate differences in BPD or death. The dexamethasone treatment had large effects on the lungs, however, and successful extubation was more frequent (**Table 2**). This small trial demonstrates that postnatal corticosteroids do improve lung function in surfactant-treated

Table 2
Responses of ventilator-dependent preterm infants randomly assigned to a 10-day tapered course of dexamethasone begun at a median age of 23 days

Values at 10 Days	Placebo	Dexamethasone	P-Value
N	35	35	—
Failure to extubate	88%	40%	<.01
Mean airway pressure (cm H_2O)	10.2	7.6	<.01
Peak airway pressure (cm H_2O)	19.6	16.7	<.01
Inspired oxygen	43.5%	34.7%	<.04
Mean blood pressure (mm Hg)	45.7	52.5	—

Data from Doyle LW, Davis PG, Morley CJ, et al. Low-dose dexamethasone facilitates extubation among chronically ventilator-dependent infants: a multicenter, international, randomized, controlled trial. Pediatrics 2006;117:756.

infants exposed to antenatal corticosteroids and managed by contemporary techniques.

A recent retrospective report compared oral prednisolone (2 mg/kg/d for 5 days and tapered for 9 days) in 131 oxygen-dependent infants at 38 weeks' gestation who had BPD and a matched group of 254 infants.[10] Among the infants who had P_{CO_2} values lower than 49 mm Hg, those treated with prednisolone were weaned from oxygen more readily than infants in the comparison group. This use of corticosteroids differs from that in other trials, because the infants were off ventilators and simply were treated with oxygen. This retrospective report does suggest physiologic responses of BPD lungs late in the clinical course. Despite concerns about outcomes, neonatologists continue to use corticosteroids in some infants because the short-term improvements in lung function can be remarkable.

HOW DO POSTNATAL CORTICOSTEROIDS WORK?

How postnatal corticosteroids work is not a simple question. Corticosteroids are potent anti-inflammatory agents, and there is a clear rationale for the use of an anti-inflammatory agent to treat BPD. Perhaps more than 50% of infants at risk for BPD have been exposed to the chronic indolent chorioamnionitis associated with very preterm birth, and those infants have inflamed lungs at birth.[11,12] Oxygen exposure and mechanical ventilation also induce inflammatory responses.[13] Multiple proinflammatory mediators and inflammatory cells are seen in airway samples from infants progressing toward BPD.[14] Postnatal corticosteroids decrease these indicators of inflammation.[15] Indomethacin also is an anti-inflammatory agent, however, and it does not decrease BPD.[16] Corticosteroids decrease edema as part of their anti-inflammatory effect, and this decrease may contribute to improved gas exchange and lung mechanics. Particularly in VLBW infants, corticosteroid treatments increase blood pressure and treat adrenal insufficiency.[17] The different types of corticosteroid—hydrocortisone or dexamethasone—also may have different actions that contribute to clinical responses. A better understanding of the mediators that promote BPD at each stage of disease progression is needed to develop therapies that are more targeted than corticosteroids.

DRUG, DOSE, AND DURATION OF CORTICOSTEROID TREATMENTS

An analysis of corticosteroid treatments in infants is bedeviled by the different steroids and variable dosing schedules used.[6–8] The early trials designed to prevent BPD used a "standard" initial dose of 0.5 mg/kg dexamethasone that was tapered slowly over 42 days; this regimen is referred to as the "42-day treatment." More recent trials have used lower initial doses of 0.2, 0.15, or 0.1 mg/kg dexamethasone with weaning schedules over 7 to 10 days and with apparently good acute effects on lung function.[4,9,18] In the United States, betamethasone phosphate is not available, but it has been used and dosed similarly to dexamethasone elsewhere in the world. These two synthetic corticosteroids are 25 times more potent than hydrocortisone, but they are not equivalent. Although the genomic effects are similar, nongenomic effects such as acute changes in membrane function and ion transport are very different.[19] Betamethasone may be more effective and safer than dexamethasone for antenatal treatment of women at risk of preterm delivery.[20] Betamethasone may have fewer effects on the fetal brain. Hydrocortisone is being used more frequently for treatment of hypotension in VLBW infants, and hydrocortisone has been used outside randomized, controlled trials to treat BPD in Europe. Hydrocortisone is the natural hormone, which may be safer to use than the synthetic corticosteroids,[21] but randomized trials of lung responses or complications are not available. Prednisolone also has been used but has not been evaluated in randomized trials.[10] Without good trial data, clinicians are using lower doses of dexamethasone or hydrocortisone for shorter treatment periods. Treatment schedules of 0.2 mg/kg of dexamethasone or less tapered over 7 to 10 days seem to avoid the hyperglycemia and hypertension frequently encountered with the higher doses and longer treatment schedules.[9] Because toxicity from corticosteroids is related to dose and treatment duration in patients of all ages, the use of lower-dose, shorter-duration treatments makes intuitive sense. Aerosolized corticosteroids are used frequently in some neonatal units, but not in others, to treat the progression of BPD. There is very little evidence that aerosolized steroids have much efficacy.[22,23] Aerosolization of steroids may be ineffectlve because very little drug gets into the lungs of preterm infants by aerosolization.[24]

CORTICOSTEROIDS AND NEURODEVELOPMENTAL OUTCOMES

A Perspective

Cortisol is a potent agent that regulates development and normally increases before term birth. Cortisol also increases with preterm birth, but to lower blood levels than found after term birth (**Fig. 1**). The fetus is protected from maternal cortisol by placental 11β hydroxysteroid dehydrogenase, which converts cortisol to the inactive cortisone as it passes from maternal to the fetal circulation. Fetal cortisol synthesis is regulated tightly so that the fetus makes minimal cortisol until late in gestation. Stressed preterm fetuses and fetuses exposed to chorioamnionitis can "induce" cortisol synthesis and secretion.[25] The unstressed preterm fetus has low blood cortisol levels and is unable to increase adrenal synthesis and secretion rapidly. Therefore, many VLBW infants have low blood cortisol values and may be functionally adrenal insufficient.[17] The preterm newborn between 26 weeks and term has an endogenous cortisol exposure much greater than that of the fetus for the 14 weeks after birth (**Fig. 1**). Therefore, brain growth in the preterm infant occurs in a high-cortisol

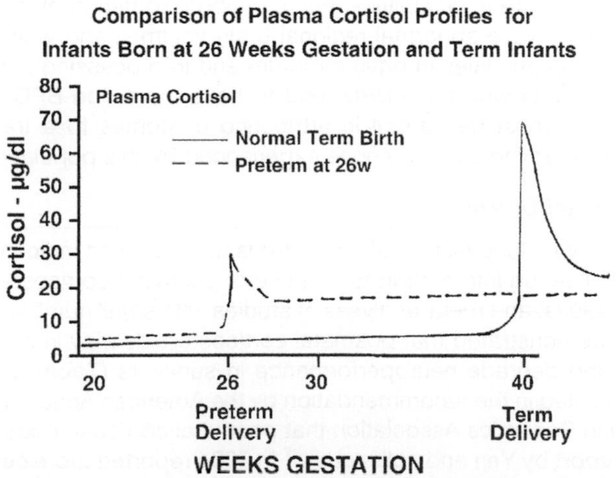

Fig. 1. Idealized plasma cortisol profile for a normal fetus that delivers at 40 weeks' gestation and for a preterm fetus that delivers at 26 weeks' gestation. The preterm infant has lower cortisol levels at delivery than the term infant. Following delivery, however, the preterm has higher cortisol levels than the fetus from 26 weeks to 40 weeks.

environment relative to brain growth in the fetus, independent of any antenatal or postnatal corticosteroid treatments.

Fetal rodents are exquisitely sensitive to fluorinated corticosteroids such as betamethasone or dexamethasone that cross the placenta from mother to fetus. Fetal or neonatal exposures cause fetal growth restriction and lung maturation, as well as programming effects that result in behavioral abnormalities and hypertension as adults.[26] Two recent reports demonstrate that neonatal dexamethasone treatments reduce life expectancy and cause sustained atherogenic plasma lipid profiles in rats.[27,28] In sheep, a brief period of exposure to corticosteroids at early gestation alters kidney anatomy, kidney function, and blood pressure regulation in adulthood.[29] Are these quite striking (and frightening) effects relevant to postnatal corticosteroid treatments for preterm infants? A reasonable way to think about possible relevance is to ask how corticosteroids might affect fetal or newborn weights in different species. At 80% gestation, the weight of the rat fetus increases by 65% in 1 day, and the weight of the mouse fetus increases by almost 100% over 1 day. A single dose of betamethasone arrests growth in the fetal sheep for several days.[30] At 80% gestation, however, the weight of the human fetus increases by 1.6% over 1 day. Thus, corticosteroids have much less effect on growth in humans than in shorter-gestation mammals. The experimental research can be used to frame the questions that should be asked in humans. One cannot assume, however, that corticosteroid effects map from rodent models to humans.

Another perspective about possible effects of postnatal corticosteroids relates to the outcomes of the infants at risk. Postnatal corticosteroids are given to the sickest VLBW infants who are on ventilators and are progressing toward BPD. VLBW infants have multiple complications and neurodevelopmental problems independent of corticosteroid use. Population-based studies from the United Kingdom showed that at school age the Mental Development Index (MDI) and Psychomotor Development Index (PDI) scores of children who had been born at gestational ages of less than 26 weeks were about 20 points lower than those of children who had been born at term.[31] Infants who have BPD have more neurodevelopmental problems than matched infants who do not have BPD.[32,33] The inflammation associated with BPD or the recurrent respiratory instabilities may contribute to neurodamage. Also, "normal" preterm infants have abnormal regional brain volumes and white matter injury at term.[34] These abnormalities in brain structure and in processing persist to school age.[35] Because infants who have BPD tend to have more non-BPD complications of prematurity, one must be careful in attributing outcomes to a treatment rather than to the multiple adverse occurrences experienced by this population of infants.

Neurodevelopmental Outcomes

Neonatologists have a long history of using drugs for unverified indications and without follow-up. Follow-up information for the use of postnatal corticosteroids became available in the 1990s, and meta-analyses of studies with small numbers of patients in 2000 and 2001 demonstrated that postnatal corticosteroids may increase the rate of cerebral palsy and degrade neuroperformance in survivors (**Table 3**).[6–8,36] In 2002 these reports resulted in the recommendation by the American Academy of Pediatrics and the Canadian Pediatrics Association that postnatal corticosteroids not be used.[2] A subsequent report by Yeh and colleagues[37] in 2004 reported more cerebral palsy in infants treated with the 42-day course of dexamethasone. Another finding of concern was that postnatal dexamethasone given for a mean of 22 days decreased gray matter volume as measured by MRI.[38] The report by Le Flore and colleagues[39] using a multivariate analysis noted that MDI and PDI scores were lower for infants who had BPD

Table 3
Follow-up of infants treated with postnatal corticosteroids

Time of Treatment	# Studies	# Patients	Relative Risk	Significance
<96 hours				
MDI < 2 SD	2	482	1.24 (.90–1.71)	—
PDI < 2 SD	2	482	1.18 (.81–1.72)	—
Cerebral palsy	9	991	1.69 (1.2–2.38)	*
7–14 days				
Cerebral palsy	4	204	1.03 (.47–2.24)	—
>3 weeks				
Abnormal Neuro	3	164	1.90 (1.08–3.33)	*

Data from Refs.[6–8]

treated with dexamethasone than for comparison infants. Recently Parikh and colleagues[40] measured smaller total and regional brain tissue volumes at term in preterm infants who had received dexamethasone after 28 days of age for a mean duration of only 6.8 days (cumulative dose, 2.8 mg/kg). These last two studies were not based on randomization to postnatal corticosteroid use.

A number of recent reports, however, find either no adverse outcomes or benefits in follow-up of infants exposed to postnatal corticosteroids. Although O'Shea and colleagues[41] reported an increased risk for cerebral palsy at 1 year of age in infants randomly assigned to the 42-day course of dexamethasone (with no cross-over dexamethasone treatments in the control group), their composite outcomes of death or major neurodevelopmental impairment were not different from controls at school age.[42] Furthermore, this same cohort of infants had higher expiratory flows than controls and no adverse effects on lung function at school age.[43] These infants also did not differ from controls in growth, fat mass, or blood pressure at school age.[44] Another experience with the outcomes of a small number of infants randomly assigned to the 42-day course of dexamethasone was improved neurodevelopmental outcomes relative to controls.[45] A comparison of outcomes of infants randomly assigned to dexamethasone or inhaled budesonide demonstrated no differences in neuroperformance, cerebral palsy, or growth.[46] The author interprets the budesonide treatment group as being equivalent to a no-treatment group.[23] Lower-dose dexamethasone given after the first week of life also did not effect 2-year outcomes adversely in another small, randomized trial.[47] These reports are in contrast to mostly older reports of adverse effects of dexamethasone on neurodevelopment.

Reports of outcomes following the use of hydrocortisone also have appeared since the recommendation against the use of postnatal corticosteroids.[2] In a randomized study hydrocortisone was used shortly after birth to treat adrenal insufficiency and to decrease BPD.[5] At 2 years, infants randomly assigned to hydrocortisone had improved neurodevelopmental outcomes relative to controls.[48] In a cohort of infants who received hydrocortisone for the treatment of BPD, Rademaker and colleagues[49] found that, relative to an older, heavier, and less sick group of comparison infants, hydrocortisone was associated with no adverse effects on multiple neurodevelopmental or MRI assessments at school age. Similar neurocognitive and MRI outcomes were reported for 8-year-olds treated with hydrocortisone for BPD.[50] A retrospective, matched-cohort analysis of infants given dexamethasone or hydrocortisone suggested that the infants exposed to dexamethasone exposed had more problems with neurodevelopmen,[21] and had altered endocrine and immune function at school age.[51]

An Approach to Postnatal Corticosteroids

There are justified concerns about the use of postnatal corticosteroids for any indication, but especially for BPD. Those concerns, however, must be balanced against the clear acute physiologic effects on lung function that can allow infants to come off mechanical ventilation. Shinwell and colleagues[52] recently reported for the Israel Neonatal Network that a decreased use of postnatal corticosteroids in VLBW infants, from 23.5% in 1997 and 1998 to 11% in 2002 and 2003, was associated with an increase in BPD (oxygen use at 36 weeks) from 12.9% to 18.7%. This report suggests that the price one pays for decreased corticosteroid use is more BPD. The author considers the critical analysis to be the meta-regression analysis reported by Doyle and colleagues,[53] which shows that postnatal corticosteroids decrease the risk of death or cerebral palsy in populations of infants who have a 50% or greater risk of BPD (**Fig. 2**). Treatment of low-risk populations may increase the risk of adverse outcomes. The DART trial demonstrated acute effects on the lungs of ventilated infants progressing toward BPD with an initial dose of 0.15 mg/kg/d.[9] The general clinical experience is that some infants respond quickly to corticosteroids and others do not. Considering the information available, the author favors corticosteroid treatment of a ventilator-dependent infant who is 14 to 28 days of age and who is progressing toward BPD. An initial dose of dexamethasone of 0.1 to 0.2 mg/kg/d for 3 days may achieve the goal of extubation. If extubation can be achieved or is likely to be accomplished, the dose can be tapered over 3 to 6 days (total treatment, 6–9 days). If extubation is not possible after the initial 3 days of treatment, the treatment should be stopped. This approach is not evidence based; it is an attempt to maximize benefit and minimize

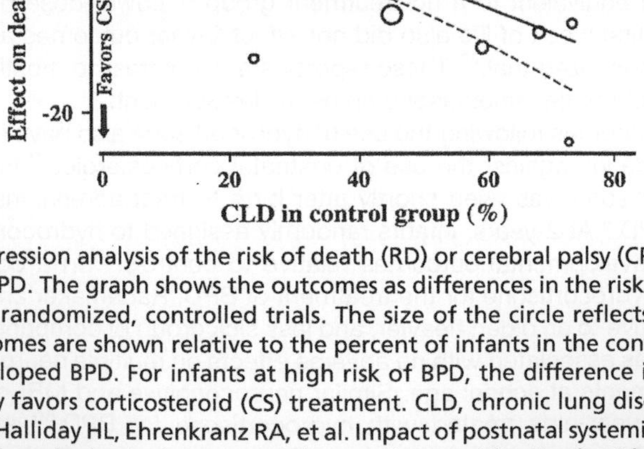

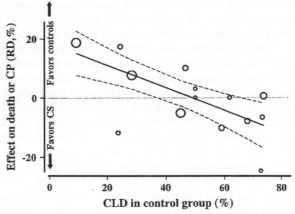

Fig. 2. Meta-regression analysis of the risk of death (RD) or cerebral palsy (CP) relative to risk of developing BPD. The graph shows the outcomes as differences in the risk for death or cerebral palsy for randomized, controlled trials. The size of the circle reflects the size of the study. The outcomes are shown relative to the percent of infants in the control arm of each study who developed BPD. For infants at high risk of BPD, the difference in risk for death or cerebral palsy favors corticosteroid (CS) treatment. CLD, chronic lung disease. (*Reprinted from* Doyle LW, Halliday HL, Ehrenkranz RA, et al. Impact of postnatal systemic corticosteroids on mortality and cerebral palsy in preterm infants: effect modification by risk for chronic lung disease. Pediatrics 2005;115:655; with permission. Copyright © 2005 by the AAP.)

the risk of postnatal corticosteroids. Betamethasone or hydrocortisone might be better choices than dexamethasone, but neither has been evaluated in trials for this indication.

Clinicians have moved beyond Galen because they now know a fair bit about the treatment: it can work, and it has risks. The follow-up data are particularly confusing, because bad or good outcomes have been reported with early or late treatment and with higher or lower exposures. Other aspects of care may interact with corticosteroids and contribute to these inconsistent outcomes. Clearly, the use of corticosteroids and indomethacin together soon after birth increases gastrointestinal perforations.[4,5] For example, good nutrition might blunt adverse effects of postnatal corticosteroids. Following the lead of Doyle and colleagues,[53] the very selective use a low-dose (but what dose?) corticosteroid (but which one?) for as short a duration as possible (presently undefined) in the infants at highest risk is the best treatment that can be offered now. The recommendation to limit postnatal corticosteroid use should not discourage careful studies of postnatal corticosteroids in high-risk VLBW infants.

REFERENCES

1. Walsh MC, Yao Q, Horbar JD, et al. Changes in the use of postnatal steroids for bronchopulmonary dysplasia in 3 large neonatal networks. Pediatrics 2006;118: e1328–35.
2. American Academy of Pediatrics - American Academy of Pediatrics Committee on Fetus and Newborn and Canadian Paediatric Society, Fetus and Newborn Committee. Postnatal corticosteroids to treat or prevent chronic lung disease in preterm infants. Pediatrics 2002;109:330–8.
3. Finer NN, Powers RJ, Ou CH, et al. Prospective evaluation of postnatal steroid administration: a 1-year experience from the California Perinatal Quality Care Collaborative. Pediatrics 2006;117:704–13.
4. Stark AR, Carlo WA, Tyson JE, et al. Adverse effects of early dexamethasone in extremely-low-birth-weight infants. National Institute of Child Health and Human Development Neonatal Research Network. N Engl J Med 2001;344:95–101.
5. Watterberg KL, Gerdes JS, Cole CH, et al. Prophylaxis of early adrenal insufficiency to prevent bronchopulmonary dysplasia: a multicenter trial. Pediatrics 2004;114:1649–57.
6. Halliday HL, Ehrenkranz RA, Doyle LW. Moderately early (7–14 days) postnatal corticosteroids for preventing chronic lung disease in preterm infants. Cochrane Database Syst Rev 2003:CD001144.
7. Halliday HL, Ehrenkranz RA, Doyle LW. Delayed (>3 weeks) postnatal corticosteroids for chronic lung disease in preterm infants. Cochrane Database Syst Rev 2003:CD001145.
8. Halliday HL, Ehrenkranz RA, Doyle LW. Early postnatal (<96 hours) corticosteroids for preventing chronic lung disease in preterm infants. Cochrane Database Syst Rev 2003:CD001146.
9. Doyle LW, Davis PG, Morley CJ, et al. Low-dose dexamethasone facilitates extubation among chronically ventilator-dependent infants: a multicenter, international, randomized, controlled trial. Pediatrics 2006;117:75–83.
10. Bhandari A, Schramm CM, Kimble C, et al. Effect of a short course of prednisolone in infants with oxygen-dependent bronchopulmonary dysplasia. Pediatrics 2008;121:e344–9.

11. Watterberg KL, Demers LM, Scott SM, et al. Chorioamnionitis and early lung inflammation in infants in whom bronchopulmonary dysplasia develops. Pediatrics 1996;97:210–5.
12. Andrews WW, Goldenberg RL, Faye-Petersen O, et al. The Alabama Preterm Birth Study: polymorphonuclear and mononuclear cell placental infiltrations, other markers of inflammation, and outcomes in 23- to 32-week preterm newborn infants. Am J Obstet Gynecol 2006;195:803–8.
13. Coalson JJ. Pathology of new bronchopulmonary dysplasia. Semin Neonatol 2003;8:73–81.
14. De Dooy J, Colpaert C, Schuerwegh A, et al. Relationship between histologic chorioamnionitis and early inflammatory variables in blood, tracheal aspirates, and endotracheal colonization in preterm infants. Pediatr Res 2003;54:113–9.
15. Speer CP. Inflammation and bronchopulmonary dysplasia. Semin Neonatol 2003; 8:29–38.
16. Schmidt B, Roberts RS, Fanaroff A, et al. Indomethacin prophylaxis, patent ductus arteriosus, and the risk of bronchopulmonary dysplasia: further analyses from the Trial of Indomethacin Prophylaxis in Preterms (TIPP). J Pediatr 2006;148:730–4.
17. Watterberg KL. Adrenocortical function and dysfunction in the fetus and neonate. Semin Neonatol 2004;9:13–21.
18. Durand M, Mendoza ME, Tantivit P, et al. A randomized trial of moderately early low-dose dexamethasone therapy in very low birth weight infants: dynamic pulmonary mechanics, oxygenation, and ventilation. Pediatrics 2002;109:262–8.
19. Buttgereit F, Brand MD, Burmester GR. Equivalent doses and relative drug potencies for non-genomic glucocorticoid effects: a novel glucocorticoid hierarchy. Biochem Pharmacol 1999;58:363–8.
20. Lee BH, Stoll BJ, McDonald SA, et al. Neurodevelopmental outcomes of extremely low birth weight infants exposed prenatally to dexamethasone versus betamethasone. Pediatrics 2008;121:289–96.
21. Karemaker R, Heijnen CJ, Veen S, et al. Differences in behavioral outcome and motor development at school age after neonatal treatment for chronic lung disease with dexamethasone versus hydrocortisone. Pediatr Res 2006;60:745–50.
22. Shah SS, Ohlsson A, Halliday H, et al. Inhaled versus systemic corticosteroids for the treatment of chronic lung disease in ventilated very low birth weight preterm infants. Cochrane Database Syst Rev 2003:CD002057.
23. Cole CH, Colton T, Shah BL, et al. Early inhaled glucocorticoid therapy to prevent bronchopulmonary dysplasia. [see comments]. N Engl J Med 1999;340:1005–10.
24. Dubus JC, Montharu J, Vecellio L, et al. Lung deposition of HFA beclomethasone dipropionate in an animal model of bronchopulmonary dysplasia. Pediatr Res 2007;61:21–5.
25. Watterberg KL, Scott SM, Naeye RL. Chorioamnionitis, cortisol, and acute lung disease in very low birth weight infants. Pediatrics 1997;99:E6.
26. Jobe AH, Ikegami M. Fetal responses to glucocorticoids. In: Mendelson CR, editor. Endocrinology of the lung. Totowa (NJ): Humana Press; 2000. p. 45–57.
27. Kamphuis PJ, de Vries WB, Bakker JM, et al. Reduced life expectancy in rats after neonatal dexamethasone treatment. Pediatr Res 2007;61:72–6.
28. Liu Y, Havinga R, Bloks VW, et al. Postnatal treatment with dexamethasone perturbs hepatic and cardiac energy metabolism and is associated with a sustained atherogenic plasma lipid profile in suckling rats. Pediatr Res 2007;61:165–70.
29. Wintour EM, Moritz KM, Johnson K, et al. Reduced nephron number in adult sheep, hypertensive as a result of prenatal glucocorticoid treatment. J Physiol 2003;549:929–35.

30. Ikegami M, Jobe AH, Newnham J, et al. Repetitive prenatal glucocorticoids improve lung function and decrease growth in preterm lambs. Am J Respir Crit Care Med 1997;156:178–84.
31. Marlow N, Hennessy EM, Bracewell MA, et al. Motor and executive function at 6 years of age after extremely preterm birth. Pediatrics 2007;120:793–804.
32. Short EJ, Klein NK, Lewis BA, et al. Cognitive and academic consequences of bronchopulmonary dysplasia and very low birth weight: 8-year-old outcomes. Pediatrics 2003;112:e359.
33. Ehrenkranz RA, Walsh MC, Vohr BR, et al. Validation of the National Institutes of Health consensus definition of bronchopulmonary dysplasia. Pediatrics 2005; 116:1353–60.
34. Inder TE, Warfield SK, Wang H, et al. Abnormal cerebral structure is present at term in premature infants. Pediatrics 2005;115:286–94.
35. Constable RT, Ment LR, Vohr BR, et al. Prematurely born children demonstrate white matter microstructural differences at 12 years of age, relative to term control subjects: an investigation of group and gender effects. Pediatrics 2008;121: 306–16.
36. Barrington KJ. The adverse neuro-developmental effects of postnatal steroids in the preterm infant: a systematic review of RCTs. BMC Pediatr 2001;1:1.
37. Yeh TF, Lin YJ, Lin HC, et al. Outcomes at school age after postnatal dexamethasone therapy for lung disease of prematurity. N Engl J Med 2004;350:1304–13.
38. Murphy BP, Inder TE, Huppi PS, et al. Impaired cerebral cortical gray matter growth after treatment with dexamethasone for neonatal chronic lung disease. Pediatrics 2001;107:217–21.
39. LeFlore JL, Salhab WA, Broyles RS, et al. Association of antenatal and postnatal dexamethasone exposure with outcomes in extremely low birth weight neonates. Pediatrics 2002;110:275–9.
40. Parikh NA, Lasky RE, Kennedy KA, et al. Postnatal dexamethasone therapy and cerebral tissue volumes in extremely low birth weight infants. Pediatrics 2007; 119:265–72.
41. O'Shea TM, Kothadia JM, Klinepeter KL, et al. Randomized placebo-controlled trial of a 42 day tapering course of dexamethasone to reduce the duration of ventilator dependency in very low birth weight infants: outcome of study participants at 1 year adjusted age. Pediatrics 1999;104:15–27.
42. O'Shea TM, Washburn LK, Nixon PA, et al. Follow-up of a randomized, placebo-controlled trial of dexamethasone to decrease the duration of ventilator dependency in very low birth weight infants: neurodevelopmental outcomes at 4 to 11 years of age. Pediatrics 2007;120:594–602.
43. Nixon PA, Washburn LK, Schechter MS, et al. Follow-up study of a randomized controlled trial of postnatal dexamethasone therapy in very low birth weight infants: effects on pulmonary outcomes at age 8 to 11 years. J Pediatr 2007;150: 345–50.
44. Washburn LK, Nixon PA, O'Shea TM. Follow-up of a randomized, placebo-controlled trial of postnatal dexamethasone: blood pressure and anthropometric measurements at school age. Pediatrics 2006;118:1592–9.
45. Gross SJ, Anbar RD, Mettelman BB. Follow-up at 15 years of preterm infants from a controlled trial of moderately early dexamethasone for the prevention of chronic lung disease. Pediatrics 2005;115:681–7.
46. Wilson TT, Waters L, Patterson CC, et al. Neurodevelopmental and respiratory follow-up results at 7 years for children from the United Kingdom and Ireland enrolled in a randomized trial of early and late postnatal corticosteroid treatment,

systemic and inhaled (the Open Study of Early Corticosteroid Treatment). Pediatrics 2006;117:2196–205.
47. Doyle LW, Davis PG, Morley CJ, et al. Outcome at 2 years of age of infants from the DART study: a multicenter, international, randomized, controlled trial of low-dose dexamethasone. Pediatrics 2007;119:716–21.
48. Watterberg KL, Shaffer ML, Mishefske MJ, et al. Growth and neurodevelopmental outcomes after early low-dose hydrocortisone treatment in extremely low birth weight infants. Pediatrics 2007;120:40–8.
49. Rademaker KJ, Uiterwaal CS, Groenendaal F, et al. Neonatal hydrocortisone treatment: neurodevelopmental outcome and MRI at school age in preterm-born children. J Pediatr 2007;150:351–7.
50. Lodygensky GA, Rademaker K, Zimine S, et al. Structural and functional brain development after hydrocortisone treatment for neonatal chronic lung disease. Pediatrics 2005;116:1–7.
51. Karemaker R, Kavelaars A, ter Wolbeek M, et al. Neonatal dexamethasone treatment for chronic lung disease of prematurity alters the hypothalamus-pituitary-adrenal axis and immune system activity at school age. Pediatrics 2008;121:e870–8.
52. Shinwell ES, Lerner-Geva L, Lusky A, et al. Less postnatal steroids, more bronchopulmonary dysplasia: a population-based study in very low birthweight infants. Arch Dis Child Fetal Neonatal Ed 2007;92:F30–3.
53. Doyle LW, Halliday HL, Ehrenkranz RA, et al. Impact of postnatal systemic corticosteroids on mortality and cerebral palsy in preterm infants: effect modification by risk for chronic lung disease. Pediatrics 2005;115:655–61.

The Role of Genomics in the Neonatal ICU

Karen Maresso, MPH*, Ulrich Broeckel, MD

KEYWORDS

• Genetics • Genomics • Neonatal

The completion of the Human Genome Project in 2003 and the subsequent work of the International HapMap Project have provided the technology and resources necessary to enable fundamental advances through the study of DNA sequence variation in almost all fields of medicine, including neonatology. Novel developments in technology leading to advances in the understanding of disease affect the manner in which patients are diagnosed and subsequently treated. The rapidly expanding field of genomics serves as an example: technological developments allow the complete analysis of an individual's genome to determine one's risk of various complex diseases, with the goal of personalized medicine. For example, recently published reports of genome-wide association (GWA) studies, in which hundreds of thousands to millions of genetic variants across the genome are tested for association with a particular phenotype in thousands of individuals, have identified replicable genetic loci that increase the risk for myocardial infarction, type II diabetes, and various other complex traits.[1–4] Such studies offer the possibility of identifying clinically useful genetic markers and also basic science insights into disease mechanisms.

With the technology for high-resolution DNA sequence analysis now available, polygenic, multifactorial diseases, such as those commonly encountered in the neonatal ICU (NICU), are now amenable to high-throughput genetic dissection. To date, the study of common DNA sequence variation in neonatology has been quite limited. A number of candidate-gene studies have been performed, but the sample sizes have been small, and results generally have not been replicable. Nevertheless, well-designed genomic studies of the effect of DNA sequence variation on neonatal health and disease offers substantial opportunities to improve the diagnosis and treatment of vulnerable preterm and sick neonates. This ability is particularly relevant, because the rate of preterm births in the United States continues to rise, and prematurity is the second leading cause of infant deaths.[5,6]

This article provides an overview of the technology and study design issues relating to GWA studies and summarizes the current state of association studies in NICU

Section of Genomic Pediatrics, Children's Research Institute, Medical College of Wisconsin, TBRC/CRI, 2nd floor, 8701 Watertown Plank Road, Milwaukee, WI 53226, USA
* Corresponding author.
E-mail address: kmaresso@mcw.edu (K. Maresso).

Clin Perinatol 36 (2009) 189–204
doi:10.1016/j.clp.2008.09.015 perinatology.theclinics.com

populations with a brief review of the relevant literature. Future recommendations for genomic association studies in this highly vulnerable population are offered also.

THE TECHNOLOGY OF GENOMICS

The field of genetics focuses on individual genes; the field of genomics is concerned with the study of an entire genome. Association studies focus on one aspect of the genome, static DNA sequence information and its relation to various phenotypic outcomes. The newer field of functional genomics attempts to capitalize on the wealth of genomic data now available to annotate function in the genome by focusing on its more dynamic aspects, such as transcription and translation. This article focuses on large-scale association studies, including GWA studies. Ultimately, the combination of genomic-based studies, including association, expression, and proteomic analyses, will afford a detailed molecular view of complex, polygenic diseases, with subsequent enhancements of molecular diagnostic tools and identification of targets for improved patient care. The next sections briefly review the technological components and issues in the design of large-scale association studies, followed by a summary of the relevant literature relating to association studies in neonatology and NICU outcomes.

Analysis at the DNA level involves associating types of genetic variants, such as single-nucleotide polymorphisms (SNPs) and copy number polymorphisms, with various health and disease outcomes. In the past, before the advent of abundant variants that could be typed easily and inexpensively, linkage analyses with hundreds of multiallelic microsatellites were performed to identify regions of the genome "linked" to a particular trait of interest. The interest in using linkage analysis to dissect the genetics of complex traits grew from its success in identifying Mendelian disease genes. Typing microsatellites was laborious and time-consuming, however, and the methodology of linkage analysis, although appropriate for mapping single genes that had large effects, had very limited resolution in identifying the genes with small-to-moderate effects that are believed to contribute to multifactorial, polygenic traits. With advances in microarray technology and SNP discovery, both driven in large part by the completion of the Human Genome Project, coupled with advances in statistical methodology, large-scale association studies became feasible. As these developments have matured, GWA studies have become possible and are the most powerful method for identifying the genes with small-to-moderate effect believed to be responsible for multifactorial, polygenic diseases, such as those encountered in the NICU. **Fig. 1** represents a workflow of genome-wide association studies. These studies assess hundreds of thousands to millions of genetic variants across the genome for association with a particular trait or outcome in sample sizes of thousands of individuals. GWA scanning builds critically on technological platforms for high-throughput genotyping. Previously, access to affordable whole-genome SNP-typing technology was a limitation to performing GWA scans, but platforms now are commercially available and are affordable for many investigators. In addition to overall cost, the coverage, efficiency (coverage per SNP genotyped), and redundancy of a platform must be considered when selecting products offering random panels of SNPs or the tagging panels offered by different suppliers.

Tagging panels consist of SNPs chosen based on linkage disequilibrium (LD). LD occurs when two or more markers segregate together with significantly different frequencies than would be expected if they segregated independently from each other. LD is generally greater for SNPs in close physical proximity. Because LD tends to reduce the number of possible haplotypes, or set of alleles, present in a population, it is

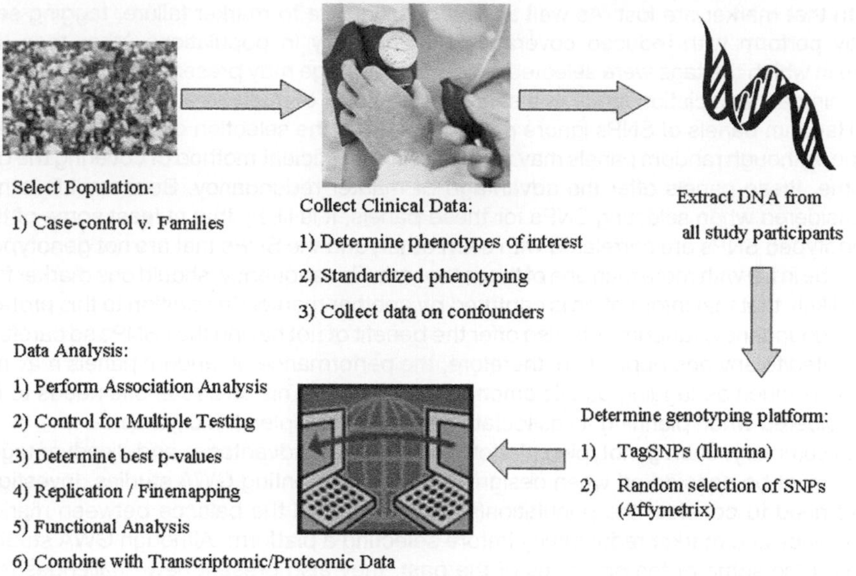

Fig. 1. Workflow of a genome-wide association study.

useful for association mapping: knowing the genotype of one marker enables one to predict the genotype of another marker in LD with it (**Fig. 2**). SNPs that are in strong LD with the greatest number of other SNPs are selected for genotyping and serve as proxies for the SNPs that are not selected. These panels offer the greatest overall genomic coverage and efficiency,[7] but they are susceptible to marker failure because all redundancy has been intentionally eliminated.[7] If one marker fails, all SNPs in LD

Possible Allelic Combinations of Two SNPs in the Absence of LD

SNP1(T/C) *SNP2 (G/A)*

AC **T** GGTACGTACCC **A** ATGTTGCATACGTT

AC **T** GGTACGTACCC **G** ATGTTGCATACGTT

AC **C** GGTACGTACCC **A** ATGTTGCATACGTT

AC **C** GGTACGTACCC **G** ATGTTGCATACGTT

Possible Allelic Combinations of Two SNPs in Presence of LD

SNP1(T/C) *SNP2 (G/A)*

AC **T** GGTACGTACCC **A** ATGTTGCATACGTT

AC **C** GGTACGTACCC **G** ATGTTGCATACGTT

Fig. 2. The principal of linkage disequilibrium (LD). A set of DNA sequences illustrating two SNPs (each shown in bold). (*Top*) The two SNPs are not in LD with each other and segregate independently. With two SNPs in linkage equilibrium, four possible allelic combinations are possible. (*Bottom*) Two SNPs in the presence of LD are illustrated. Notice that LD reduces the number of possible allelic combinations, because the SNPs no longer segregate independently. Here the T allele of SNP1 segregates only with the A allele of SNP2, and the C allele of SNP1 segregates only with the G allele of SNP2. It is necessary to genotype only one of these two SNPs , because the genotype at one SNP provides the genotype information for the other.

with that marker are lost. As well as being vulnerable to marker failure, tagging sets may perform with reduced coverage and efficiency in populations other than the one in which the tags were selected. This disadvantage may present difficulties in performing an association study in a sample consisting of multiple ethnic groups.

Random panels of SNPs ignore patterns of LD in the selection of markers to genotype. Although random panels may not be the most efficient method of covering the genome, these panels offer the advantage of marker redundancy. Because LD is not considered when selecting SNPs for these panels, it is likely that at least some of the genotyped SNPs are correlated with each other; and the SNPs that are not genotyped may be in LD with more than one of those that are. Consequently, should one marker fail, it is likely that that information is captured by another marker. In addition to this protective redundancy, random sets also offer the benefit of not having their SNPs so carefully targeted to any one population; therefore, the performance of random panels may not vary as much as tagging panels among populations.[7] This characteristic needs to be considered when planning an association study in multiple ethnic groups.

In summary, each genotyping platform has inherent advantages and disadvantages that must be considered when designing and implementing GWA studies. Investigators need to consider the population(s) of interest and the balance between marker efficiency and marker redundancy before selecting a platform. Although GWA studies overcome some of the obstacles of the past, they also present new challenges that must be considered. A primary concern when performing a GWA study is addressing the large number of statistical tests that are carried out. Using a simple Bonferroni correction, which stipulates a significance level of 10^{-7} for a study incorporating 500,000 markers, may be overly conservative, because it does not take into account LD. Controlling the false-discovery rate and permutation testing are two additional methods that address multiple testing. This area should see further development as more GWA datasets become available. Additional important issues that must be considered when designing and executing a genome-wide study include the inability of current GWA platforms to capture adequately low-frequency variants, which some argue are involved in complex diseases, and the need for replication of results in different populations.

Recently, the results of several GWA studies have been published. Four independent groups have identified an interval on chromosome 9 that affects the risk of coronary artery disease and myocardial infarction.[2,8,9] Consistent loci also have been identified for type II diabetes, age-related macular degeneration, and a number of other complex phenotypes.[1,3,10] These studies demonstrate the ability of the GWA approach to identify meaningful associations between genetic variants and polygenic, multifactorial outcomes.

The lack to date of GWA studies based on NICU populations, or even of comprehensive candidate-gene screens sufficiently powered to detect small effects, probably results from the lack of infrastructure supporting the interinstitutional and even international collaborations required to collect well-powered sample sizes, to phenotype those samples uniformly, and to store and analyze the massive amounts of data generated by such large genomic studies. Almost all GWA screens have been performed in adult populations. Although some GWA studies surely will be performed in children, NICU populations represent a special subset of children: many are premature and may have particular genetic variants that predispose them to various diseases that would be clinically insignificant in infants born at full term.[11] Because the environmental exposures in a NICU population are likely to differ substantially from those in a population of infants born at full term, separate GWA studies of NICU babies are warranted.

Although no GWA studies in a NICU population have been published, numerous candidate-gene association studies have been undertaken in NICU populations. These studies are discussed in depth later in this article. As an example, one of the best-studied candidate-gene associations in neonatology is the association of polymorphisms in the surfactant protein A gene (*SP-A*) with prematurity-related respiratory distress syndrome (RDS). A number of investigators have demonstrated associations of certain genotypes in the *SP-A* gene, namely alleles $6A^2$ and $1A^0$, with an increased risk of RDS.[12–14]

Data such as that generated from GWA studies need to be integrated with data from both the RNA and protein levels to inform fully the molecular understanding, and hence prevention, diagnosis, and treatment, of the types of complex diseases encountered in the NICU.

GENOMICS IN THE NEONATAL ICU

Advances in medical technology are continually lowering the limits of viability for premature infants. Within the first few days to months of life, however, these infants are vulnerable to a host of complex diseases that threaten their development and continued survival. Because premature birth remains the leading cause of neonatal morbidity and mortality,[15] and because premature birth is on the rise in the United States,[5] the proper diagnosis and management of diseases associated with prematurity are critical issues facing the field of neonatology. The proper incorporation of genomics into this field offers great opportunities for advances in the care and treatment of this extremely vulnerable patient population. The types of advances offered by genomics and its functionally related areas of transcriptomics and proteomics include more individualized prevention and treatment strategies based on an infant's genotype(s), more specific disease classification and prognostic criteria based on a newborn's gene expression profile, and the identification of novel, clinically significant biomarkers.

A genetic component has been identified for a number of the diseases to which NICU babies are susceptible.[11,16,17] This section briefly reviews the published association studies for some of the more common problems affecting preterm neonates, including RDS, bronchopulmonary dysplasia (BPD), acute renal failure (ARF), retinopathy of prematurity (ROP), and sepsis. **Table 1** lists these diseases and their associated genes and polymorphisms. The following discussion summarizes the findings overall and proposes recommendations for future directions of such studies.

Respiratory Distress Syndrome and Bronchopulmonary Dysplasia

The phenotype of RDS can be complex. Respiratory failure does occur in term infants, but its cause and clinical course often are distinct from that of RDS presenting in preterm babies. RDS in term infants is associated with rare mutations leading to surfactant deficiency.[18–20] This form of RDS is extremely rare compared with RDS of prematurity. Although the genetic variations behind inherited surfactant deficiency are relatively rare, they are highly penetrant, reflecting a Mendelian form of inheritance. In the case of RDS of prematurity, the variations identified generally are more common but less penetrant, without a clear form of inheritance. This form of RDS is the focus of this section.

In neonatology, RDS is perhaps the best-studied disease in relation to genetics, because it is one of the most prevalent diseases of the neonatal period. It is a complex disease, with multiple factors influencing susceptibility and outcome. It has long been established that a greater degree of prematurity, white ethnicity, and male gender are risk factors for RDS.[21–23] Epidemiologic studies also have demonstrated that genetics

Table 1
Diseases frequently diagnosed in the NICU and their associated genes

Disease	Gene(s)/Loci	Polymorphisms	Comments
Respiratory distress syndrome	*SFTPA1*	$6A^2$-$1A^0$ haplotypes[28,29,46,71]	
	SFTPA2		
	SFTPB	Ile131Thr T/C SNP[29,60]	
	SFTPC	SP-Bi4 insertion/deletion[29,46]	
Bronchopulmonary dysplasia)	*SFTPB*	SP-Bi4 insertion/deletion[69,74]	
	SP-A–SP-D haplotypes	Various haplotypes[69]	
	MBL2	rs1800450 and −221 variant[41]	
	Factor VII	323 insertion/deletion[34]	
	ACE	I/D allele[48]	
	TNFα	−238 SNP[47]	
Retinopathy of prematurity	*VEGF*	−634 G/C SNP[16,89]	Some ND variants are detected in very small numbers of ROP cases and not seen in controls. One group could not detect association with such variants[31] and another could not identify such variants in their ROP cases.[51]
	ND gene	Various polymorphisms[30,42,78,85]	
Sepsis	*IL-6*	−174 G/C SNP[5,8,33]	A recent meta-analysis of the *IL-6* gene did not detect association of the *IL-6–174* SNP with sepsis.[14]
	TNFα	−308 G/A SNP (sepsis mortality)[36]	
	CD14	59 C/T SNP (multiple blood-stream infections)[8]	
	Factor XIII	Val34Leu SNP[34]	
Acute renal failure	*HSP72*	1267 C/G SNP[24]	
	TNFα-IL6 haplotype	Haplotype of TNFα high- producing allele and IL-6 low- producing allele[87]	

Abbreviations: ACE, angiotensin I-converting enzyme; HSP72, heat shock protein 72; IL-6, interleukin-6; MBL2, mannose-binding lectin; ND Norrie disease; ROP, retinopathy of prematurity; *SFTPA1*, surfactant, pulmonary-associated protein A1 gene; *SFTPA2* surfactant, pulmonary-associated protein A2 gene; *SFTPB* surfactant, pulmonary-associated protein B gene; TNFα, tumor necrosis factor alpha; VEGF, vascular endothelial growth factor.

has a role in the risk of RDS. Nagourney and colleagues[24] showed an increased relative risk of RDS in second siblings born to women who had successive preterm pregnancies; and a 2002 study of premature twins by van Sonderen and colleagues[25] demonstrated that RDS occurred more frequently in monozygotic than in dizygotic twins (67% versus 29%). Following these reports, a number of polymorphisms have been identified in the various surfactant genes that are associated with RDS of prematurity. Most of this evidence comes from candidate-gene association studies in case-control samples.

Because earlier work had identified a surfactant deficiency as the cause of congenital RDS in term infants, the five surfactant genes, *SFTPA1*, *SFTPA2*, *SFTPB*, *SFTPC*, and *SFTPD*, became logical candidates to examine in the setting of prematurity-associated RDS. These five genes, encoding the four surfactant proteins SP-A through SP-D, have become the primary focus of numerous studies examining the genetics of RDS. Much work in this area comes from Finnish populations. Two risk-associated alleles in the *SP-A* genes, each made up of four nonsynonymous SNPs ($6A^2$ in *SFTPA1* and $1A^0$ in *SFTPA2*), have been associated with a risk of RDS in very premature infants in independent populations.[13,26,27] A study by Marttila and colleagues,[28] however, demonstrated that these same haplotypes conferred protection from RDS in near-term infants. Using a family-based approach, Haataja and colleagues[12] demonstrated that the $6A^2$-$1A^0$ haplotype was transmitted more often than expected from parents to affected infants and was seen less often in families of infants born earlier than 32 weeks' gestation who did not have RDS. These risk-associated haplotypes have population frequencies greater than 50%.[29,30]

One SNP in the *SFTPB* gene, a T to C (Ile131Thr) nonsynonymous change, has also been associated with risk of RDS in preterm infants, although only in the presenting twin.[31] In addition, this polymorphism has been shown to interact with the $6A^2$ haplotype of the *SFPTA1* gene. In premature neonates born before 32 weeks' gestation and carrying the *SFTPB* Thr/Thr genotype, the 6A2 allele was significantly overrepresented in the neonates who developed RDS compared with those who did not.[13] These gene–environment and gene–gene interactions demonstrate the complexity of the genetic architecture of RDS. An insertion/deletion polymorphism (SP-B i4) also has been identified within this gene, but its association to RDS remains controversial, with findings differing depending on the population studied.[13,26,32]

Within *SFPTC*, two common nonsynonymous SNPs also have been associated with RDS and very premature birth (< 28 weeks' gestation) in a group of infants born earlier than 34 weeks' gestation.[33] The strength of the association in this study was modified by gender, again demonstrating the complexity of RDS genetic etiology.

Unlike the other surfactant genes, variations within the *SFPTD* gene have not been reported to be associated with RDS in preterm infants.

Because the risk of BPD increases with the severity of RDS, candidate genes that affect risk of RDS also are likely to affect the risk of BPD. Rova and colleagues[32] examined all surfactant genes for an association with BPD in a cohort of 365 Finnish infants born at 32 weeks' gestation or earlier. They found that the SP-B i4 deletion variant was associated with BPD even after adjustment for other known confounding variables. None of the other genes demonstrated an association with this phenotype. A small family-based study by Pavlovic and colleagues[34] also demonstrated association with BPD for various markers in the *SFPTB* gene, as well as with haplotypes in the *SP-A* through *SP-D* genes.

Most recently, a handful of studies have demonstrated an association of BPD with polymorphisms in nonsurfactant genes. A 2007 report showed that mannose-binding lectin was associated with BPD in 284 preterm infants.[35] A high prevalence of mannose-binding lectin deficiency was demonstrated previously in preterm neonates.[36] A 2006 study by Hartel and colleagues[37] documented an association of the factor VII-323 del/ins polymorphism with BPD. Kazzi and colleagues[38] reported an association with increased risk and severity of BPD for the deletion allele of the *ACE* gene in very low birth weight (VLBW) infants, but this finding was not seen in another study of a similar group of infants.[39] Because inflammatory mechanisms have been implicated in the development of BPD, inflammatory genes also have become candidates for association. The A allele of the -238 polymorphism within the tumor necrosis alpha (*TNFα*) gene, which associates with decreased TNFα production, has been associated with protection from BPD.[40] Other cytokine polymorphisms have been tested, and association with BPD has not been demonstrated,[41–43] but it is not clear if these findings represent false negatives resulting from the limited sample sizes of these studies.

Retinopathy of Prematurity

ROP is a vascular disorder characterized by hyperoxia-induced vasocessation immediately after preterm birth and followed by a shift to hypoxia-induced vasoproliferation. ROP is one of the leading causes of blindness in pediatric populations, occurring in 5% of babies born with a birth weight of 1250 g or less.[44] Despite treatment, 10% to 15% of affected newborns become blind.[45] Although the disease regresses spontaneously in 80% to 85% of cases, distinguishing the infants in whom ROP will regress from those in whom it will not remains a challenge. The identification of genetic factors that predispose to or modify the ROP phenotype would assist in identifying newborns at risk for developing the disease and/or those at increased risk for severe ROP and blindness.

A 2006 study of premature twins estimates that 70% of the variance in the liability for ROP is caused by genetic factors.[46] Most of the genetic investigation in this area has focused on three functional candidate genes: vascular endothelial growth factor (*VEGF*), insulin-like growth factor 1 receptor (*IGF-1R*) and the Norrie disease (*ND*) gene. *VEGF* is an angiogenic mediator that has been implicated in the pathogenesis of ROP.[47] Many of the numerous variants of this gene impact *VEGF* mRNA and protein expression levels in various health and disease states.[48,49] Recently, a number of small, case-controlled association studies of ROP examined SNPs within this gene, particularly the -634G/C promoter polymorphism.[50–52] The results to date have been conflicting. Cooke and colleagues[50] demonstrated an increased risk for threshold ROP in those carrying the G allele of this SNP, whereas Vannay and colleagues[52] found an increased risk for those who had the C allele. Shastry and Qu[51] did not find evidence supporting a significant association with this variant. The reason for these discrepancies is not clear, but it has been suggested that differential LD between the -634G/C polymorphism and another potentially functional SNP may exist among the populations examined and cause the contrasting findings.[50]

The second candidate, *IGF-IR*, is a receptor for insulin-like growth factor 1 (IGF-1), which has been shown to be critical for normal retinal vascularization through its regulation of VEGF.[53,54] Low levels of IGF-1 have been implicated in ROP.[55,56] The +3174G/A polymorphism within the IGF-1 receptor has been associated with decreased IGF-1.[57] Two studies examining this SNP in relation to ROP were unable to document a significant association, however.[58,59]

The gene most studied in relation to ROP is the *ND* gene, which is the causative gene in Norrie disease, a rare X-linked recessive disorder characterized by early childhood blindness caused by retinal changes similar to those seen in ROP. Because of the phenotypic similarities observed between ND and ROP, the *ND* gene has been extensively studied as a ROP candidate gene. As with the *VEGF* gene, however, findings for a role of *ND* gene polymorphisms in ROP are conflicting. In 1997, Shastry and colleagues[60] first reported the identification of two missense mutations in the *ND* gene in 4 of 16 ROP patients that were not identified in 50 control subjects. Since then, additional groups have reported finding novel *ND* mutations and polymorphisms in small numbers of ROP patients.[61–63] Mutations were not identified in a Korean population of infants who had ROP,[64] however, and although Haider and colleagues[65] documented the occurrence of some of the previously identified point mutations, no significant associations with ROP were detected in a Kuwaiti cohort of 102 premature newborns. It has been estimated that approximately 3% of severe ROP cases may be caused by *ND* variants.[66] Two recent studies suggest that *ND* mutations may play a minor role in the pathogenesis of ROP in some populations but that additional genetic factors probably are involved.[66,67]

Sepsis

Sepsis remains a significant cause of mortality in the NICU. The mortality rate in VLBW infants who have sepsis is more than twice that in VLBW infants who do not.[68,69] Challenges in the diagnosis and treatment of sepsis relate to the substantial amount of interindividual variation seen in the response to infection and the subsequent development of sepsis and in therapeutic outcome.[70] Markers that correlate with the clinical course of infection, the development of sepsis, and/or the response to therapy are urgently needed within this population. Such markers would allow earlier identification and more rapid treatment of VLBW infants at increased risk of death from infection.

Numerous lines of evidence support a role for host genetics in the clinical course and ultimate outcome of infectious diseases.[16] Innate immunity genes are obvious candidates to examine in the context of infectious diseases and their sequelae, particularly in premature infants, who do not yet have fully developed immune systems. These genes have been the focus of a number of candidate-gene association studies examining sepsis in preterm infants.

The −174G/C promoter polymorphism of the interleukin 6 (*IL-6*) gene has been tested in many of these studies.[71–75] This SNP has been shown to influence IL-6 production in neonates, although findings in adults are inconsistent.[76–78] Initial reports suggested that the −174C allele was protective against sepsis in VLBW infants,[71,74] but later reports found conflicting results.[72,73,75] Recently, a meta-analysis combined data from 1323 VLBW infants across six independent cohorts.[79] Based on their analysis, the authors concluded that the *IL-6* 174G/C SNP is not associated with neonatal sepsis in VLBW infants. Other polymorphisms exist within this gene, and it may be that certain haplotypes of particular *IL-6* SNPs, rather than one SNP alone, actually affect the risk of sepsis or poor sepsis outcome in preterm infants. Such an effect for *IL-6* haplotypes has been demonstrated for mortality in critically ill adult patients.[80]

Another frequently studied variant in relation to sepsis is the *TNF-α* 308G/A polymorphism, which has been shown to affect gene transcription in vitro.[81] Although this variant has not been demonstrated to have an effect on the occurrence of sepsis in neonates,[75] Hedberg, and colleagues[82] demonstrated a threefold increase in mortality for ventilated VLBW carriers of the 308A allele compared with homozygotes of the 308G allele. Large-scale studies are needed to substantiate these findings. Interestingly, this polymorphism seems to be in LD with two SNPs in the *LTA* gene, one of which has been shown to be functional[83] and one of which was associated with higher mortality in a small cohort of children who had positive blood cultures.[84] These findings need to be taken into account in any future studies of any of these variants. Again, as for *IL-6*, it may be the combined effect of various SNPs across these two genes that determines risk or outcome of neonatal sepsis.

Other genes and SNPs that have been examined in the context of sepsis in preterm infants include the *TLR-4G* and *TLR2* Arg753Gln variants, the *NOD2* 3020insC polymorphism and the *MBL B/C/D* alleles, but no associations could be established.[71] An association has been documented for the *CD14* 159C/T SNP with multiple blood stream infections in a retrospective cohort of 293 African American VLBW infants receiving ventilation[72] but was not associated with culture-proven sepsis in a white cohort of 356 VLBW infants.[71] These disparate findings may result from race and/or differences in ventilation; large-scale studies in racially and phenotypically homogenous cohorts are needed to clarify the role of the *CD14* 159C/T variant. Sequence variations in coagulation factors, including the factor V Leiden variant, the prothrombin G20210A SNP, the factor VII-121del/ins polymorphism, and the factor XIII-Val34Leu change, also have been examined as potential risk factors for sepsis.[37] Only carriers of the factor XIII-Val34Leu polymorphism had higher sepsis rates than noncarriers.[37] No associations with sepsis were seen for the other variations.

Acute Renal Failure

ARF is quite common in the NICU, with estimates of prevalence ranging from 8% to 24%.[85,86] Depending on the underlying pathology, mortality can be high, estimated at 10% to 61%.[85] Risk factors for ARF include sepsis, cardiac failure, intracerebral bleeding, RDS, patent ductus arteriosus, mechanical ventilation, and indomethacin treatment.[87] To date, only a handful of studies have examined sequence variants in relation to the development and/or outcome of ARF in NICU infants. Nobilis and colleagues[88] studied the *ACE* and *AT1* receptor genes, because as members of the rennin-angiotensin-aldosterone system they play a role in regulating systemic blood pressure and renal hemodynamics. The *ACE* insertion/deletion (I/D) SNP is a common known polymorphism, and lower ACE activity has been associated with the homozygous insertion genotype.[89] The C^{1166} variant in the *AT1* receptor gene has been associated with an enhanced effect of angiotensin II.[90] No association for either of these variants with neonatal ARF could be identified, however.[88] Subsequently, Treszl and colleagues tested interleukin gene variants in relation to ARF, because various cytokines have been implicated in ARF, and a number of functional SNPs within these genes have been documented.[91–93] Examining *TNF-α*, *IL-1β*, *IL-6*, and *IL-10* in 92 VLBW neonates with severe systemic infection, the authors could not identify an association with any of the variants when tested individually; however, they showed the prevalence of a haplotype consisting of the high *TNF-α*–producing and the low *IL-6*–producing alleles to be significantly higher in the ARF group than in the non-ARF group.[93] Finally, an association between the 1267 C/G variant of the heat shock protein 72 (*HSP72*) gene, which has been shown to correlate with HSP72 expression levels, was documented in 130 preterm VLBW infants.[94] The frequency of the *HSP72* 1267GG genotype, which correlates with decreased HSP72 expression, was higher in the infants who developed ARF than in those who did not.[94] This finding is significant, because in premature animals a temporal correlation between peak expression of HSP72 protein and protection of from hypoxic renal insult has been documented.[95]

Summary of Literature and Recommendations for Future Association Studies in Neonatology

Although the findings from the studies demonstrating an association of various gene polymorphisms with common diseases found in the NICU are supported by a strong biologic plausibility, given the known functional role of many of the tested genes, and although many of the SNPs tested are functionally relevant, in that many are nonsynonymous coding changes, a number of limitations still exist. Sample sizes in most of the studies in this area are very limited, corrections for multiple testing often are not made even though multiple tests are performed, and many of the reported p-values are borderline. Consequently, type I errors in these studies cannot be ruled out. In addition, the documented gene–gene and gene–environment interaction in a number of these disorders complicates risk estimates and requires large sample sizes. The establishment of bio-banks and the combining of samples by networks of investigators with a common research question would help increase sample sizes.

Some investigators within the field of neonatology have called for increased collaboration and the establishment of bio-banks.[11] Meta-analysis of previously conducted association studies is another method for increasing the statistical power to detect an effect. A meta-analysis of the IL-6 promoter polymorphism and sepsis in VLBW infants was published recently.[79] It is hoped that more meta-analyses for additional commonly studied variants in NICU outcomes will follow soon.

Along with issues relating to sample size, many studies have not surveyed the variation in a particular gene comprehensively, instead genotyping only one or a few variants. This approach ignores the patterns of LD within and around a gene and may lead to premature conclusions regarding the role of a particular variant and gene in disease risk. There also is a need for more precise phenotype definitions to ensure phenotypic homogeneity within and between studies of a particular phenotype. A better selection of control infants is required also. Controls should be population based to avoid selection bias. Standardizing case and control selection for a given disease would allow more informative comparisons to be made among studies. Furthermore, in case and control selection, racial homogeneity is essential for meaningful association results. Because the frequency of genetic markers can differ by ethnicity, studies should consist of an ethnically homogenous group, or, alternatively, in studies involving more than a single ethnicity, the study design must take these allelic differences into account.

Finally, there has been a focus in the literature on selecting genes based on known or presumed function and their relation to implicated disease pathways. Genes outside these pathways also may contribute to disease risk, severity, and response to treatment. Although these genes may not be amenable to identification through a strict functional or disease biology approach, GWA studies can assist in identifying such novel gene targets, because GWA studies are hypothesis free with regard to the underlying genetic correlates of a disease. Ultimately, the successful implementation of GWA studies of the clinical outcomes affecting NICU infants will depend on strong interinstitutional and even international investigator networks and collaborations to build the required sample sizes and to mine the wealth of data such studies generate.

REFERENCES

1. Duerr RH, Taylor KD, Brant SR, et al. A genome-wide association study identifies IL23R as an inflammatory bowel disease gene. Science 2006;314(5804):1461–3.
2. McPherson R, Pertsemlidis A, Kavaslar N, et al. A common allele on chromosome 9 associated with coronary heart disease. Science 2007;316(5830):1488–91.
3. Salonen JT, Uimari P, Aalto JM, et al. Type 2 diabetes whole-genome association study in four populations: the DiaGen consortium. Am J Hum Genet 2007;81(2): 338–45.
4. Wellcome Trust Case Control Consortium. Genome-wide association study of 14,000 cases of seven common diseases and 3,000 shared controls. Nature 2007;447(7145):661–78.
5. National Center for Health Statistics. Period linked birth/infant death data. 2004. Available at: www.marchofdimes.com/peristats. Accessed July 21, 2008.
6. National Center for Health Statistics. . Final natality data. 2005. Available at: www.marchofdimes.com/peristats. Accessed July 21, 2008.
7. Barrett JC, Cardon LR. Evaluating coverage of genome-wide association studies. Nat Genet 2006;38(6):659–62.
8. Helgadottir A, Thorleifsson G, Manolescu A, et al. A common variant on chromosome 9p21 affects the risk of myocardial infarction. Science 2007;316(5830):1491–3.

9. Samani NJ, Erdmann J, Hall AS, et al. WTCCC and the Cardiogenics Consortium. Genomewide association analysis of coronary artery disease. N Engl J Med 2007; 357(5):443–53.
10. Klein RJ, Zeiss C, Chew EY, et al. Complement factor H polymorphism in age-related macular degeneration. Science 2005;308(5720):385–9.
11. Cotten CM, Ginsburg GS, Goldberg RN, et al. Genomic analyses: a neonatology perspective. J Pediatr 2006;148(6):720–6.
12. Haataja R, Marttila R, Uimari P, et al. Respiratory distress syndrome: evaluation of genetic susceptibility and protection by transmission disequilibrium test. Hum Genet 2001;109(3):351–5.
13. Haataja R, Rämet M, Marttila R, et al. Surfactant proteins A and B as interactive genetic determinants of neonatal respiratory distress syndrome. Hum Mol Genet 2000;9(18):2751–60.
14. Hallman M, Haataja R, Marttila R. Surfactant proteins and genetic predisposition to respiratory distress syndrome. Semin Perinatol 2002;26(6):450–60.
15. Esplin MS. Preterm birth: a review of genetic factors and future directions for genetic study. Obstet Gynecol Surv 2006;61(12):800–6.
16. Cooke GS, Hill AV. Genetics of susceptibility to human infectious disease. Nat Rev Genet 2001;2(12):967–77.
17. Parker RA, Lindstrom DP, Cotton RB. Evidence from twin study implies possible genetic susceptibility to bronchopulmonary dysplasia. Semin Perinatol 1996; 20(3):206–9.
18. Nogee LM, de Mello DE, Dehner LP, et al. Brief report: deficiency of pulmonary surfactant protein B in congenital alveolar proteinosis. N Engl J Med 1993; 328(6):406–10.
19. Nogee LM, Garnier G, Dietz HC, et al. A mutation in the surfactant protein B gene responsible for fatal neonatal respiratory disease in multiple kindreds. J Clin Invest 1994;93(4):1860–3.
20. Shulenin S, Nogee LM, Annilo T, et al. ABCA3 gene mutations in newborns with fatal surfactant deficiency. N Engl J Med 2004;350(13):1296–303 [see comment].
21. Farrell PM, Wood RE. Epidemiology of hyaline membrane disease in the United States: analysis of national mortality statistics. Pediatrics 1976;58(2):167–76.
22. Hulsey TC, Alexander GR, Robillard PY, et al. Hyaline membrane disease: the role of ethnicity and maternal risk characteristics. Am J Obstet Gynecol 1993;168(2):572–6 [see comment].
23. Khoury MJ, Marks JS, McCarthy BJ, et al. Factors affecting the sex differential in neonatal mortality: the role of respiratory distress syndrome. Am J Obstet Gynecol 1985;151(6):777–82.
24. Nagourney BA, Kramer MS, Klebanoff MA, et al. Recurrent respiratory distress syndrome in successive preterm pregnancies. J Pediatr 1996;129(4):591–6.
25. van Sonderen L, Halsema EF, Spiering EJ, et al. Genetic influences in respiratory distress syndrome: a twin study. Semin Perinatol 2002;26(6):447–9.
26. Kala P, Ten Have T, Nielsen H, et al. Association of pulmonary surfactant protein A (SP-A) gene and respiratory distress syndrome: interaction with SP-B. Pediatr Res 1998;43:169–77.
27. Ramet M, Haataja R, Marttila R, et al. Association between the surfactant protein A (SP-A) gene locus and respiratory distress syndrome in the Finnish population. Am J Hum Genet 2000;66:1569–79.
28. Marttila R, Haataja R, Ramet M, et al. Surfactant protein A gene locus and respiratory distress syndrome in Finnish premature twin pairs. Ann Med 2003;35:344–52.

29. Floros J, Fan R, Matthews A, et al. Family-based transmission disequilibrium test (TDT) and case-control association studies reveal surfactant protein A (SP-A) susceptibility alleles for respiratory distress syndrome (RDS) and possible race differences. Clin Genet 2001;60:178–87.
30. Ramet M, Haataja R, Marttila R, et al. Human surfactant protein A gene locus for genetic studies in the Finnish population. Dis Markers 2000;16:119–24.
31. Marttila R, Haataja R, Ramet M, et al. Surfactant protein B polymorphism and respiratory distress syndrome in premature twins. Hum Genet 2003;112:18–23.
32. Rova M, Haataja R, Marttila R, et al. Data mining and multiparameter analysis of lung surfactant protein genes in bronchopulmonary dysplasia. Hum Mol Genet 2004;13(11):1095–104.
33. Lahti M, Marttila R, Hallman M. Surfactant protein C gene variation in the Finnish population—association with perinatal respiratory disease. Eur J Hum Genet 2004;12(4):312–20.
34. Pavlovic J, Papagaroufalis C, Xanthou M, et al. Genetic variants of surfactant proteins A, B, C, and D in bronchopulmonary dysplasia. Dis Markers 2005; 22(5–6):277–91.
35. Hilgendorff A, Heidinger K, Pfeiffer A, et al. Association of polymorphisms in the mannose-binding lectin gene and pulmonary morbidity in preterm infants. Genes Immun 2007;8(8):671–7.
36. Frakking FN, Brouwer N, Zweers D, et al. High prevalence of mannose-binding lectin (MBL) deficiency in premature neonates. Clin Exp Immunol 2006;145(1): 5–12.
37. Hartel C, Konig I, Koster S, et al. Genetic polymorphisms of hemostasis genes and primary outcome of very low birth weight infants. Pediatrics 2006;118(2): 683–9.
38. Kazzi SN, Quasney MW. Deletion allele of angiotensin-converting enzyme is associated with increased risk and severity of bronchopulmonary dysplasia. J Pediatr 2005;147(6):818–22 [see comment].
39. Yanamandra K, Loggins J, Baier RJ. The angiotensin converting enzyme insertion/deletion polymorphism is not associated with an increased risk of death or bronchopulmonary dysplasia in ventilated very low birth weight infants. BMC Pediatr 2004;4(1):26.
40. Kazzi SN, Kim UO, Quasney MW, et al. Polymorphism of tumor necrosis factor-alpha and risk and severity of bronchopulmonary dysplasia among very low birth weight infants. Pediatrics 2004;114(2):e243–8 [see comment].
41. Adcock K, Hedberg C, Loggins J, et al. The TNF-alpha −308, MCP-1 −2518 and TGF-beta1 +915 polymorphisms are not associated with the development of chronic lung disease in very low birth weight infants. Genes Immun 2003;4(6): 420–6.
42. Lin HC, Su BH, Chang JS, et al. Nonassociation of interleukin 4 intron 3 and 590 promoter polymorphisms with bronchopulmonary dysplasia for ventilated preterm infants. Biol Neonate 2005;87(3):181–6.
43. Lin HC, Tsai FJ, Tsai CH, et al. Cytokine polymorphisms and chronic lung disease in small preterm infants. Arch Dis Child Fetal Neonatal Ed 2005;90(1):F93–4.
44. Palmer EA, Flynn JT, Hardy RJ, et al. Incidence and early course of retinopathy of prematurity. The Cryotherapy for Retinopathy of Prematurity Cooperative Group. Ophthalmology 1991;98(11):1628–40.
45. Early Treatment for Retinopathy of Prematurity Cooperative Group. Revised indications for the treatment of retinopathy of prematurity: results of the early

treatment for retinopathy of prematurity randomized trial. Arch Ophthalmol 2003; 121(12):1684–94.
46. Bizzarro MJ, Hussain N, Jonsson B, et al. Genetic susceptibility to retinopathy of prematurity. Pediatrics 2006;118(5):1858–63.
47. Alon T, Hermo I, Itin A, et al. Vascular endothelial growth factor acts as a survival factor for newly formed retinal vessels and has implications for retinopathy of prematurity. Nat Med 1995;1:1024–8.
48. Renner W, Kotschan S, Hoffmann C, et al. A common 936 C/T mutation in the gene for vascular endothelial growth factor is associated with vascular endothelial growth factor plasma levels. J Vasc Res 2000;37(6):443–8.
49. Watson CJ, Webb NJ, Bottomley MJ, et al. Identification of polymorphisms within the vascular endothelial growth factor (VEGF) gene: correlation with variation in VEGF protein production. Cytokine 2000;12(8):1232–5.
50. Cooke RW, Drury JA, Mountford R, et al. Genetic polymorphisms and retinopathy of prematurity. Invest Ophthalmol Vis Sci 2004;45(6):1712–5.
51. Shastry BS, Qu X. Lack of association of the VEGF gene promoter (−634 G->C and −460 C->T) polymorphism and the risk of advanced retinopathy of prematurity. Graefes Arch Clin Exp Ophthalmol 2007;245(5):741–3.
52. Vannay A, Dunai G, Bányász I, et al. Association of genetic polymorphisms of vascular endothelial growth factor and risk for proliferative retinopathy of prematurity. Pediatr Res 2005;57(3):396–8.
53. Hellstrom A, Carlsson B, Niklasson A, et al. IGF-I is critical for normal vascularization of the human retina. J Clin Endocrinol Metab 2002;87(7):3413–6.
54. Smith LE, Shen W, Perruzzi C, et al. Regulation of vascular endothelial growth factor-dependent retinal neovascularization by insulin-like growth factor-1 receptor. Nat Med 1999;5(12):1390–5.
55. Hellstrom A, Engstrom E, Hard AL, et al. Postnatal serum insulin-like growth factor I deficiency is associated with retinopathy of prematurity and other complications of premature birth. Pediatrics 2003;112(5):1016–20 [see comment].
56. Hellstrom A, Perruzzi C, Ju M, et al. Low IGF-I suppresses VEGF-survival signaling in retinal endothelial cells: direct correlation with clinical retinopathy of prematurity. Proc Natl Acad Sci U S A 2001;98(10):5804–8.
57. Bonafè M, Barbieri M, Marchegiani F, et al. Polymorphic variants of insulin-like growth factor I (IGF-I) receptor and phosphoinositide 3-kinase genes affect IGF-I plasma levels and human longevity: cues for an evolutionarily conserved mechanism of life span control. J Clin Endocrinol Metab 2003;88(7):3299–304.
58. Balogh A, Derzbach L, Vannay A, et al. Lack of association between insulin-like growth factor I receptor G(+3174)A polymorphism and retinopathy of prematurity. Graefes Arch Clin Exp Ophthalmol 2006;244(8):1035–8.
59. Shastry BS. Assessment of the contribution of insulin-like growth factor I receptor 3174 G->A polymorphism to the progression of advanced retinopathy of prematurity. Eur J Ophthalmol 2007;17(6):950–3.
60. Shastry BS, Pendergast SD, Hartzer MK, et al. Identification of missense mutations in the Norrie disease gene associated with advanced retinopathy of prematurity. Arch Ophthalmol 1997;115(5):651–5.
61. Hiraoka M, Berinstein DM, Trese MT, et al. Insertion and deletion mutations in the dinucleotide repeat region of the Norrie disease gene in patients with advanced retinopathy of prematurity. J Hum Genet 2001;46(4):178–81.
62. Talks SJ, Ebenezer N, Hykin P, et al. De novo mutations in the 5′ regulatory region of the Norrie disease gene in retinopathy of prematurity. J Med Genet 2001; 38(12):E46.

63. Haider MZ, Devarajan LV, Al-Essa M, et al. A C597->A polymorphism in the Norrie disease gene is associated with advanced retinopathy of prematurity in premature Kuwaiti infants. J Biomed Sci 2002;9(4):365–70.
64. Kim JH, Yu YS, Kim J, et al. Mutations of the Norrie gene in Korean ROP infants. Korean J Ophthalmol 2002;16(2):93–6.
65. Haider MZ, Devarajan LV, Al-Essa M, et al. Missense mutations in Norrie disease gene are not associated with advanced stages of retinopathy of prematurity in Kuwaiti Arabs. Biol Neonate 2000;77(2):88–91.
66. Dickinson JL, Sale MM, Passmore A, et al. Mutations in the NDP gene: contribution to Norrie disease, familial exudative vitreoretinopathy and retinopathy of prematurity. Clin Experiment Ophthalmol 2006;34(7):682–8.
67. Hutcheson KA, Paluru PC, Bernstein SL, et al. Norrie disease gene sequence variants in an ethnically diverse population with retinopathy of prematurity. Mol Vis 2005;11:501–8.
68. Makhoul IR, Sujov P, Smolkin T, et al. Epidemiological, clinical, and microbiological characteristics of late-onset sepsis among very low birth weight infants in Israel: a national survey. Pediatrics 2002;109(1):34–9.
69. Stoll BJ, Hansen N. Infections in VLBW infants: studies from the NICHD Neonatal Research Network. Semin Perinatol 2003;27(4):293–301.
70. Hartel C, Schultz C, Herting E, et al. Genetic association studies in VLBW infants exemplifying susceptibility to sepsis—recent findings and implications for future research. Acta Paediatr 2007;96(2):158–65.
71. Ahrens P, Kattner E, Köhler B, et al. Genetic Factors in Neonatology Study Group. Mutations of genes involved in the innate immune system as predictors of sepsis in very low birth weight infants. Pediatr Res 2004;55(4):652–6.
72. Baier RJ, Loggins J, Yanamandra K. IL-10, IL-6 and CD14 polymorphisms and sepsis outcome in ventilated very low birth weight infants. BMC Med 2006;4:10.
73. Göpel W, Härtel C, Ahrens P, et al. Interleukin-6-174-genotype, sepsis and cerebral injury in very low birth weight infants. Genes Immun 2006;7(1):65–8.
74. Harding D, Dhamrait S, Millar A, et al. Is interleukin-6 −174 genotype associated with the development of septicemia in preterm infants? Pediatrics 2003;112(4):800–3.
75. Treszl A, Kocsis I, Szathmari M, et al. Genetic variants of TNF-[FC12]a, IL-1beta, IL-4 receptor [FC12]a-chain, IL-6 and IL-10 genes are not risk factors for sepsis in low-birth-weight infants. Biol Neonate 2003;83(4):241–5.
76. Bennermo M, Held C, Stemme S, et al. Genetic predisposition of the interleukin-6 response to inflammation: implications for a variety of major diseases? Clin Chem 2004;50(11):2136–40.
77. Endler G, Marsik C, Joukhadar C, et al. The interleukin-6 G(−174)C promoter polymorphism does not determine plasma interleukin-6 concentrations in experimental endotoxemia in humans. Clin Chem 2004;50(1):195–200.
78. Kilpinen S, Hulkkonen J, Wang XY, et al. The promoter polymorphism of the interleukin-6 gene regulates interleukin-6 production in neonates but not in adults. Eur Cytokine Netw 2001;12(1):62–8.
79. Chauhan M, McGuire W. Interleukin-6 (−174C) polymorphism and the risk of sepsis in very-low-birth-weight infants: meta-analysis. Arch Dis Child Fetal Neonatal Ed 2008;93(6):F427–9.
80. Sutherland AM, Walley KR, Manocha S, et al. The association of interleukin 6 haplotype clades with mortality in critically ill adults. Arch Intern Med 2005;165(1):75–82.

81. Wilson AG, Symons JA, McDowell TL, et al. Effects of a polymorphism in the human tumor necrosis factor alpha promoter on transcriptional activation. Proc Natl Acad Sci U S A 1997;94(7):3195–9.
82. Hedberg CL, Adcock K, Martin J, et al. Tumor necrosis factor alpha – 308 polymorphism associated with increased sepsis mortality in ventilated very low birth weight infants. Pediatr Infect Dis J 2004;23(5):424–8.
83. Knight JC, Keating BJ, Kwiatkowski DP. Allele-specific repression of lymphotoxin-alpha by activated B cell factor-1. Nat Genet 2004;36(4):394–9.
84. McArthur JA, Zhang Q, Quasney MW. Association between the A/A genotype at the lymphotoxin-alpha+250 site and increased mortality in children with positive blood cultures. Pediatr Crit Care Med 2002;3(4):341–4.
85. Andreoli SP. Acute renal failure in the newborn. Semin Perinatol 2004;28(2): 112–23.
86. Stapleton FB, Jones DP, Green RS. Acute renal failure in neonates: incidence, etiology and outcome. Pediatr Nephrol 1987;1(3):314–20.
87. Vasarhelyi B, Toth-Heyn P, Treszl A, et al. Genetic polymorphisms and risk for acute renal failure in preterm neonates. Pediatr Nephrol 2005;20(2):132–5.
88. Nobilis A, Kocsis I, Toth-Heyn P, et al. Variance of ACE and AT1 receptor gene does not influence the risk of neonatal acute renal failure. Pediatr Nephrol 2001;16(12): 1063–6.
89. Rigat B, Hubert C, Alhenc-Gelas F, et al. An insertion/deletion polymorphism in the angiotensin I-converting enzyme gene accounting for half the variance of serum enzyme levels. J Clin Invest 1990;86(4):1343–6.
90. Duncan JA, Scholey JW, Miller JA. Angiotensin II type 1 receptor gene polymorphisms in humans: physiology and pathophysiology of the genotypes. Curr Opin Nephrol Hypertens 2001;10(1):111–6.
91. Jaber BL, Pereira BJ, Bonventre JV, et al. Polymorphism of host response genes: implications in the pathogenesis and treatment of acute renal failure. Kidney Int 2005;67(1):14–33.
92. Liangos O, Balakrishnan VS, Pereira BJ, et al. Cytokine single nucleotide polymorphism. Role in acute renal failure. Contrib Nephrol 2004;144:63–75.
93. Treszl A, Toth-Heyn P, Kocsis I, et al. Interleukin genetic variants and the risk of renal failure in infants with infection. Pediatr Nephrol 2002;17(9):713–7.
94. Fekete A, Treszl A, Toth-Heyn P, et al. Association between heat shock protein 72 gene polymorphism and acute renal failure in premature neonates. Pediatr Res 2003;54(4):452–5.
95. Vicencio A, Bidmon B, Ryu J, et al. Developmental expression of HSP-72 and ischemic tolerance of the immature kidney. Pediatr Nephrol 2003;18(2):85–91.

Index

Note: Page numbers of article titles are in **boldface** type.

Clin Perinatol 36 (2009) 205–214
doi:10.1016/S0095-5108(08)00129-2 perinatology.theclinics.com

N

O

P

R

S

Printed and bound by CPI Group (UK) Ltd, Croydon, CR0 4YY

03/10/2024

01040447-0003